# EXTREME TRANSFORMATION

## CHRIS POWELL
### AND
## HEIDI POWELL

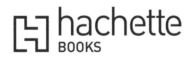 hachette
BOOKS

NEW YORK   BOSTON

Hachette Books
Hachette Book Group
1290 Avenue of the Americas
New York, NY 10104
www.HachetteBookGroup.com

Printed in the United States of America

LSC-C

First trade edition: December 2016
10 9 8 7 6 5 4 3 2 1

Hachette Books is a division of Hachette Book Group, Inc.

The publisher is not responsible for websites (or their content) that are not owned by the publisher.

LCCN: 2016304790

ISBN 978-0-316-33950-6 (pbk.)

Heidi's Dedication:

*To my best friend. If people only knew the highs and lows we have endured together. Through it all, you've shown me generous acts of love and kindness even when I feel like I least deserved it. You make me want to be the best version of myself possible. Sometimes I have to pinch myself to make sure I'm really living this life as your other half. You are most definitely my better half. You've taught me more than you will ever know by your shining example. I can't wait to grow old with you, Chris.*

Chris's Dedication:

*To my best friend, Heidi. My world changed forever the day we met. You have taught me the most valuable lessons in this life. Our ride has certainly been a wild one. But when it is all said and done here, I cannot wait to look into your eyes, hand in hand, and know in our hearts that we did it all.*

# CONTENTS

Love It!                                                              96

Live It!                                                             137

Phase One's Done: Now What?                                          175


PART THREE

**YOUR NEW LIFE**                                                    177

PART FOUR

**THE METABOLIC MOVEMENTS**                                          191

# INTRODUCTION

**CREED OF THE PHOENIX**

*I found myself*
*Lost in the depths*
*Of darkness and despair,*
*Blinded by confusion*
*That was dwelling everywhere.*

*No matter how many times I tried*
*I couldn't find my way.*
*But when I opened up my eyes*
*A whole new life awaited.*

*Through hope and heart and promises,*
*Integrity and dignity,*
*My life is now my masterpiece.*
*I control my destiny.*

*I am a Phoenix now*
*From ash I rise above*
*As I climb, step-by-step*
*The path to true self love.*

The Phoenix is a mythical bird that, near the end of its lifetime, crashes into the earth in a ball of flames—and then reincarnates itself to begin life anew.

It has been six years since we started our show *Extreme Weight Loss*—six seasons, over 70 incredible transformations on camera, and millions of lives changed in more than 140 countries! So much has happened in that short span of time—our family has expanded, our passion for helping others continues to grow, and our insight into how people can effectively lose weight and get in shape has deepened. But one of the biggest transformations of all is how we finally understand the necessary steps to keeping it off forever.

Since Heidi became even more visible on the show, the response has been overwhelming. People want more of her—on the show and via her blog, HeidiPowell.net. But what many don't realize is that Heidi and I have worked side by side from day one, helping our people change their lives for the better. As Heidi's role on the show has increased, I've been super excited—but not a bit surprised—to see how our viewers have responded to her amazing spirit, energy, and wisdom. They seem to relate to her emotionally charged, dig-in approach; instead of backing off when things get tough, Heidi helps them through some of the tough inner parts of their struggle to lose weight and hold steady to their transformation journey…and ultimately their lifelong dreams.

It turns out that my strengths as head cheerleader and chief educator dovetail nicely with Heidi's more emotional approach. Don't get me wrong: We are both tough, but in different ways, and we came to realize that the most successful of the people we work with need just that: cheerleader, educator, and counselor. They also have relied upon us as trusted friends—and that's what we want to be to you, friends you can depend on—to be honest with you, and to help guide you to your best life.

Together, we have always felt like a formidable team, but now with so many people responding to us as a couple (and family), we realize that yes, two is better than one…and our differences support our approach. And that's what we want to give you in this third—our most comprehensive and complete—book: a combination of both our approaches through a 21-day lifestyle shift that will put you on course to change your body and your life, forever.

Since our last book, we have made some influential discoveries—influential on *us*! Taking in the experience of the hundreds of courageous women and men we have guided through the weight loss journey, we've learned *so* much more about the struggles, and how to overcome them for continued success. We have dug deep with our people over the years, and now deliver to you the fastest, most convenient, most balanced way to achieve profound weight loss. Over the years we have set out to identify the reasons why it is so difficult for many to not just lose the weight, but to continue losing weight over time, and ultimately maintain a lifestyle of success. Why? Why do we lose motivation? Why do we fall off of the wagon time and again? How can we finally lose the weight for good? These are the questions that we have obsessed over for years and have sought tirelessly to find the solutions.

The answer is simple: Most diets are just that—diets. They are simple plans to follow for weight loss. Some even come with an exercise component. But they don't provide the inner compass, the knowledge, and the realistic expectations of what the journey is *really* like, to make a diet into what it's meant to be—*a transformation*. Before, there was no real *guide* to transformation. And that's our promise to you: a complete road map that will lead to long-term success—once and for all.

Our guide to Extreme Transformation is a product of over 14 years of experience on a journey that we've taken with hundreds of people. Nearly every individual we have transformed is like family to us. We talk, we laugh, we cry, and we have totally open and authentic communication about their struggles and triumphs—and through this experience we have gleaned *so* much about the pitfalls and how to prevent them, during both the weight loss journey and maintenance.

The weight loss technique we use for Extreme Transformation is the most complete and powerful nutrition and exercise plan we have ever designed. It is based upon our insight into the people who not only lose the weight, but also keep it off. Within each of the 21 days is a fundamental lesson that we have discovered to have a lasting impact upon every single transformation achieved. This approach leads to true, lasting success—the kind we are all interested in. We give them the tools to not only maximize their weight loss but also *stay* active and fit. These tools and fundamental lessons make this possible and set them apart from the millions of yo-yo dieters out there. They continue to practice these simple 21 lessons every day.

We have analyzed exactly what makes these *most* successful people do so well on our program. You're about to meet many of them, hear their stories, and see their remarkable transformations in their before-and-after photos.

When you witness their journeys of success, you will be inspired and motivated to declare your own dream as well—because if *they* can do it, you can, too—whether you're trying to lose just 20 pounds, or well over 100.

If you, your client, your family member, or your loved one wants Extreme Transformation and wants to change life forever, this is your guide. We are ready to give full transparency to our whole approach, and give you real-life expectations of what is to come. Woven into these 21 days are rules, tips, tricks, and shortcuts that we will share with you—from tactics that can accelerate your weight loss, to shifting the way you think about yourself and about weight loss forever.

This same method that we use to take 50 to 200 pounds off our participants in less than a year is the *same* one we've effectively used for hundreds of other clients who want to lose just 10 to 15 pounds! Not only does it help them achieve their weight loss goals, but it also sets them up for lifelong success. Early on, we'll help you see and understand the hidden path of transformation, which usually coincides with a big "a-ha" moment, and once you "get it," you will never see life or the weight loss journey the same way again. Whether it's the final 20 pounds or more than 200 that you want to lose, just follow the program, apply the lessons, and the results will be phenomenal. Best of all, along the way we'll show you how to control the throttle, so you can drop weight at a slower, more comfortable pace, or accelerate to get to your goal in record time.

We applied the science behind behavior and habits, alongside our own personal experience, with our participants: what is necessary to break a bad habit and how we can lay down new, positive habits. We found what worked and didn't work in their real-life situations, and have filtered it down to the most effective, tangible steps toward lifelong change.

You may have heard that it takes 21 days to change a habit, and while many of us can change a habit in 21 days, recent research by such behavioral scientists as Ann M. Graybiel has shown that, for some of us, it can take longer. We're not telling you this to worry you but instead to educate you and give realistic expectations of the journey ahead. The good news is that we have planned around this. We have structured our nutrition and exercise method in 21-day phases so that you learn how to change the bad habits that led to your weight gain and replace them with new, empowering habits that help you lose weight and feel much better. You can repeat the 21-day phase until you've reached your goal weight and replaced those destructive habits with new routines to "anchor in" your new body and mind-set.

As you can see, this is *the* guide to total transformation. These are *all* of our secrets. This transformation you are about to embark upon will lead to a whole new you. It is a kind of change that is deep and life altering. It is not superficial. It is not just physical change; it is an emotional, mental, social, and even spiritual change. It's the kind of change that takes all of you—your thoughts and your feelings, your body and your brain. All of you.

Now, we aren't just going to sit here, telling everyone else to follow these 21 lessons. No, we actually practice and follow them ourselves. We are so passionate about this process because these steps have enriched and changed *our* lives! Yes. We live Extreme Transformation on a daily basis. So when we teach you the lessons of transformation, we are sharing with you not just as your coaches, but also as your equals—your teammates on this journey. These steps are lessons that we'll never master—but to live our best life, we must continually practice them! We're all in this together. While you are living Extreme Transformation, know that we, and hundreds of thousands of other people are, too!

We've also included tips—some from Heidi, and some from me. You'll know who's talking to you by these clever little icons that tag them:

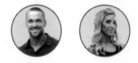

When you follow the 21 days of the Extreme Carb Cycle (our nutrition plan) and Metabolic Missions (our exercise plan), you will see and feel your body change rapidly. But when you learn and apply the lessons within the 21 Days to Transformation, you will feel a whole new sense of control over your life and your destiny. Finally, after years of feeling lost, depressed, or frustrated, you will come to a place where you feel hopeful and optimistic. You will see your life and your future with clarity. You will wake up in the morning with enthusiasm. You will go through your day confident and self-assured. You will turn out the light at night feeling successful, satisfied, and in control.

The 21 Days to Transformation fall into three weeks, each week covering one of the three components to create your own Extreme Transformation. Your days begin with good ol' delicious nutrition and a workout challenge, followed by one transformation lesson and activity that creates a deeper understanding of who you are and how you can unlock your true potential.

Week One: Days 1–7 help you **Learn It**

Week Two: Days 8–14 help you **Love It**

Week Three: Days 15–21 help you **Live It** for the rest of your life!

This is our promise to you: We will show you how to lose weight, get fit, and discover a part of you that you never knew existed. You will feel confident and energetic—able to take on life's challenges with vigor. You will feel happier and more in control than ever before. You will love yourself. That's what Extreme Transformation can do for you.

Let the journey begin...

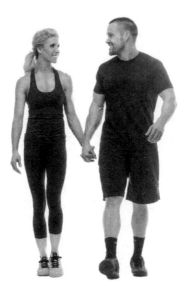

# The Method

Chapter One

# WHY EXTREME TRANSFORMATION?

**O**ur hit show *Extreme Weight Loss* has inspired millions of men and women around the world to change their lives for the better. In the show, we guide our courageous participants through a year-long journey of transformation. Although they lose hundreds of pounds in the process, the most rewarding part is what they gain: confidence, self-esteem, love, courage, and the know-how to control their bodies for the rest of their lives.

Our goal for this book is to share every component, every lesson, every aspect of transformation that will enable you to reach your weight loss goals and live enthusiastically—for the rest of your life. Though we've designed this 21-day guide around the exact method that we use with our participants, we have fine-tuned it so that whether you are here to lose those pesky 10 pounds that you put on and take off like a yo-yo, the last 20 pounds of post-baby weight, or 100 pounds or more, you can consider these 21 action-packed days your personal transformation boot camp—your guide to lifelong weight loss. We feel that this is the most effective method to date because it builds on our previous strategies and successes over the years, and includes new improvements that can deliver significant weight loss (as much as 1.5 percent of your body weight per week if you choose).

The 21-day plan is built upon a simple but powerful carb-cycle approach to eating, a once-a-day brief exercise *mission* that will stimulate your muscles and activate your body for weight loss, a fun activity of your choosing to accelerate your weight loss, and a simple yet powerful lesson and mental activity. This may sound routine, but let us assure you—the transformation journey you are about to embark upon is anything but!

We know that most diets can work—at least in the short term. Heck, a quick Internet search will find literally hundreds of plans that will most likely get you to take off weight if you follow them correctly. Unfortunately most diets don't take into account the necessary mental strategies, tactics, and know-how to control your weight for the rest of your life. So what happens? You lose weight in the short term, but then inevitably you go back to your old habits and patterns and gain it all back.

This is why Extreme Transformation is nothing like a diet. Instead, our no-nonsense approach to transformation contains within it our 21 simple but crucial lessons that clear the way for you to change your relationship with food and alter the habits that led to your weight gain to begin with. In these pages, we will lay out the entire journey for you—the good, the bad, and the ugly. We don't want to sugarcoat what lies ahead. Changing deeply engrained habits will get you out of your comfort zone and you will have moments—or days—of uneasiness and challenges. But we believe that if you face this inevitable discomfort head-on, you will find a sense of personal strength you never thought possible. So if you are ready to lose the weight forever, look no farther. But be prepared: There is some tough love ahead!

We realize that if you've picked up this book, you are already open to this process. You've taken an essential step toward a better life. But listen closely: True and lifelong transformation digs much deeper than diet and exercise. The process of losing excess pounds? That's the easy part. Really. And that's where we are going to start. We are going to show you the very simple, straightforward way to eat and exercise that will help you lose all the weight you want to lose. We'll show you how and why it works. We'll give you the exact method we use to help people lose up to hundreds of pounds in less than a year. You are going to be eating delicious foods (and we have included dozens of easy-to-prepare recipes for each day of the 21-day cycle) and discovering just how easy and rewarding the Metabolic Missions and Accelerators are.

As soon as you shift into this weight loss mode, you will begin to lose weight, feel lighter, and be more energetic! And that's just the beginning.

After one week, your body will begin to shed unwanted water weight and fat, and show signs of a more efficient metabolism. In two weeks you will see and feel a significant change in your body, and by the third week you will begin to feel more confident and clear about reaching your goals...and your life. You'll begin to see and believe that you really *can* do this.

We give you all that you need to do—a day-by-day road map that will get you to your weight loss goals (see chapter 2 for more details on how the carb cycle works). Each day offers five meals, a quick 5- to 20-minute Metabolic Mission, a weight loss Accelerator, and a fundamental lesson and mental activity to stoke your motivation and create a deeper understanding of yourself so that you can keep the weight off forever. All your meals—breakfast, lunch, snacks, and dinner—are laid out for you so you don't have to do any thinking! And we've also included some "Clean Cheat" snacks and meals for your reward days, too! Just follow the path!

These days are set up so that we can all go through the plan together. Day 1 through Day 4 we rev up our metabolism and burn fat with healthy carbs, Metabolic Missions, and Accelerators. Come Day 5, we all switch to low-carbs, turbocharging our weight loss for two days so we can all step on the scale the morning of Day 7 and see our amazing progress. If you want the same experience our participants go through on the show, this is it. In fact, as you are going through this *right now*, our participants and thousands of people around the world are, too!

Of course, if your work or living schedule doesn't match up with a Monday-through-Sunday schedule, no problem. You can start your Extreme Cycle on any day of the week—just choose what best fits with you. The 21-day cycle is flexible and adaptable to you, your goals, and your lifestyle.

But the beauty is that in just 21 days, you will begin a powerful and effective way to lose weight and get in shape. You will lose a number of pounds weekly and feel lighter, more fit, and more confident in just 21 days. You will maximize your metabolism so that your body can mobilize and oxidize fat effectively. You will also become more finely attuned to your body's response to food so that you feel satisfied, balanced, and no longer at the mercy of out-of-control cravings. And if you ever do experience a craving, we show you all of the tricks of the trade to curb it instantly, so that you always remain in control.

Our new exercise plan is part of this metabolic remake: These 15 Metabolic Missions will challenge you to explore your physical capabilities of running, jumping, pushing, crunching, and squatting so that you boost metabolism, and shape and develop lean muscle. You will begin to see an entirely new, more slender and cut silhouette. Just look at the dozens of before-and-after photos of our peeps in the pages ahead, and see what they created for themselves through Extreme Transformation! Best of all, you will repeat the 15 Metabolic Missions every three weeks, and when you perform them again you will perform more reps and more rounds than before. Every 21 days, you will see quantitative proof that you are getting fitter! These missions are designed to turn you into a badass.

Each Metabolic Mission is simple and easy to work into your daily routine. You will not have to carve out huge sections of time to fit in a complicated fitness program. You don't need any equipment. And you don't even need to go to a gym if you prefer exercising at home! You will be able to do a quick, effective workout in less than 15 to 20 minutes a day, five days a week. Accelerators are an added bonus that are included to boost your metabolism and burn even more fat. These longer-duration exercises (think cardio) are optional—but once you learn how they actually accelerate your weight loss, we won't need to convince you. Ultimately, they can lead to your record-breaking weight loss!

Eating and exercising are just the beginning of your transformation journey. In fact, they're the easy part. The secret ingredient to your life of transformation lies in the motivational lessons that accompany each of the 21 Days to Transformation.

## HOW EXTREME TRANSFORMATION
## REALLY WORKS

We do things a little differently around here. Yes, you are going to follow the exact diet and exercise plan that we use for all of our remarkable transformations, but we have found that when you are able to "see" weight loss from a different perspective, you will focus on something totally different than the diet and exercise, and actually embrace this process with *enthusiasm*. Anybody can reluctantly follow a diet plan and lose weight…but think about what we're actually saying here: Imagine going through this weight loss journey and arriving into maintenance, without ever having to fixate on diet and exercise. That's right. Granted, we will teach you diet and exercise, but you're going to feel so good focusing on the true components of transformation, the weight loss just happens. We are going to show you how to radically shift your thinking to do just that, which is why your results will be so extraordinary!

In the process, you will identify different aspects of your life that have been holding you back, preventing you from achieving an extraordinary life. We understand how overwhelming and uncomfortable it can feel to begin yet another attempt at weight loss…when those in the past never really worked. Don't worry. We will show you the way.

You may have encountered advice and tips from positive psychology or other forms of self-help. What we've designed here is different: It's a path that is physical, emotional, and mental; one that is backed by the latest neuroscience and research into habit formation, our reward pathways, and getting at the root of addictive behaviors. It's also supported by some of the most advanced research in nutrition and exercise physiology. We take all of the science and bundle it up with some good old-fashioned common sense and real-life experience, and deliver it to you in this guide. Extreme Transformation is real, and it's yours.

## THE TRIAXIOM: THREE PRINCIPLES OF EXTREME TRANSFORMATION

While the new Extreme Cycle is a potent combination of high- and low-carb days to give you effective and reliable *weight loss* results, the real secret to life-long *transformation* is lying underneath the diet. Extreme Transformation is not just about how you eat and how you exercise. It's about changing habits and replacing them with a whole new way of thinking and being. It's rehabilitation.

Over the past few years, we've distilled down our observations of those who have become truly and permanently successful in their weight loss and maintenance, as well as reflections on our own experience, plus a deep dive into the most current research in the areas of integrative nutrition, exercise physiology, and neuroscience. We've simplified everything into three principles that encompass all that we do for people—focusing on their bodies, their hearts, and their minds. For lifelong change and weight loss, no single principle can exist without the others. They all must happen together. You'll feel amazing, and best of all, you'll know how and why you feel amazing.

These three principles consist of 21 lessons, which fall into the three weeks of transformation:

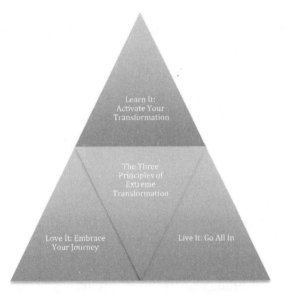

## Week One: Learn It

The first seven lessons will teach you what it takes to make the radical shift in thinking that is necessary at the beginning of your journey of transformation. You will dig deep and find two critical components for lifelong change: your *what* and your *why*. You'll identify exactly *what* it is that you want to achieve, and *why;* the motivating factors that will lead you to these goals. Then we will help you discover the true path to transformation that has been there all along. This path is in all of us, but it often lies hidden. Seeing the true path will completely shift our focus off the diet and exercise and place it where it belongs for lifelong change. We then teach you the crucial lessons of setting up your environment and your support system for success, tracking your progress, and best of all—making the journey fun!

The steps in this section will have you rethinking every weight loss program you've ever done. We will show you a path to the lifelong transformation that you have always wanted. It has always been there; you just didn't know how to see it!

## Week Two: Love It

In Week Two, you will go from learning the process of Extreme Transformation into mental and emotional action—actually taking the steps toward believing in yourself, your true abilities, and the process that leads directly to success. You will find a place that is honest and vulnerable so that you can peel away all the excuses that you've used in the past. You will learn how to unload the *real* weight—to finally be at peace with any unresolved emotional trauma you have experienced in the past—that is holding you back from living your life to the fullest.

You will take responsibility for your actions, you will learn how to identify and banish the negative self-talk that has held you back, and ultimately embrace a whole new identity—one built on self-love, integrity, and dignity!

Finally, you will address your fears. We know and understand these fears, and we are going to teach you tactics to conquer them once and for all. We'll take you through some tough situations that will help you get inside yourself— maybe to a place that you've never let yourself go before. Don't be afraid.

We have seen it all, and nearly every individual who begins to Love It— embrace their journey with enthusiasm—will tell you that it is one of the greatest accomplishments of their life. In the end, you will feel powerfully free from those chains that have held you back in the past.

## Week Three: Live It

The lessons in Week Three prepare you to handle the challenges ahead, and set you up to live a life of transformation. You will learn how to become a priority in your own life, and you will know how to defend your priorities aggressively so that no one will stand in the way of your success. We will lay out inevitable obstacles ahead that will try to derail your progress. When you do fall off track, we will teach you the tried-and-true method to getting right back on. And we will shine a spotlight on your current triggers, so that you can identify them and navigate safely around or through them.

These lessons will help you uproot deeply engrained behaviors that have kept you fixed in patterns of coping with triggers by eating foods that not only add weight, but are most likely making you sick. You will learn how to replace these bad habits, addictions to food, and routines that have been sabotaging you, with a new way of living so that you can continue to lose weight and maintain that weight loss—forever.

## Janey's Story

Janey's story has inspired thousands of followers on my blog HeidiPowell.net. Check out how this single mom lost 36 pounds, going from 158 to 122, and got into the best shape of her life!

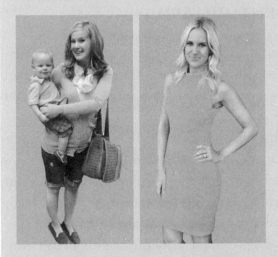

"Health and fitness have not always been my forte. Just a few years ago I couldn't run to the end of my block without feel-ing winded and the only veggies in my life were the limp celery slices that came with my Buffalo wings. I was over 30 pounds heavier, unhealthy, unhappy, out of shape, *and* freshly divorced. At 21, with a toddler in tow, I was about to start my life over, and just the thought of facing the world after that kind of pain and heartbreak was enough to keep me in bed with only a large cheese pizza to keep me company... seri-ously, I once ate an entire cheese pizza in an attempt to drown my sorrows! It was time for a change, and the day I signed divorce papers was also the day I com-mitted to leading a healthy lifestyle for the rest of my life. That's when I met Heidi and Chris. I started slow and began to see small changes happening in my body, and I loved it. Just three months after I had made it my goal to change my life, I crossed the finish line of my very first 10K. Best. Feeling. Ever. Ironically, it was on this exact same day that I told my boyfriend (now husband), Kyle, that I loved him for the first time, another huge feat I never imagined possible.

"About a year ago, almost exactly three years after deciding to start my life over, my husband and I crossed off one of the final "to-do's" on my fitness bucket list and completed a half marathon together, crossing the finish line hand in hand. It was so symbolic of all of the changes I had made in my life to get to this point, and was easily one of the most emotionally raw moments of my life. So grateful to have my husband alongside me in this journey!"

## IT'S YOUR LIFE. NOW LIVE IT
## WITH ENTHUSIASM!

Throughout this guide, you will read about and see the amazing transformations we have helped others achieve. The results speak for themselves. We are confident in our methodology because time and time again we have proven firsthand its life-changing power.

The 21 days and their accompanying lessons are crucial to your transformation. They are the stepping-stones to the grander path that you will be achieving and accessing. What you are in for is so much bigger, so much more powerful, so much more fulfilling than anything you've ever imagined. Yes, your weight loss will be amazing and fitness will improve—they are goals that keep on giving and giving. But the empowered heart and clarity of mind that come from understanding and finally appreciating yourself—are priceless.

We're so excited for you.

Now here we go!

POWELL

# Chapter Two

# HOW THE EXTREME CYCLE WORKS

During the last three seasons of *Extreme Weight Loss* we used an innovative new approach to carb cycling to see if, as predicted, it would help our people lose their desired weight in a more sustainable way. This cycle, which we call the Extreme Cycle, is made up of five high-carb days, followed by two low-carb days.

This flow worked wonders for all of our participants. They not only lost weight easily and immediately and without feeling rocked by big changes to their eating habits, but also felt strong and stable enough to continue eating this way when they went home after 90 days of boot camp with us and beyond.

As Jeff told us, "Ever since I truly committed to Chris and Heidi's Extreme Cycle, I am finally feeling amazing. I eat something delicious and filling every three hours. I set aside time for myself every day to train—and I want to. I'm seeing results every week. I like who I am and how I feel. I even got a tattoo on my arm that says THIS IS MY LIFE NOW. This experience saved my family and my life."

We are going to share a lot more about Jeff's transformation—his story is an amazing ride of highs and lows and ultimately true transformation (see page 128). But we are sharing his testimonial because we want to give you a sense of just how passionately our participants respond to the Extreme Cycle and how amazing it feels to lose weight with confidence and control.

In a nutshell, we have designed our Extreme Cycle so that it:

- Gives you a way to eat that is convenient, simple, delicious, and satiating.
- Enables you to continuously lose at least one percent of your body weight each week.
- Increases your body awareness (we will explain why this is so important to continued weight loss and commitment to your goals).

So what does this all mean? If you are 5'6" and weigh 275 pounds now, you can lose upwards of seven or more pounds per 21-day cycle; if you weigh 155 pounds at 5'2" you can lose up to five or more pounds per 21-day cycle. Or if you weigh 350 pounds at 6', you can feasibly lose over ten or more pounds per 21-day cycle. And keep in mind, you can accelerate these numbers even more to lose weight as fast as the participants on the show if you choose—we'll show you how. The beauty and brilliance of Extreme Transformation is that once you establish your goals, you can repeat the 21-day cycle for as long as you need to reach them.

The point is that Extreme Transformation is both realistic and successful. It requires changes, but it doesn't wreak havoc on your daily life and make you feel like you have to live in a bubble of deprivation and restriction. You are at home, at work, living your life—*losing weight and getting fit*.

## MASTERING YOUR METABOLISM AND CREATING WEIGHT LOSS

The number of calories you burn each day varies according to how active you are. If you follow the same routine every day, eating and moving around (or not) in pretty much the same ways, you'll burn roughly the same number of calories every day. The proportion of calories used by each of your body's three energy consumers—digestion, maintenance, and movement—will also stay pretty constant.

So, how many calories are we talking about? That depends on some factors: your gender, your height, your weight, and your age. Generally, a bigger body needs more calories than a smaller one does, and a younger body needs more calories than an older body does.

All these numbers are swell, but you're reading this book because you want to slim down, not because you want to study science. Let's put the facts and figures together into tools that will help you get the body you want. The arithmetic of weight loss is super-simple:

- Each day that you eat more calories than your metabolism burns, your body stores the extra energy as body fat. You gain weight.
- Eat the same number of calories as your metabolism burns, and your body neither builds nor uses up its stores of fat. You maintain your weight.
- Eat fewer calories than your metabolism burns, and your body makes up the energy shortfall by tapping into your fat. You lose weight. This is what fitness professionals call a *calorie deficit,* and it's the key to weight loss.
- The calorie deficit is what weight loss is all about. If you want to drop the pounds, you have to run your metabolism at a deficit. How big a deficit? Here's the magic number: To lose one pound of fat in a given window of time—say, a week—you've got to burn 3,500 more calories than you take in. That doesn't mean you have to cut out 3,500 calories a day (you probably don't even eat that much!). But to lose weight you do have to eat less. Most carb-cyclers find that they get the best results by creating a 500- to 1,000-calorie deficit through their diet daily—then boost the deficit even more through Accelerators!

Keeping your own metabolism in mind as you work the 21-day cycle is an important tool to keep you focused on your calorie intake. If you begin to plateau, for instance, check in and make sure that your calories didn't spike.

## WHAT IS CARB CYCLING?

Carb Cycling is an alternating, patterned way of eating to maximize the ability to manipulate your body for fat loss. High-carb days consist of predominantly high-protein, *high*-carb, low-fat meals. Low-carb days consist of predominantly high-protein, *low*-carb, high-fat meals.

During high-carb days, there is a moderate to high insulin response after the meals, triggering a temporary anabolic state—driving nutrients into the muscles and boosting metabolic rate. During low-carb days, there is a minimal insulin response after the meals, keeping the body in a mostly catabolic state—breaking down and oxidizing fat. Long story short, high-carb days boost your metabolism (while still losing fat), and low-carb days turbocharge your fat loss.

Carb Cycling has actually been used in the fitness industry for decades as a powerful way to positively alter body composition by maximizing fat burn while maintaining muscle mass. With the Extreme Cycle, we just put a real-life twist on it, and the results speak for themselves: Incredible weight loss, eating foods that you enjoy, without crashing your metabolism.☺

## WHAT IS THE *EXTREME* CYCLE?

The Extreme Cycle is a continuous pattern of four high-carb days followed by two low-carb days, then a Reset day. Because of the strategic way the high-carb and low-carb days are structured, you lose weight more steadily, and in a way that makes you feel balanced and controlled. You'll learn how to truly manipulate your body to maximize fat loss and turn good numbers on the scale every week. With each passing week, you will feel stronger and more agile. As you integrate the daily Metabolic Missions, you will increase your lean muscle mass and tone your body. When you add the weight loss Accelerators, you'll see the numbers on the scale drop even faster.

### Extreme Cycle Weekly Schedule

Here's a broad overview of what a week of the Extreme Cycle looks like:

Day 1: Monday: High-Carb Day

Day 2: Tuesday: High-Carb Day

Day 3: Wednesday: High-Carb Day

Day 4: Thursday: High-Carb Day

Day 5: Friday: Low-Carb Day

Day 6: Saturday: Low-Carb Day

Day 7: Sunday: Weigh-In and Reset Day

## How the Extreme Cycle Works on the Inside: The Science

Before we go any further, we feel it's helpful for you to understand how the Extreme Cycle is specifically designed to maximize your weight loss experience—both physically and psychologically.

We're going to drop some science on you here. If you're a physiology and psychology geek like us, then enjoy! ☺ If not, don't worry…we'll break it all down for you in "normal" terms beyond this section. You'll see that there is a specific purpose to every component of the Extreme Cycle design. We developed the cycle this way for a multitude of physiological and psychological reasons:

1. The calorie ranges are designed so that for six days of the week you will be in an overall calorie deficit—which means that the body will spend more time breaking down fat stores (mobilizing) and using them for energy (oxidizing). As long as the calorie deficit is maintained, the laws of physics remain on your side—and always work. When you consume less energy than your body burns, you lose weight. That's the beauty of physics. Even on high-carb days, the total of your meals is designed to result in a calorie deficit, so you will consistently lose weight. On low-carb days, the weight loss process is turbocharged even more.

2. Starting with four high-carb days in a row gives a type of "normalcy" to a structured way of eating every day. It creates mental comfort and allows you to get into

a groove with meals and preferences that work for you. Alternating between high- and low-carb days is effective, but switching between days can be confusing and disruptive to our habitual patterns. The beauty and ease of this Extreme Carb Cycle pattern allows for the powerful nature of carb cycling, without the discomfort of significantly uprooting your eating patterns.

3. Carbs are *necessary* for weight loss! Carbohydrates are the "92-octane fuel" that powers our brain, our muscles, and the rest of the organs of our body. Fueling the body with carbs puts more fuel into the muscles, yielding greater intensity and effort during workouts—which then results in a greater metabolic afterburn (more calories burned at rest) and stronger stimulus for muscle development and growth.

4. Carbs in the diet are directly linked to more effective thyroid conversion in the liver—therefore keeping metabolic rate up. Low-carb diets blunt thyroid conversion and ultimately result in metabolic slowdown. Four high-carb days in a row get the metabolic furnace burning red-hot, priming the body for maximum fat loss when switching over to the low-carb days.

5. Breakfast always includes a carbohydrate and a fat—in addition to a protein—for a couple of reasons. The carbohydrates are designed to replace liver glycogen lost during the overnight fast (glycogen was used to fuel the heartbeat and diaphragm during sleep). Since the liver is one of the main controlling organs of the body, filling up its store of glycogen puts the body into a "fed" state—which essentially signals the body to "wake up" and increase metabolic processes. The fats are designed to slow digestion, keeping you fuller well into the morning and just in time for your midmorning snack (meal 2).

6. Starchy carbohydrates are a no-no at dinner. While there are still carbs included in the form of fibrous vegetables (leafy greens or cruciferous veggies), all sugars and starches are out. This is to prevent a rise in blood sugar in the evening. Instead, by pulling starchy and sugary carbs, the body is more likely to have a minor insulin response, remaining in a catabolic state into the overnight fast, which keeps your body mobilizing (breaking down) and oxidizing (burning) fat well into the night…when the body experiences a metabolic slowdown. Basically, when done right, you don't store fat at night this way—you actually burn it while you are sleeping!

7. After four high-carb days, we drop into two low-carb days. This is where the *real* control over your weight loss starts to take place. Pulling carbs from your meals and snacks flips the switch to turbocharge

the rate at which your body burns fat. However, because you don't have starchy carbs in your system, your body does not release as much insulin, triggering your body to burn fat instead—you go into maximized fat mobilization and oxidation.

8. The two low-carb days are also designed to help remove any excess water retention and bloating in the body. Starchy carbs are like magnets for water. Therefore, removing sugary and starchy carbs from the diet for two days results in a natural release of water—revealing a more true weight on the scale.

Imagine being a sculptor in this process. You put a light blanket of water over your body during the four high-carb days. During this time you chisel away under the blanket with good nutrition, Metabolic Missions, and Accelerators—carving the body you want. After four days, you drop into two low-carb days, pulling the blanket off and revealing the progress so far. The next week you do it again…and again…each week putting the blanket over the sculpture and working away, revealing the latest results every weigh-in…until you are finally finished with your masterpiece.

This is the beauty of the Extreme Cycle and makes you the true artist here. You're in total control the whole way!

9. Every seventh day, you will weigh yourself in the morning, then reset your metabolism, rest your body, and give yourself a reward. Physiologically, the increase in calories boosts metabolism significantly. Psychologically, the Reset day gives us something to look forward to, so we don't feel deprived on this journey. This is your chance to satisfy any cravings you may have, relieving any feelings of restriction. On Reset days, you eat high-carb meals and snacks, but you can also reward yourself with a Clean Cheat snack or meal (see page 86 for a complete list of Clean Cheats). Rest and reward are a huge part of avoiding feelings of deprivation and preventing overwhelming cravings.

So there you have it: a broad overview of *how* the Extreme Cycle works to help you reach your weight loss goals quickly and comfortably.

As you will soon see, we have designed the 21-day cycle so that your meal planning is fast and enjoyable. We've laid it all out for you with quick-and-easy recipes. In fact, several of these recipes were inspired by gourmet chef David Rushing, who lost over 200 pounds during Season 4 of *Extreme Weight Loss*. Through his journey of transformation, he took his extensive knowledge of the culinary arts and weight loss experience, and helped us to create many of the delectable meals you will enjoy in this book!

We've also provided simple, go-to meal suggestions, and a three-step plan to creating your own meals if you don't want to bother with the recipes. Those are all listed on page 72.

## WHAT DO I EAT?

Contrary to popular belief that we need to restrict certain nutrients to lose weight and to nourish our bodies for optimum weight loss, we need *all* of the main macronutrients—proteins, carbohydrates, *and* fats. The secret is in how we combine them in our meals to manipulate our bodies to do what we want them to do—lose fat!

In order to create the powerful meal combinations in the Extreme Cycle, we must categorize foods into different macronutrients based upon their predominant nutrient content. For example, lean ground turkey is predominantly made of protein; however, it may have 2 or 3 grams of fat. Therefore, lean ground turkey falls into the protein category. Most foods are not exclusively *one* macronutrient, but have trace amounts of other macros in them. We have done all of the footwork for you, and have categorized them for the most effective meal combinations!

### Protein

Protein is vital to the proper functioning of our muscles, brain, organs, and other tissues, and is the foundation macronutrient used in the Extreme Cycle. We eat it with every meal. Protein is the building block for the most active metabolic tissues of our body—our muscles—and we need to make sure they are nourished with every meal. In addition, protein is a quickly satiating nutrient, meaning that it makes us full when we eat it. Because of this, we prefer to eat protein first at every meal to make us immediately full. It's a quick and easy rule that we have used for years, and it works like a charm to curb cravings and prevent overeating carbs or fats later!

Some of the proteins you will enjoy include:

- Protein shakes and smoothies
- Lean beef
- Fat-free and low-fat dairy such as cottage cheese, Greek yogurt, and egg whites
- Chicken, turkey, and pork tenderloin
- Fish and shellfish
- Soy protein sources such as tofu and tempeh
- Other vegetarian protein options such as hemp, bean, and pea protein
- And many more…check out Appendix D for the full list!

## Carbohydrates

Carbohydrates have been demonized over the past couple decades as a main cause of the obesity epidemic, but when you eat the right carbs at the right times, they can actually be one of your greatest allies in the weight loss battle. All carbs are broken down into the sugar called glucose—which is the high-octane fuel our cells are designed to function on. In short, carbs nourish our body! When we get the right amount of glucose in our system, it nourishes our liver, our muscles, our brain, and all of our other organs. It naturally boosts our metabolism and primes our body for maximum weight loss. In fact, there's a saying in the physiology world that "fat burns in a carbohydrate fire."

However, too much glucose in our system is not a good thing. That's why when losing weight we want to avoid carbohydrates that are broken down quickly in our system. These carbs are the highly processed, starchy, or sugary carbs found in snacks, junk foods, or baked goods. Instead, when following the Extreme Cycle, we nourish our body regularly with quality carbs that are broken down slowly, to trickle the glucose into our bloodstream. These are the real, clean, natural carbohydrates found in foods like:

- Whole grains (rice, breads, pastas, cereals, popcorn)
- Beans and legumes

- Root vegetables (potatoes, yams, squash, et cetera)
- Fruit

(A full list of all the healthy foods is in Appendix D.)

These carbs are packed with vitamins and minerals, high in fiber, and digested easily by your body so that it feels satisfied, and you feel energetic.

While protein is mandatory at each meal, there is an optional food on the Extreme Cycle that you can add to, or remove from your meals, based upon your customized needs—vegetables! Whereas vegetables are technically a carbohydrate, most are rich in fiber and extremely low in any calorie impact. Because of this, we classify these in their own special category and consider them a so-called "free food": They can be enjoyed in limitless portions, and are one of the most powerful tools for feeling full and satiated.

Veggies are high in fiber, water, and valuable antioxidants, and we highly advise you to eat as many as possible in your meals—although it is not mandatory. We make veggies an optional food because oftentimes the amount of mandatory food you are already eating in your meals can have such volume, it can be difficult to consume so much food. However, if you struggle with cravings, adding veggies to your meals will be an incredibly powerful tactic to curb any cravings and keep you feeling full and satisfied throughout the day.

We're going to show you some amazing ways to volumize your meals to gigantic proportions using delicious vegetables. Follow our list of veggies, and they're yours to enjoy in limitless amounts. You are approved to eat all the veggies you want—anytime!

- Broccoli
- Cauliflower
- Green beans
- Carrots
- Onions
- Spinach
- And many more...

## Fats

Fats are the third main macronutrient—and a powerful one at that! Our brains rely on fats—especially the essential fatty acids such as omega-3s and omega-6s—to maintain proper cellular function and hormonal balance. These fats are enormously important to how our brain and bodies manage the hormones that regulate our body temperature, our moods, and our digestion.

However, following the Extreme Cycle, we use fats to trick your body and your mind to make weight loss SO much easier. Fats have a powerful effect on slowing digestion and keeping our stomachs full. When we use the right fats at the right time, we can curb cravings and maximize fat loss at the same time. Keep reading and we'll show you how!

Often people worry when they think about cutting out carbs for two days, but adding in some tasty fats *really* opens up the food options for delicious meals! Check out the kinds of dietary fats you can have on these low-carb days. You're going to start looking forward to these days!

- Egg yolk
- Butter
- Heavy Cream
- Cheese
- Bacon
- Olives
- Avocado
- Nuts and seeds
- Olive and flaxseed oil
- Nut butters such as peanut butter and almond butter
- And many more...

As you can see, you will be eating an array of delicious, enjoyable foods. Just wait until you see the meals and recipes we lay out for you—it only gets better! Now, let's take a look at the different meal combinations we use following the Extreme Cycle, to maximize your fat loss results:

# BREAKFAST:
# IGNITE YOUR DAY

Our parents were right. Breakfast really *is* the most important meal of the day. It helps "*break* the *fast*" from not eating for many hours, and helps jump-start your metabolism from its overnight slumber (slowdown). No matter whether it is a high- or a low-carb day, your breakfast breakdown is always the same: Protein + Carbohydrate + Fats.

## High-Carb Days

After breakfast things change a little bit:

For Meals 2, 3, and 4 on high-carb days, you will be eating carbohydrates with each meal and cutting out the dietary fats, so it looks like this:

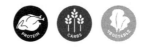

For Meal 5 on a high-carb day, we will remove the carbohydrate and replace it with a healthy fat to flip the fat-burning switch. It will look like this:

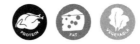

## Low-Carb Days

After breakfast on the low-carb days, we cut carbs and instead eat fats with each of the last 4 meals, so it looks like this:

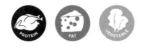

### *Reset Days*

Once a week on your weigh-in day, you get to reset your metabolism and reward yourself for a job well done! Your Reset day is neither a high-carb nor a high-fat day…it's more of a high-*calorie* day. Reset day is incredibly important for a few reasons: Physiologically, the increase in calories boosts your metabolic rate for more effective fat loss the following days. Mentally, it satisfies any psychological or emotional cravings that you may be experiencing, so that you will never feel deprived and risk straying from your weight loss journey. We have even designed some incredible Clean Cheat recipes (see page 269) to help you bump up your calories for your Reset day, while indulging in some of your favorite delicacies. However, instead of cheap junk food, you'll be eating high-quality foods that will nourish your body and prepare you for the best weight loss results. Some of these recipes include:

- Hootenanny Pancakes
- BLT Burger and Sweet Potato Fries
- Barbecue Chicken Pita Pizza
- Spinach Artichoke Dip
- Peanut Butter Chocolate Chip Cookie Dough
- Mac and Cheese with Bacon
- And *many* more…

As you can see, there is a *lot* to look forward to with this program. You are in for some delicious new dishes. Who said dieting had to be bland?!

## WHEN DO I EAT?

With the Extreme Carb Cycle, you will be eating every three hours. Think of your metabolism as a furnace for your body. Eat less often and your metabolism cools down; eat more often and it heats up. The hotter your furnace gets, the more fuel it burns, including the stored fat that hasn't been doing anything but weighing you down!

Following the Extreme Cycle, we always eat breakfast within 30 minutes of waking, then eat a meal every three hours after. A typical Extreme Cycle meal schedule (whether high-carb or low-carb) looks like this:

Wake up at 6:30 a.m.
Meal 1: Breakfast at 7:00 a.m.

Meal 2: Morning snack at 10:00 a.m.
Meal 3: Lunch at 1:00 p.m.
Meal 4: Afternoon snack at 4:00 p.m.
Meal 5: Dinner at 7:00 p.m.

Of course, you would adjust this schedule depending on when you wake up. If you are a very early riser, you might be starting your breakfast at 6:00 a.m. and finishing your dinner around 6:00 p.m. Even if you work the midnight shift and wake up at 7:00 p.m. every day, the rules still apply: Eat within 30 minutes of waking and approximately every three hours thereafter!

## Reality Check

Look, we know that life has all kinds of unexpected twists and turns, especially when it comes to the daily grind. The timing of your meals does not have to be *exactly* every three hours; just try to get it as close as possible. Sometimes you may eat every two and a half hours, sometimes every four hours. If your days run long and you find yourself hungry after your final meal, try spacing out your meals to every three and a half hours, so you eat closer to the time you go to bed. With the Extreme Cycle, *you* create the meal timing that works best in your life!

## WATER, WATER, WATER

We cannot stress enough the importance of drinking a *lot* of water when on the weight loss journey. Fact of the matter is that if you don't drink enough water, you will not lose the weight at your fastest potential. Why? Water is the main ingredient in the majority of the metabolic processes of the body—which is the driving force behind weight loss! Proper hydration keeps metabolism high, increases mental clarity and energy, and is a powerful influencer for curbing cravings. In addition, living the Extreme Transformation lifestyle, you will be exercising more, so you will lose fluids faster through perspiration and breathing, making hydration even more important.

Did you know that nearly 90 percent of Americans are chronically dehydrated? And unfortunately, most of us go through our days without realizing it, causing us to suffer from unnecessary fatigue and increased cravings. Early on your journey, we are going to ask you to drink an extra quart of water every day. However, ultimately we would like you to work up to drinking at least a gallon of water every day. This will be critical in maximizing your results!

## Take the Hydration Test

Pinch the skin on the back of your hand and let go. If your skin stays puckered for any length of time then you are more than likely dehydrated. Also, keep an eye on your urine. If the color is slightly yellow or darker, your body is telling you that it needs fluid. And since water is the safest fluid, we suggest sticking to drinking water. Drink until your urine is consistently clear or just slightly yellow. Then you'll know your body's hydration is primed for fat loss!

## Reality Check

Let's get real. Like many of you, we don't like to drink regular water. It is bland, especially when trying to push a gallon or more every day! If we're going to get that much water in, we need to *want* to drink it. We need flavor! There are some *amazing* low- and no-calorie sweeteners out there for water these days. Feel free to grab some (or a lot) at the supermarket, and flavor away to stay well hydrated during your transformation journey. Carry a huge water bottle around with you every day (from 1 liter to 1 gallon), flavored however you choose!

## Chris Tip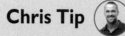

To make sure you get all the water you need, follow our 10-gulp rule:

Every time the water bottle touches your lips, take 10 gulps before putting it down...
and you will stay well hydrated all day long!

## Heidi Tip
## Vitamins, Minerals, and Fiber

Even though following the Extreme Cycle will have you eating highly nutritious foods, anytime you are eating fewer calories than you are burning, your body is most likely at a slight deficit in its necessary vitamins, minerals, and fiber as well. You may want to supplement the Extreme Cycle with a good multivitamin to make sure your body is getting the vitamins and minerals it needs to perform at its best. In addition, we recommend adding at least 1 tablespoon of psyllium fiber to your daily meals (it's usually added to a protein shake or some other liquid) to ensure proper fiber intake. A healthy body begins with a healthy gut—which is where all of our nutrients are absorbed! Fiber is nature's "scrub brush" for the intestines; if you add at least an extra tablespoon of fiber daily, your body and bowels will thank you for it!

## HOW MUCH DO I EAT?

Any weight loss plan inevitably begs the question: How much do I eat if I want to lose weight? Science dictates that fat is lost only when we take in fewer calories than our body burns. A lot of different plans use different methods to accomplish this goal: points, portion plates, hand portions, pre-planned recipes, and so on. In previous books, we taught quick-and-easy portion sizing using your hand as a measure. While this works for most people in reducing their calorie intake and teaches appropriate portions, Extreme Cycling is a precision program. Yes, all of the recipes are dialed in to maximize your weight loss, but we are going to show you what's happening behind the curtain—so that you have the power to create your own meal combinations, and customize your own menu if you choose!

We have designed our calorie guidelines and portion sizes to work for most people who are seeking to optimize the way they feel during the days, and optimize the weight they see on the scale every week. In most cases, the recipes are tailored for women at 1,500 calories, and 2,000 calories for men—in our experience, these are typical calorie allotments that enable weight loss and quick-and-easy troubleshooting when combined with an exercise plan. In general, men tend to have more muscle mass, so they are allotted more calories than women. You will want to pay attention to these calorie differences when you prepare your meals and follow the recipes. All the recipes contain adjustments for men and women.

## Chris Tip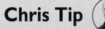

You will find that even though we talk about eating low dietary fat on high-carb days, it is impossible to go a full day without eating at least *some* dietary fats. You actually need some fat every day for proper metabolic function, and fats are bound to be present, even in low-fat, high-carbohydrate foods. That's why typically on a high-carb day, around 20 percent of your calories consumed will come incidentally from dietary fat.

Same goes for low-carb days. Carbohydrates are going to occur naturally in some of your foods—much of them as fiber on these days—but still there will be some light starches that may find their way into your meals to the tune of about 20 or so percent. Not to worry. The structure is designed for this.

Just as with everything in life—*nothing* is perfect. You are not expected to hit these exact numbers for every meal. You'll even see that the recipes we have designed for you don't hit the numbers perfectly—but overall they come darn close. With most things in life, "close enough" doesn't cut it. So be grateful that this diet is so beautifully structured that as long as you come close on your portions, you win.

## Quick Meals on the Go

Realistically speaking, we know that you will not always have a chance to prepare your own meals. When you find yourself eating elsewhere, a quick-and-easy rule of thumb to get close to appropriate portions for you would be to follow the hand-portion guide:

**Proteins:** Palm-size portion
**Grainy, starchy carbs & fruit:** I clenched fist
**Veggie carbs:** 2 clenched fists
**Fats:** I thumb
**Sauces:** I thumb

## Josh's Story

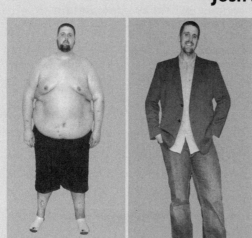

Josh tried out for *Extreme Weight Loss* but did not make the cut. At 6'9" he had gained 300 pounds, tipping the scales at 585 pounds at only 25 years old. Not being selected for the show, however, was just the beginning of Josh's transformation story. He was so committed to his own process that he buckled down and did the Extreme Cycle on his own. Within a year, he had lost 233 pounds. As he described, "I was so unhappy. I knew that this life wasn't the one I imagined. I stopped talking to girls. I stopped going out with my friends. I was a shut-in—always so sick and tired. I realized that I didn't need the TV show to make the change. And in the very first week, I lost 26 pounds. I never looked back."

Josh said that learning the Extreme Cycle and eating every three hours "just worked. I never ever felt hungry. I didn't have to ever feel deprived. Eating like this is now just second nature." Josh has now lost over 300 pounds and is currently a personal trainer, helping others achieve their dreams of living happy and healthy lives.

Know this: As soon as you switch to the Extreme Cycle, your brain and body awareness will reconnect, and your hormonal signals will right themselves. Extreme Cycling is a livable, convenient, satisfying way to eat. You won't feel like you're dieting or depriving yourself, but instead you'll feel like an artist, sculpting your new body each week under total control. Designing your meals for weight loss, eating every three hours, and drinking adequate amounts of water will open your eyes to a whole new quality of life.

Onward and upward!

POWELL

# Chapter Three

# METABOLIC MISSIONS AND ACCELERATORS

The Extreme Cycle nutrition lays down the foundation for your weight loss, but it's exercise that accelerates the results: Exercise is how you control the throttle of your weight loss journey. If you choose, you can lose weight slowly over time with just the Extreme Cycle alone. However, if you want to speed up your weight loss and nearly double your results, then you'll want to add in daily movement to see your body change faster than ever. When you exercise regularly—even if it's only 5 or 15 minutes a day—you stimulate your body's muscles, hormones, and other systems to incinerate more calories. That's why nutrition controls the fat-burning switch—and exercise turbocharges it! And with our Metabolic Missions and Accelerators, we are going to show you how we get our participants to drop extraordinary amounts of weight in record time. Now it's your turn!

## WHAT METABOLIC MISSIONS DO FOR YOU

We have designed 15 different Metabolic Missions to be completed during your 21 days of Extreme Transformation. Each Metabolic Mission is a short-duration, high-intensity circuit, designed for maximum metabolic afterburn, as well as to stimulate the muscles for shape and development. As you know, your body is made to move—to push, pull, squat, crunch, run, and jump! So all of the exercises in the missions reflect those basic, natural movements your body is meant to do.

The high-intensity nature of each Metabolic Mission elicits a strong neuro-endocrine response—to release catecholamines, increase oxygen uptake, increase lactic acid in the body, and raise body temperature. Sounds like a lot of blah, blah, science stuff… but this is why it's so awesome: When you train hard and fast, your brain is stimulated to increase the release of growth hormone—this stuff is like liquid gold. Growth hormone is one of the most lipolytic (fat-burning) hormones in the human body, and increases the rate at which the cells replenish themselves. So basically, high-intensity exercise increases fat loss and makes you look and feel younger. Doing the Metabolic Missions is the true path to the fountain of youth!

The Metabolic Missions don't require any equipment and can be done anywhere—at home, in a gym, and outside—whatever works in *your* life and is enjoyable for you! Now, these Metabolic Missions might seem simple, but that doesn't mean they aren't going to test your mettle. These rapid challenges will raise your heart rate, make your muscles burn, and get you the results you want—a slender, more toned body. An added benefit? Once you do them, you help your body burn even *more* calories throughout the day!

The Metabolic Missions are totally scalable by ability and can be done by anyone—whether you haven't worked out in 10 years, or you're already a gym rat. As long as you push yourself, you will take your fitness to new levels.

And to make this process even more forgiving, if you are just starting, you can cut the Metabolic Missions in half until you feel ready to take on a full mission.

## Metabolic Mission Code

For our Metabolic Missions, we use five different types of challenges. Each day of the work week (Monday through Friday, or whatever five days work in your schedule), you will embark upon one of these missions… and will not stop until the mission is accomplished!

1. **Stepladders**—These are circuits that either ascend or descend in repetitions. With the ascending stepladders, it's fun to see how far you can get in an allotted amount of time. The descending ladders are awesome because as you progress, the rep counts get smaller and you see an end in sight!

2. **RFT**—This acronym stands for "rounds for time." See how long it takes you to do a set number of rounds of the prescribed circuit!

3. **Chipper**—These circuits have a *lot* of reps of each exercise. It can seem daunting at first, but rep after rep you will "chip away" at the total circuit. See how long it takes to complete one round of the entire circuit!

4. **AMRAP**—This acronym stands for "as many rounds as possible." Whenever you see AMRAP next to a Metabolic Mission, do as many rounds of the circuit in the allotted time as you can!

5. **Tabata**—Tabata was developed by a brilliant physiologist from Japan. It indicates a four-minute exercise routine in which you perform as many repetitions of an exercise as possible for 20 seconds, then take a 10-second rest, then begin again with another 20-second round, followed by a 10-second rest, until you reach four minutes (8 rounds total). When you see Tabata next to one or more exercises, you know what to do: Just Tabata each of the exercises in the list for an amazing workout!

**NOTE:** Each Mission is a competition, either with yourself or with others. As with any game, it is important to have movement standards—ways to measure if the rep counts! For all of the Metabolic Mission Movements and their competition standards, refer to the detailed instructions in Part Four.

## ACCELERATORS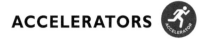

Following the Extreme Cycle and doing Metabolic Missions alone will put you on the path to steady, sustainable weight loss and greater fitness. However, many folks want faster results. We understand. When working with our participants during a one-year transformation, we have 365 days to get these individuals to lose between 100 and 300 pounds. So to accelerate the process and give them the results we all want, we add an Accelerator to their daily program. An Accelerator is a cardio-based exercise or activity that, when added to your normal routine, will aggressively burn body fat and accelerate weight loss. Accelerators are not super-quick high-intensity circuits like the Metabolic Missions. They are activities that raise and maintain an elevated heart rate, that last longer than the missions, and are much less intense. So if you want to accelerate your weight loss, add an Accelerator such as walking, running, soccer, racquetball, biking, or swimming into your routine six days of the week.

An Accelerator keeps your muscles moving and raises your heart rate for a prolonged period of time. The concept is pretty simple: The longer you move, the more calories you burn. Here's the best part about Accelerators: You get to choose the one that works best for you. It can be anything from basketball to rowing, hiking to mixed martial arts. The only major rule is that it has to be fun! If a fun exercise seems far-fetched right now, then for the time being, choose the *most* fun way you can think of to move your body...or maybe something you've always wanted to do. We have no doubt that over time as you begin to explore the capabilities of your body, you really will find *fun* in these activities! We've created a go-to guide to help you find the best Accelerator for you in Lesson 6—Make It Your Own!

What's the most effective Accelerator for fat loss? The quick-and-easy answer is running. You don't have to run *fast*...just run. If you can't run, then jog. If you can't jog, then walk. In our history of extreme transformations, those who began running, jogging, or walking (or any combo of the three), dropped the most weight, the fastest.

However, when it comes to the *best* Accelerator for you, the correct answer is: the one you love to do the most! You have freedom to choose in this journey. If you don't love running, jogging, or walking, then select a fun Accelerator that you love to do!

For those starting out, you will want to ease into your Accelerators. This slow start is done for a multitude of reasons. In the beginning, less is more. If your body has not been exposed to exercise for a long period of time, simply doing a Metabolic Mission and five minutes of Accelerating is more than enough to get some stellar results! But even more important, it's about learning to carve out that time for *you* during the day. Make sure that you can set that daily appointment and keep that promise to yourself every day. (You will read more about putting yourself first in Lesson 17—Be Beneficially Selfish.)

If you want to jump right into an hour-long class or a competitive sports league, then go for it. However, if you are starting out with an individual exercise like walking, jogging, running, rowing, cycling, and so on, you will begin your Accelerator with just 5 minutes. You'll do 5 minutes the first week, then add 5 more minutes for the second week. Then add 5 more minutes for the third. If at *any* time you feel you are unable to increase the duration of your Accelerators, stick with the current duration until you are ready to add the next 5 minutes. It is more important that you keep your commitment to completing a *shorter* period of time rather than commit to accelerating for longer and not do it! Again, we'll go into those very important commitments soon. ☺ In the meantime, here's an idea for how we structure Accelerators for Extreme Transformation:

| Intensity | Time spent breaking a sweat (120 bpm minimum)* | | |
|---|---|---|---|
| Cycle 1 | Week 1: 5 minutes | Week 2: 10 minutes | Week 3: 15 minutes |
| Cycle 2 | Week 4: 20 minutes | Week 5: 25 minutes | Week 6: 30 minutes |
| Cycle 3 | Week 7: 35 minutes | Week 8: 40 minutes | Week 9: 45 minutes |
| Cycle 4 | Week 10: 50 minutes | Week 11: 55 minutes | Week 12: 60 minutes |
| *To take HR, take pulse (on neck or wrist) for 6 seconds and multiply by 10. | | | |

Please know that this schedule is what it would look like in a perfect world. In reality, an individual may start off doing 5 minutes and remain at 5 minutes for several weeks until he or she is *ready* to move up to 10 minutes. And again, be realistic—this increase in duration may not happen for a while. It may take several 21-day Extreme Transformation cycles to hit 25 or 30 minutes daily—it is all about how much time you are willing to commit to yourself and your health. As your Accelerators get longer, feel free to split them into two or even three different bouts of exercise, if it is more convenient for you.

For our one-year transformations, we encourage our peeps to aim for at least 60 minutes of daily Accelerators starting off, and ultimately they increase to 90 to 120 minutes every day (split into 45- to 60-minute bouts each)! How much weight you want to lose, and how fast you want to lose it…are up to you!!

## Make Accelerators Fun with Intervals!

"Cardio sucks." "I hate running." "It's so boring." We've heard it all, and we understand. Heck, we sometimes feel the same way. But what if cardio was actually fun and entertaining, and the time flew by? When sports are your Accelerators, it's pretty easy to get wrapped up in the game…but how can we make those individual sports like jogging, running, rowing, and cycling more entertaining? Intervals! Not only do they break up the monotony of steady-state cardio, they actually burn fat at an even faster rate—both during and after the bout of exercise! Any Accelerator can quickly pass when you're chipping away with these high- and low-intensity challenges! We use five different intervals for our peeps:

Thrilling Thirties: :30 low intensity / :30 high-intensity
Mighty Minutes: 1:00 low intensity / 1:00 high-intensity
Nasty Nineties: 1:30 low intensity / 1:30 high-intensity
Tenacious Twos: 2:00 low intensity / 2:00 high-intensity
Dirty Two-Thirties: 2:30 low intensity / 2:30 high-intensity

For example, if you're jogging and doing "Mighty Minutes," you will slow to a walk/ jog for 60 seconds, then speed up to fast jogging/running for 60 seconds, then slow back down to the walk/jog for 60 seconds, then speed back up for 60 seconds. Repeat until your Accelerator duration is completed! The high and low intensity is completely up to you, but be sure to challenge yourself and don't let your heart rate drop below 120 beats per minute (bpm) during the low-intensity intervals!

Most of our peeps love these intervals that we do; however, some prefer to play with other interval types, like:

- Playlist intervals: One song high-intensity, one song low intensity
- Distance intervals: One lap around the block fast, one lap slow—or walk to one light post, run to the next, etc.

No matter how you interval, you win! During the 21 days, we will prescribe different intervals each day for you to play with.

Check out Step 6: Make It Your Own! for other fun ways to accelerate your weight loss and get phenomenal results!

# HOW AND WHEN TO DO YOUR METABOLIC MISSIONS AND ACCELERATORS

## When to Exercise

We both prefer to wake up in the morning and do our workout right away. It's a great way to start the day, plus the majority of the calories you eat after exercise will be partitioned into repairing and building muscle. In addition, the high-intensity Metabolic Mission spikes metabolism for hours afterward, so your body will continue to burn calories at a faster rate than it would without exercise. Most important, and we're sure this will resonate with many of you, we have four kids. Life gets busy really quickly around our home. Most days, if it doesn't happen first thing in the morning, it doesn't happen at all!

But here's the deal. *Any* time you can find to exercise is a "win" in our book. If you can't exercise first thing in the morning, find a time that you trust in your schedule and stick to it. That's the main point: Carve out that time for you every day—and do it. Regardless of whether you train in the morning or at night, as long as you *train*, you are going to get phenomenal results!

## Heidi Tip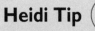

We are all too busy to work out, but part of your new transformation lifestyle is finding time every day to move your body. Here are two of my favorite—and most popular—tips for carving out time to work out:

1. Wake up 15 minutes earlier than you normally do. Not an hour, not even 30 minutes. All it takes to jump-start your metabolism is 5 to 15 minutes of moving.

2. Take advantage of nap time! For those of you who are moms with little kids, when it's time for the little people to sleep, it's time for you to move! And if the kids don't nap, let them join in. My two youngest love nothing more than to follow me around, imitating my workout!

## Days to Exercise

We've designed a full schedule of Metabolic Missions and Accelerators into your 21-day sequence of Extreme Transformation. We do Metabolic Missions and Accelerators on Days 1 through 5 of each week, and do an extra Accelerator on Day 6—to maximize your weigh-in on Day 7. It is critically important that you do not work out every day of the week. You *must* have a rest day. Five days of Metabolic Missions and six days of Accelerators will put some physical stress on the body—and it needs at least one day to rest, recover, and reset itself for the week ahead!

## When to Eat

If you train in the morning, there are several ways to eat around your Metabolic Mission. If you have an iron stomach, feel free to eat beforehand. However, if you find yourself a bit queasy working out on a full stomach, either eat half your breakfast before and half after, or simply eat breakfast when the mission is complete.

As you will soon see, the 21-day plan in the pages ahead is set up so you can simply follow the Extreme Cycle nutrition, Metabolic Mission, and Accelerator described for each day.

---

### Summary: The Five Rules of Extreme Transformation

To sum it all up, here are the Extreme Transformation five rules of weight loss—the key to taking control of your metabolism so that you can lose the weight you want and keep it off forever:

1. Eat within 30 minutes of waking and every 3 hours after.

2. Follow the Extreme Cycle daily meal combinations.

3. Drink lots of water all day long.

4. Build muscle and spike your metabolism through Metabolic Missions 5 days a week.

5. Accelerate your weight loss daily through fun cardio options 6 days a week.

# 21 Days to Extreme Transformation

WARNING: Transformation is an active physical, mental, and emotional process.

Each of the 21 days has an adjoining lesson with psychological and emotional activities that will help you lay down daily habits and create the mental awareness to keep the weight off forever. From learning the shortcuts of effective meal prep to identifying what your motivating force is, your level of involvement with these lessons will absolutely reflect your potential for long-term success. We highly advise you to focus on these lessons and follow through with the mental activities. They are simple and take very little time, but they provide you with the tools to make a radical shift in your life.

Knowing the path of transformation and having realistic expectations for the journey ahead is critical to your success. Before beginning the journey, we advise you to read, or at least skim, through the following 21 days so that you can see what lies ahead for you. You will find that many of the steps are intertwined and work off each other. Many of the lessons in the later days may be helpful to your journey *now*, so don't feel like you must wait until later in the process to complete the lessons. Read ahead. You can do one a day, or do them all today. There may be information in Day 4 that is pertinent to the beginning of your journey now. Or perhaps Day 17 is a chapter that you need to review on a regular basis to help you move forward with your life. Whatever works for you. This is your journey.

This book is written to be your guide. Don't just go over the lessons and be done with them. They are here to read and re-read...to practice for the rest of your life.

As you embark upon the day-to-day nutrition and exercise components of the next 21 days, review the lesson for that day, revisit it, and re-explore that area of your life and mind further. It will anchor you in your transformation—forever.

POWELL

# LEARN IT!

You are here: at a momentous time and place in your life. You are at the beginning of a journey that will change your life forever.

The first seven days of Extreme Transformation are all about learning how to embrace the process and make it yours. You get to be the artist here. Over the next seven days you will identify what *you* want, discover *your* real why, learn how to set *your* goals, and discover a path within *yourself* that you never knew existed. You will learn the importance of keeping commitments to yourself—one promise at a time. You will learn how to customize your nutrition and exercise—so that they work for you—and you will put together your Transformation Team to rally you along the way. These early lessons are critical to getting a feel for how this process truly works. Before beginning this first week, we highly encourage you to read these first seven lessons ahead of time so you are well prepared starting out.

Oh, and last but not least, have fun. ☺

This is going to be awesome!

## DAY 1

### Before You Begin

Before Day 1 (or the morning of), do your first weigh-in. Record your weight in a daily tracker, in your journal, or on your smartphone. (You will also find a 21-Day Daily Tracker in Appendix A, which you can use as well.)

## Chris Tip
## Take Your Before Pictures
## and Memorialize This Moment

One of the most wonderful gifts you can give yourself during this transformation is *proof of progression*. Not only will this memorialize where exactly you came from (serving as a constant reminder never to go back), but it also will give you a more objective perspective of your own body—so you can see the true results. Naturally, our eyes play tricks on us—*what we see in the mirror is not reality. What we see in pictures is much more objective!* Remember that these pics are just for *you*—unless, of course, you want to share them. And trust us, when this journey is over, these pics will give you some major bragging rights!

Here are a few photo pointers to help you out:

**Tip 1**—Wear clothing that will give you a *full* view of your body so you can see where the transformation is happening! Since you will be the only one seeing these, *shorts* and a *sports bra* may do the trick for you. You'll want to see your shoulders, arms, abdomen, thighs, and calves.

**Tip 2**—Snap shots from a few different angles—we personally prefer a front shot and a side/profile shot.

**Tip 3**—Take a beginning picture and *weekly front and side* pictures after that. You won't be able to see the changes on a day-to-day basis, but when the weekly pictures are lined up, you will be *amazed* at the transformation you are achieving. Use these pictures as *daily reminders* by placing printed copies of the pictures in a visible spot. Try inside your fridge, on your bathroom mirror, in your room, or in the bottom of a drawer that you use often. And if you're *really* proud to show them off, use one as your screensaver!

For your convenience, we have included weekly shopping lists for the delicious recipes in this book (see Appendix B). You'll notice there are separate lists for men and women to help you determine the amount of food *you* will need. Clean Cheat shopping lists are also included there, but we recommend NOT purchasing these foods until the day before Reset day to help keep temptation out of the house throughout the week.

## Day 1: High-Carb Day

Meal 1: Breakfast
    Recipe: Cinnamon French Toast

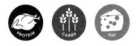

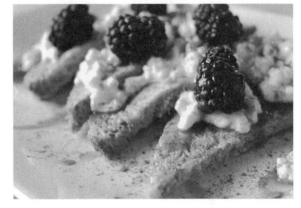

Meal 2: High-Carb Meal
    Recipe: Chocolate Peanut Butter and Banana Smoothie

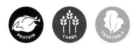

Meal 3: High-Carb Meal
    Recipe: Three-Bean Salad with Chicken and Kale

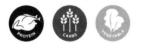

Meal 4: High-Carb Meal
    Recipe: Sweet Potato Chips, Celery Sticks, and Shake

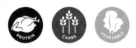

Meal 5: Low-Carb Meal
    Recipe: Creamy Cauliflower Soup

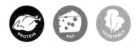

## Fitness Testing Day

Just like stepping on the scale to get a measure for your current weight, we need to get a measure for your fitness level. Don't worry, this won't take long—only 4 minutes total. However, if you haven't been active for quite some time, you may feel a little soreness tomorrow! At the end of the 21 Days to Extreme Transformation we will test you again, and you will be blown away at the difference! The challenge here is to set a clock for one minute and perform as many repetitions of the following exercises as you can 3—2—1...go!

See Part 4, The Metabolic Movements, for step-by-step instructions on the following exercises. Set a running clock and do as many reps as you can in 1 minute. Record your time in the Daily Tracker to complete the mission!

Push-Ups
Sit-Ups
Squats
Burpees

## Day 1: Metabolic Mission: Go the Distance (Stepladder)

Your mission is to start at 3 reps each of the movements below and increase 3 reps every circuit (for example 3, 6, 9, 12, 15, 18...). How many circuits can you do in 12 minutes of these three exercises? Record how far you make it in your tracker!

**Kickbacks**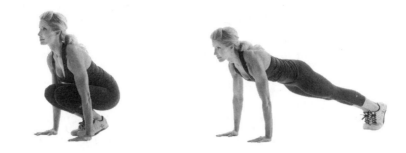

**Push-Ups**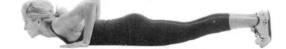

**Back Lunges**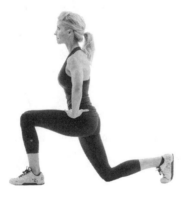

Get ready...3—2—1...go!!

## Day 1: Accelerator: 5 minutes (minimum)

Select any activity of your choosing (see page 89 for a list of activities), and keep your heart rate above 120 beats per minute (bpm) the entire time. Prescribed optional interval for maximum results: Mighty Minutes (1:00 low intensity / 1:00 high intensity).

# FIND YOUR *WHAT* AND YOUR *WHY*

*Life isn't about finding yourself. Life is about creating yourself.*

—George Bernard Shaw

To be successful on any journey, you *must* have a clear-cut picture of where you want to go. This journey is no exception. You *must* know ahead of time what your goal is, and why you want it. This begs the extremely important question: *What* do you want to achieve from Extreme Transformation?

Now is not the time to be vague. We are naturally programmed to give simple and nebulous answers like "I just want to be healthier" or "I want to be fitter." In transformation, these goals are absolutely unacceptable. There is no way to measure them, so you can justify reaching them at any time. We tend to make these unclear goals subconsciously so that we aren't held accountable to any true commitment.

Not this time.

One of the keys to maximizing the impact of the Extreme Transformation is setting SMART goals. Transformation cannot begin until a SMART goal is set. So what is a SMART goal? A goal that is:

1. **Specific**—What you want must be laid out in precise detail. Ask yourself the question, *What exactly will I achieve?* The next few components will help you dial in the specificity of your goal.

2. **Measurable**—What you will achieve must be able to be measured to verify whether it was achieved or not. It must be quantifiable! Pounds lost, inches lost, medical numbers, clothing sizes, and performance times are all measurable and acceptable for your goal! In addition, because your goal is measurable, you can regularly measure your progress to see if you are on track. Numbers don't lie, and they can keep you moving in the right direction or help you refocus your efforts.

3. **Attainable**—A successful goal must be attainable—not too difficult or idealistic, or you're setting yourself up for failure from Day 1. Yes, you could say your goal is to exercise five days a week for 30 minutes, but let's be honest: Sometimes life gets in the way and the best plans go out the window. What

happens then? You break a commitment and you feel like a failure. You need to make your goal attainable—one you know that you can keep every single day—and you'll be well on your way to success. You'll love those daily feelings of accomplishment so much that you might even do more than you've promised yourself you'd do (like exercising more than five minutes a day)!

4. **Relevant**—A SMART goal must be important enough to you that you'll want to make the necessary sacrifices to achieve it. It must be a major priority in your life, to the point at which it creates a sense of urgency in your life.

5. **Time-Sensitive**—A SMART goal must have a time limit so you won't get sidetracked and not accomplish it. Placing a time limit on your goal creates a sense of urgency that will make it a priority. There must be a specific window of time in which the goal is achieved. Eventually, sometime, or next year will never happen. Your goal will not be complete until you put a hard date on it.

## Call to Action: Declaring Your Dream

It's time to create your first SMART goal. Today you are going to create a goal for the transformation journey with us. For example: *I will lose 20 pounds in 60 days*. One final note before you declare your SMART goal: Our choice of words is extremely important here. We must leave no wiggle room for our goals to escape us. We *never* use the wording *I want to* or *I'll try*—that type of phrasing plants the seed of avoidance and gives you an out. In declaring your goal, use the words *I will*. This transformation is the real deal, and you *will* be held to your word.

It is time now for you. Take some time to think about it, then in the space below write it down and declare your goal. It must start with *I will* and finish with a specific date by which it will be completed. Maybe your goal with us is to lose a certain number of pounds; maybe it's something else. You are the artist...paint your picture below, and tell us what you *will* achieve:

_____

_____

_____

_____

### Find Your Why

Nice work creating such a powerful SMART goal! It isn't easy to make such a solid commitment, but those who have the courage to take these steps have what it takes to change forever. Now that we have identified where we want to go with your SMART goal, we're going to help you discover something just as important: your why. This is the motivating force that is going to keep you on track the whole way.

So why is this goal important to you? Why do you want to lose weight? Why do you want to transform? *Defining your why* is the driving force of your journey and is something that should not be taken lightly.

Pay close attention: Our why is our motivation!

Ever lose your motivation? Exactly. That's why we need to know our why, and keep it in front of us at all times. It is a main key to long-term success on this journey!

The decision to begin this journey of transformation occurs for many reasons, for many different kinds of people. Many decisions to lose weight are triggered by huge life events, sometimes even traumatic events. For some people it's a health scare—a report that delivers a diagnosis such as diabetes, the precursors of heart disease, or high blood pressure. Others are confronted by a realization that their lives are just not working anymore—that life as they know it is painful, and they desire more. Some choose to make changes because of a sudden loss or trauma in their lives, an event so cataclysmic that the desire for deep change feels like survival. Others decide to lose weight for those around them, saying to themselves, *"If I lose weight, I can be a better spouse, parent, or child."*

Many people reach a rock bottom, a point of realization that their current condition of living is so toxic and unbearable that they can no longer fathom another day in the same way. As Tony Robbins said, "Change happens when the pain of staying the same is greater than the pain of change."

For Mike, his why came in the form of hearing the news from his doctor that his heart was going to fail if he didn't radically change his habits. With an 11-year-old child, he realized that not only did his own life depend upon his becoming healthy, but his son's did as well.

For David, it was the moment walking down the street when he saw his reflection in a window and said to himself, "*Who's that fat guy?*" before he realized that he wasn't the fit young man he used to be. He wanted to be fit and healthy again.

For Merhbod, finding his why occurred when his girlfriend presented him with a tape recording of him sleeping. The tape revealed that his sleep apnea had become so bad that every few minutes he would stop breathing for 45 to 60 seconds. Mehrbod was shocked and decided at that moment that he had to change before he might literally stop breathing and die in his sleep.

For Josh, transformation began after his father died. The loss devastated him, but it brought him a crystal-clear moment when he realized that he was not living the life his father would want for him. "This was not my life," Josh remembers saying to himself. "No one knew how unhappy I was. I was closed off from everyone. But deep down I wanted more from life, and I deserved more from life. So I went out and took it because I knew that life wasn't going to hand it to me!"

Juliana wanted to walk down the halls of her high school with confidence.

Cassie wanted to look the son she'd put up for adoption in the face without feeling ashamed of herself.

Kenny wanted to feel like the proud U.S. Marine he'd once been.

Cassandra wanted to be the athlete she used to be.

Other people's whys are much less dark and complicated. Your why might simply be that you want to look good at your high school reunion. Or maybe to drop a couple sizes to fit into some smaller jeans. Some people just want to lose the baby weight to feel sexy for their significant other again! As Kristen remembers, "I've been there! After devoting nine months to growing a baby and another year to nursing, multiplied by four babies, I was simply ready to feel strong, powerful, beautiful, and sexy again. I wanted my body to feel like something I controlled for once in 10 years of the pregnancy process…not a body that was controlled by external forces any longer."

Whys don't have to be dramatic, but they do need to come from a place of passion. You've got to want it more than you want anything else and be willing to make this a priority, like you would an emergency or crisis, or you will not have the drive to do what it takes to complete the journey. What do *you* want more from this than anything else? What is your why?

### Finding the Clarity of Your Why

Our motivation to change can be boiled down to our two most primal emotions: fear (the force behind you) and love (the force in front of you). The way we see it, either there is something you are running from, or something you are running toward—or a little bit of both! Every why has one or both of these two emotions driving it: one that you are wanting to move *away* from (*fear*), and one that you are wanting to move *toward* (*love*). Which one you choose to focus on is totally up to you.

Fear-based whys tend to be the situations or feelings that we are running away from—bad health, unacceptable appearance, depression and self-loathing, upset/frustration of spouse/family members, fear of death, and so on. These emotions scare us and so we turn to transformation as a way out. Love-based whys are motivating situations or feelings that we actually run toward—that perfect beach body, the ability to run and play with your kids, the possibility of being an athlete, six-pack abs, a spouse who loves and accepts you. When your why is love-based, it's positive, affirming, and ultimately more liberating.

But that's not to discount fear-based whys: Often this is the powerful place many of us start at, and that is okay. The most important point to keep in mind is that you start—even if it is a fear-based why that helps get you to begin your journey of transformation. Eventually, you may likely shift to a love-based why.

Take a look at how some of the common ways people explain their whys to us fall into the two categories, love-based and fear-based:

**Fear**—"I have too much physical pain and discomfort—I can barely move around anymore."

**Love**—"I want to be able to move freely without pain."

**Fear**—"My relationship is getting worse and worse. My partner is going to leave me."

**Love**—"I want to love myself more, so I can be a better person for my partner—and our relationship can thrive."

**Fear**—"I don't want to be lonely anymore."

**Love**—"I want to look better so I can meet others and date with confidence."

You get it. We're either running away from something we don't want, or running toward something we do want. There is no right or wrong here. While we do hope to help you and every person ultimately find a why based on love at some point of their journey, you might not be there yet. The fact of the matter is that you are here and you are reading this book…taking that first step toward a new you!

## Call to Action: Declare It!

Looking through the lists above, take a moment to think about your why and ask yourself these two questions:

**1.** Why is your goal important to you?

_____
_____
_____
_____

**2.** Is it fear-based or love-based?

_____

Remember: If you don't want to lose motivation, you must memorialize your why. Put it in multiple places you will see every day. These are common places where our participants have placed their whys:

- Bathroom mirror
- Dashboard
- Workplace or desk
- Refrigerator
- Living room
- Cell phone home screen

Do not read any further until you have taken action. Put this book down and immediately memorialize your why. Don't risk losing your motivation ever again. Put it everywhere you can to remind yourself!

Next, share your why with others. If you are still scared of the commitment, try sharing it with one friend. If you are ready to rock, post it online for all of your friends! Better yet, post it on *our* social networks and let our community support you in achieving your why! #extremetransformation

Facebook:
RealHeidiPowell
RealChrisPowell
Twitter:
@RealHeidiPowell
@RealChrisPowell
Instagram:
@RealHeidiPowell
@RealChrisPowell

## Reality Check

You will likely forget why you're doing this every now and then. Your pictures will likely lose their impact and you will become desensitized to seeing the same pic in the same place every day. To stay motivated, keep telling others about your goals. Try putting up new pics every week or two. Change their location; do whatever it takes to keep it fresh!

In difficult times, you may try to convince yourself that you don't really want your why, or that it has changed. While it is perfectly okay for your why to shift as you get to know yourself through this process, it isn't okay to tell yourself that you never really wanted your why in the first place... and this is all too easy to do when the going gets tough. Don't lie to yourself. You want it and you know it. It's yours, so go get it!

## Heidi Tip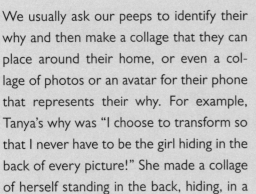

We usually ask our peeps to identify their why and then make a collage that they can place around their home, or even a collage of photos or an avatar for their phone that represents their why. For example, Tanya's why was "I choose to transform so that I never have to be the girl hiding in the back of every picture!" She made a collage of herself standing in the back, hiding, in a handful of pics. If your why has something to do with becoming more active and connected to your family, you might create a collage with some photos of you sitting with your kids and then other pics of a mom (like you!) running, jumping, swimming, or playing in the park or on the beach! The point is to choose images that inspire you!

### The Deeper Why

Often what we *think* is our why is just scratching the surface of what we *really* want. We're not saying that your why isn't valid, because whatever comes up for you is real and true. But what we've learned through the years of helping hundreds of people successfully lose excess pounds is that your first why may be just the surface of a much deeper well of understanding. So keep checking in with yourself and be aware that your first why may be a powerful stepping-stone toward a much more important why inside yourself.

As you dig deeper into yourself (and as you do the 21 steps), you very well may (and *should*!) realize that your why is actually deeper than you initially thought. As Mark explains, "I wanted more than anything to find the love of my life, and I know I couldn't do that at 650 pounds. I wanted the girl of my dreams!"

But what Mark didn't realize at the time was that his why was so much deeper than just wanting to find a wife. As he followed his own journey of transformation—as he continually focused on improving himself (and being open, honest, and vulnerable)—he "peeled back those layers" of protection that had masked his true self. How did he finally get to his deeper why? He kept asking himself why and listened to his own answers:

"Well, why do I want the girl of my dreams so bad? Because that would make me happy, whole, and complete. I've never had that before."

"Why do I need someone else to make me feel happy, whole, and complete? Because I can't seem to find happiness on my own...I am not happy."

"Why and how would another human being fill this void then?"

Well, that was the critical question that led to Mark's true why.

For Mark, his deeply rooted answer boiled down to simply trying to fill the basic human need to be loved and accepted. And while this *need* doesn't have to come from another, he felt a wife would give him the love and acceptance he craved.

After time working his inner steps, Mark ultimately realized that when he started to love and accept himself by keeping his promises and finding integrity, he was able to rely much less on validation, love, and acceptance from others and rely much more on himself—all the love and acceptance he needed was within him!

## DAY 2

### Day 2: High-Carb Day

Meal 1: Breakfast
   Recipe: Scrambled Eggs and Hash

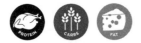

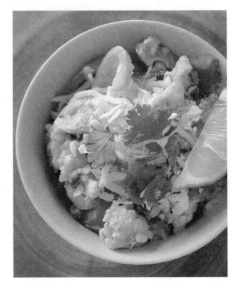

Meal 2: High-Carb Meal
   Recipe: Lemon Poppy Seed Protein Bites

Meal 3: High-Carb Meal
   Recipe: Chicken Fajita Bowl

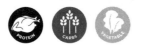

Meal 4: High-Carb Meal
   Recipe: Homemade Tortilla Chips with Tomato Salsa

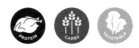

Meal 5: Low-Carb Meal
   Recipe: Shrimp and Chicken Stir-Fry

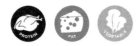

## Day 2: Metabolic Mission: The Whole 9 (RFT)

Set a running clock and do 9 rounds as fast as you can of the following circuit. Record your time in the tracker to complete the mission!

Air Squats: 9 reps
Hollow Rocks: 9 reps
Push-Ups: 9 reps

## Day 2: Accelerator: 5 minutes (minimum)

Select any activity of your choosing, and keep your heart rate above 120 beats per minute (bpm) the entire time. Prescribed optional interval for maximum results: Dirty Two-Thirties (2:30 low intensity / 2:30 high intensity)

LESSON 2

# DISCOVER THE TRUE PATH TO TRANSFORMATION

*The only journey is the one within.*

—Rainer Maria Rilke

Do a Google search for "weight loss" and within seconds you will see hundreds (if not thousands) of different diets, programs, and plans that promise a set of guidelines to help you lose weight. Guess what? *Most* of them work. So with widespread access for much of the world to this free information, why isn't everyone lean and healthy? They all tout being the "path" to your weight loss goals. So why do 9 out of 10 people fail on these diets? Why haven't we found the universal answer to weight loss?

Because we're looking in the wrong place.

There is only *one* true path to what you really want.

We have been blinded by so much confusion everywhere, with every weight loss program pitching that they have "the answer" to your problems with new diets and exercises, that we've never thought to look where the path *really* is—and what lifelong success is really all about—the journey within. Inside all of us is the secret path to our true selves, which coincides with being *at* our ideal weight. It already exists. It has been there all along. We are intrinsically programmed to follow it, but we must see the journey for what it really is…and never underestimate its power.

This path has all the answers—why you've failed in the past, why you lost belief in yourself, why you feel the way you do right now, and why you are struggling with those extra pounds. This path will lead to your goal weight and body, but ultimately it will lead you to loving and appreciating yourself. It will lead you to joy, confidence, and esteem greater than you can imagine. It's ready and waiting for you to explore it.

What we are talking about is the path of *integrity.*

Please pay close attention. When you understand the path of integrity and follow it, your whole life changes. Immediately. *This* is the secret we have used with all of our transformations over the years—and every single one will tell you that it changed their lives forever.

Before we dive in deep, let's define it.

What is integrity?

*Integrity is…*

*Doing what you say you are going to do, when you say you are going to do it.*

We are going to say something that may upset you here. We are going to be so bold as to say that you likely have *not* had integrity with yourself. You're probably reading this thinking, "Well, screw you guys. I have integrity. Anytime I tell someone I'm going to do something, darn it, I do it!"

We're sure you probably do have integrity with *other* people. Heck, if you make a commitment to someone, you've got to follow through, right? Well, try this scenario: What if you made a promise to the most important person in the world. Would you do it? Before you answer, think long and hard about it. Because there *is* one person in this world who has the greatest power to impact your life and your *quality* of life—you.

Let's try something—if you've been following the path of integrity with yourself, then how many times have you said, "The diet starts Monday"? or, "I'm going to set my clock an hour early to exercise tomorrow morning." How about, "2010—this is my year!" How about 2011? 2012? 2013? 2014? 2015?

Get the point? If you had followed the path of integrity, you would have only made the promise *once*. Right now, you'd be at your goal.

You see, we spend so much time making and breaking promises to ourselves, we reach the point that eventually when we make yet *another* promise to lose the weight, we don't believe ourselves anymore…it's just going to be another failed attempt…because we don't believe *in* ourselves anymore.

We're sure that for each of these failed attempts, there are a million reasons why it didn't work. However, understand this: Your integrity does not know excuses. You either do it, or you don't.

Engrain this truth in your mind, and it will change your life forever:

When you say you are going to do something…do it. Our promises are one of the single most powerful forces in existence. In order to make any progress in life, in order to transform ourselves, we must make promises to ourselves and keep them. However, what most of us don't realize is that *every time* we make a promise to ourselves, we are putting our most valuable asset on the line—our dignity. Our dignity is our confidence, our esteem, our self-love, our ability to believe in ourselves. If we keep the promise, our dignity grows even more. If we don't, the broken promise can trigger a catastrophic backslide. (More to come in Lesson 3!)

## Call to Action: The Feeling of Integrity

When we complete a commitment, or keep a promise, we are left with a feeling of being whole, complete, fulfilled, and satisfied.

1. List three times you've followed through with what you said you were going to do—both for yourself and for others.

_____

_____

_____

_____

_____

_____

2. How did you feel about yourself when you did it?

_____

_____

_____

Now…take that feeling and amplify it by 1,000. When you start keeping your promises to yourself, it's kind of like that... but even better. ☺

Integrity is not only the essence of once again feeling whole and loving yourself, but also the root of human change. Each time you honor your word, not just to others, but most important to yourself, you take control of your destiny and put yourself in the driver's seat of your own life. Each time you make and keep a promise to yourself, you show yourself that you have control over what you say and do.

When you follow through and do something that you said you were going to do, you become more dependable and solid to yourself. The result? You not only grow your integrity but also achieve a greater level of dignity—the quality of being worthy of honor or respect. Yes—your integrity grows your dignity. And the reward for building a life based on integrity is dignity—the love, respect, and esteem of yourself.

From this moment on, you must realize that while the nutrition of the Extreme Cycle and the power of Metabolic Missions and Accelerators will help you lose weight quickly and effectively, they are *not* the answer to your transformation. Your integrity is. Your ability to honor your word to yourself. When you do what you say you are going to do—when you say you are going to do it—you will execute the Extreme Cycle, Metabolic Missions, and

Accelerators beautifully, leading to extraordinary results. Your focus should now and forever be first and foremost on keeping your promises to yourself. When that happens, everything else falls into place. Are you starting to understand it now?

When our people stand on stage at the end of their yearlong journey, with their chest out and their chin high, they no longer care about the number on the scale. (It was simply a SMART goal that they achieved—by doing what they said they were going to do, when they said they were going to do it.) They look and feel that way because they *love* themselves. They know what the journey is *really* about. For example, if they made a commitment to do 30 minutes on a treadmill, and one of us pulled them off at 29 minutes, they would throw a punch at us. They would literally fight us to complete that last minute. Why? Will one minute on a treadmill make *any* difference in their weight loss? Nope. But they know what is on the line—their dignity—and nothing is worth jeopardizing that. If they broke their promise, it could trigger a devastating backslide of more broken promises. They know where the true value is—not in the exercise, not in the diet, but in themselves and their promises.

They became promise keepers, and it led them to the ultimate reward. And oh yeah, because of it they lost a lot of weight, too. ☺

Georgeanna recalls, "In the beginning, I really needed Chris and Heidi and the rest of the team to believe in me. It took me making and keeping my own promises to believe that I really could do it. I remember one day Chris asked me, 'Georgeanna, why is it that you can make and keep all sorts of promises to other people, but you can't keep them for yourself?'—a lightbulb went on and I just understood why it was so important for me to put myself first. That's how I began to really believe in myself."

Each day you follow this path, you walk toward a profound sense of self-love. And when you reach this place, it's not an end of a journey but rather an opening to a vast and endless source of vitality, meaning, fulfillment, and peace. This is where you will live. And this is what transformation is all about.

Take a look at the stereogram image below. This captures the essence of transformation so beautifully. Before you shift your focus, all you see is a chaotic mess of dumbbells and food. Basically, it is the confusing mess of every single diet and exercise program out there for weight loss. But once you shift your focus, the 3-D path of true transformation—and lifelong weight loss—becomes clear.

Transformation path viewing tips:

1. With your eyes about 18 to 24 inches from the image, choose a spot in the center of it and stare directly at it.
2. Continue to stare at the image and let your eyes relax. Focus your eyes as if you are trying to look through the image at something behind it.
3. Your eyes may go slightly out of focus—this is okay.
4. After a short period of time, you may start to see some depth appear on the image. If this is the case, then you are very close. Hold your eyes on the same spot and continue to let the hidden image move toward you.
5. If you do it properly, you will now start to see the hidden image.
6. If you still can't see the image, keep trying. There is a hidden image or 3-D element in this image. Don't give up!

### *The Hidden Path Stereogram*

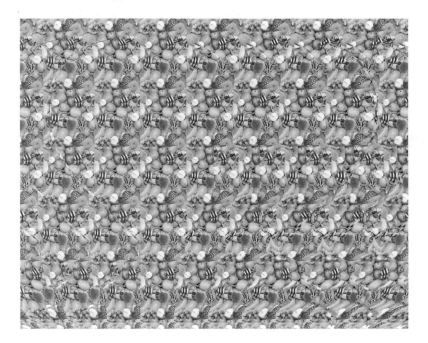

The stereogram image represents the path of integrity that lies inside each one of us. Each step up represents a promise you make and keep. These steps combine and form your goals—daily goals, weekly goals, monthly and yearly goals. Your promise-filled life is an ever-rising stairway to your best self.

As you can see the stereogram is built upon a stairway of such promises; they build on one another and head in only one direction—up, toward the top. What's at the top of this staircase? Dignity. Esteem. Confidence. Self-love. And once you have that, you have everything. The world is your oyster...you can conquer and achieve anything.

Jacqui describes her Extreme Transformation and what it felt like when she discovered her why, and connected to her inner path to integrity and self-love. "We all can get stuck in our lives, but I feel so lucky. I didn't believe I could change or had the power to change. I tried and failed time and again. This mind-set reinforced that I was not good enough, so I stayed in that cycle of broken promises and failure. I believed the lies about myself. But Chris and Heidi believed in me—for me. They showed me the true path to transformation, and it finally all made sense. I realized it was a battle with my mind and my heart, not my body."

She was looking outside herself for answers, instead of inside. And when she changed her focus to her integrity, to keeping her promises, she never looked back.

## Call to Action

The absolute essence of the shift in mindset that needs to happen throughout your transformation journey requires that you get to the realization that the power to change is within you. So if you are ready to transform, read this out loud and own it:

**"I know the hidden path to transformation lies in my integrity. I understand the extreme value of my promises and their power over my results and the way I feel about myself. From this moment on, I am a promise keeper to myself."**

## Reality Check

On the way, it is easy to forget that transformation is about integrity, and get wrapped back up in the numbers game. You'll get desperate to turn numbers on the scale and start looking for other fad diets and quick fixes to get the number you want to see. At this point, your focus will shift back to the chaos of the thousands of diet and exercise programs out there.

Keep this book close. Remember, it is your guide. Read through the lessons over and over again. And remember, your path is within you.

## DAY 3

### Day 3: High-Carb Day

Meal 1: Breakfast
   Recipe: No-Bake Oats

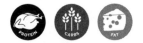

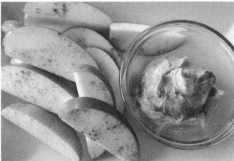

Meal 2: High-Carb Meal
   Recipe: Honey Dijon Chicken Snack Wrap

Meal 3: High-Carb Meal
   Recipe: Butternut Squash Chili

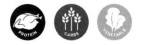

Meal 4: High-Carb Meal
   Recipe: Apple and Dip

Meal 5: Low-Carb Meal
   Recipe: Cheesy Chicken and String Beans

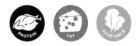

### Day 3: Metabolic Mission: Burpee Love (Chipper)

Set a running clock and see how long it takes to complete the mission. Record your time in your Daily Tracker! Ready? 3—2—1...go!

60 Burpees

**Day 3: Accelerator: 5 minutes (minimum)**

Select any activity of your choosing, and keep your heart rate above 120 beats per minute (bpm) the entire time. Prescribed optional interval for maximum results: Thrilling Thirties (:30 low intensity / :30 high intensity)

LESSON 3

## KEEP YOUR PROMISES

*The journey of 1,000 miles begins with a single step.*

—Lao Tzu

To put things into perspective: Every diet and exercise program (including this one) involves a series of promises. To make it clear for you, we have identified the three most powerful, universal promises of Extreme Transformation:

1. Eat according to the Extreme Cycle high- and low-carb days, with portions, recipes, and acceptable foods.
2. Do a Metabolic Mission five days per week.
3. Do an Accelerator six days per week.

Keeping these promises will lead to significant weight loss. If you are able to take on all of these promises all at once, that's fantastic. You will achieve your goals in record time! However, it's time for a reality check. If you cannot keep all of these promises, you *must* only commit to the ones you know you *can* do. Just as kept promises are the powerful steps toward a lean and fit body, loving yourself, and believing in yourself, broken promises are the devastating reciprocate. A single, small broken promise can trigger a catastrophic backslide of weight gain, crushed esteem, and lost belief in ourselves.

### Silent Promises

For the first few attempts at weight loss, most of us have told others our intentions and promises. Failure after failure, we lose more and more belief in ourselves, and usually feel ashamed when others question our resolve. When we lose belief in ourselves, we begin to do something dangerous—we make silent promises. Heaven forbid you commit to starting a program in front of your family, friends, or co-workers, right? Because come Thursday and you are housing a whole stuffed crust pizza in the break room, you're going to have some explaining to do, right? When we are not ready to truly commit, or don't believe in our ability to succeed, we make *silent promises* to ourselves. We whisper to ourselves that "the diet starts Monday." Our ego avoids declaring them in front of others in case we do fall—so that it avoids the shame of looking bad and weak in front of others, and possibly losing connection with them. The voice in our head tells us that if nobody heard the promise, then we can just sweep it under the rug when we break it—no harm done, right? Wrong. More harm done than had you never made the promise in the first place. Promises are promises, silent or not! You don't realize it, but you gambled with your dignity again...and you lost.

So here's where it gets nasty—when you break a promise, you don't just go back to square one. You drop twice as far. Promise after promise broken leads to more and more darkness, despair, and self-hatred. If many of you are wondering how and why you found yourself in such a dark place, *this is the answer.* You've been playing with fire all along and you never even knew it. When we meet our people for the first time, we don't see hundreds of pounds of extra weight—we see hundreds of pounds of broken promises.

Promises should never be silent. They should be said out loud. And they should be SMART! Just like your goals, you need to keep your promises simple and smart (you may want to revisit the SMART goals you declared in Lesson 1). You also want to declare them—to yourself and to others.

Keep in mind that every time you failed at weight loss in the past can be traced back to a single moment when you broke your integrity. Every backslide begins the moment you *don't* do what you said you were going to do. It doesn't matter the circumstances. Go back in your past and think about it...

Seriously...think about it.

On the course of *every* program you've followed in the past, the backslide began with one slip—one broken promise.

Not this time.

Now that you know the power of our promises and how they can cut both ways, the only promises you should ever make from this moment on are the ones that you *know* you can keep. The journey to loving yourself is done one simple promise at a time.

The beauty of the path to your true self is simple: It is uncovered as soon as you make a single promise to yourself and fulfill that promise. The bricks-and-mortar of your integrity will rise every time you keep that promise. Dignity and self-love are both by-products of integrity. Although they may seem minuscule, these small promises are the foundation to profound change.

"Starting now, I will eat breakfast every day."

"From now on, I'm going to drink flavored water instead of soda."

"I will ride the stationary bike for five minutes every morning."

When you make such simple promises to yourself and you keep them day after day, you begin to grow your trust in yourself that you can actually *keep* that promise. You begin to...wait for it...

*Believe in yourself.*

Maybe even for the first time. But over time, once you believe and trust yourself to keep a promise, you begin to wonder what else you can do. So you make another small promise—and keep it. It is a wonderful upward climb of integrity and curiosity! You feel love for yourself, you have dignity, and you build what we call "integrity momentum."

The more you keep your promises, the more you don't want to break the streak! Integrity momentum is like a freight train. It starts out slow, but once it gets moving you can't stop it. This is exactly what we do with the participants on the show. They build up so much integrity momentum, you can't stop them!

Now let's put this into weight loss perspective. When you focus on fulfilling your promises based on diet and exercise, weight loss happens! You keep the promise, goals are achieved. Period.

So how do you get started? In our second book, we offered a list of 101 Power Promises—these are a collection of effective, single promises that you can use to set the foundation and take the first step in your transformation journey. We took those 101 promises and simplified them down to the most vital 20 promises for you to choose from. For your Power Promise, you can select one of these provided, or you can choose your own!

Heather was a chronic sumo dieter—she was never hungry in the morning, so she skipped breakfast, went to work, never ate a thing until late lunch. By that time she was so hungry she could (and would) eat anything. She ended up stuffing her face for late lunch and then again when she came home from work. She was so hungry late in the day she would eat until she went to bed. Heather began her transformation journey by Power Promising that she would wake up half an hour earlier in the morning so she had time for breakfast. That was her first promise to herself and by keeping it, she learned something hugely important: She was able to show up for herself each day. We put no calorie limits on breakfast, and she could choose anything—because the promise was just to eat breakfast. It became a victory each morning to start her day. The feeling was contagious, and it spread to other aspects of her life. After a couple weeks of keeping this Power Promise, she began to grow more and more confident in her ability to actually do it...like really, truly stick to it!

Once she was so confident she could keep her Power Promise, it was time to make her second promise. Her second promise to herself? She ate every three hours. At first, this didn't feel comfortable—she felt like she was eating too much. But the result was surprising. "I felt no need to overeat; I never felt hungry. Oddly enough, the scale started going down. I simply felt great!" One year and a few more promises later, and Heather is now 140 pounds lighter and a self-proclaimed promise keeper.

Promises to ourselves are the mini steps that lead to our goals. John's first promise to himself was to stop eating at drive-thrus. As a trucker, he is on the road all the time. He eats in his truck, sleeps in his truck, and for all intents and purposes lives in his truck. Making this promise to himself meant that John had to stop, park, and move to eat. He had to get out of his truck and walk into a diner or other low-key restaurant that served non-processed foods. This required time, patience, and energy. But John believed that he could. He believed that he had the power to follow through on this one initial promise. And each day he fulfilled this promise, he began to feel differently about himself. Instead of that "inside me" voice that said he was lazy and fat, he began to hear another voice: "You're doing great, boy—keep it up!" He was becoming his own coach. As the days passed, it got easier and easier to avoid the drive-thru. In addition, because walking into a restaurant was a conscious decision based upon his new commitment, he was more aware of the foods he was eating and naturally chose to make healthier choices. Even when he was short on time, he had gone so long without giving in to temptation that to him, it wasn't even an option anymore. At the end of two months, he not only had lost thirty-six pounds, he felt better, stronger, and more confident.

### Defining Your Power Promises

Being on your path, continuing to make promises to yourself and keeping them, requires focus and energy. It asks you to make one promise at a time and fulfill it, so you can build the scaffolding of your path to self-love. That's the essence of growing integrity and, ultimately, dignity. But once your path reveals itself, you are free to choose your destiny. Now you know, and you can never unlearn it!

You may have thought that eating right and exercising are the foundation of long-term weight loss. But now you know that that's not the case. As so many of our clients will tell you, the reason they were able to drop 10 or 20 sizes or shed 50 to 200 pounds was because they changed their life one promise at a time.

The key to transformation—we tell them again and again—is this: The more you build your integrity, the more dignity you grow. Every time you make a promise to yourself, your self-esteem, the very basis of your integrity, is on the line.

So how do you get started? Of course you can name any promise you want, but we want to give you some direction on how to define your promises and how these lead to and support your goals (which you will declare in the next step). Your Power Promises can fall into multiple categories, like: food promises, body promises, and mind promises. We have identified **20 Daily Power Promises** to jump-start you.

A Power Promise is something that is committed to daily.

1. I will eat breakfast within 30 minutes of waking up.
2. I will reduce drinking alcohol to one day a week or not at all.
3. I will drink an extra quart of water every day.
4. I will drink a cup of water before each meal.
5. I will stop drinking soda.
6. I will eat five meals a day.
7. I will eat protein first at every meal.

8. I will not eat my kids' food.
9. I will not eat after my fifth meal.
10. I will not eat in the car.
11. I will not eat fast food.
12. I will not add salt to my food.
13. I will eat veggies of at least two different colors every day.
14. I will take a brisk walk every morning or lunch break every day.
15. I will exercise for at least five minutes every day.
16. I will not watch TV unless I do exercises during the commercial breaks.
17. I will set my alarm 30 minutes early every morning to make time for my exercise.
18. I will track my food every day.
19. I will not eat when watching TV or using the computer.
20. I will pay attention to my hunger and only eat when I'm physically hungry.

## Call to Action

Keep in mind that these Power Promises are suggestions. But understand the power of the promise you choose, and that your integrity and dignity (and ultimately your success) are on the line here. You can adapt these promises, replace them, and add to them. It's all up to you. What's important is that you declare a promise that you can repeat each day, stick to it, and acknowledge to yourself that you did so. This conscious awareness of your accomplishments is an important part of your motivation and growing belief in yourself.

If you read between the lines of the 20 Daily Power Promises, you might notice the outlines of the healthy lifestyle that we are introducing. (Feel free to go back and check on the exact instructions for the Extreme Cycle in chapter 2.) But for now, if you're not ready to take on the whole Extreme Cycle, Metabolic Missions, and Accelerators just use *one* of these Power Promises to get you started on the right foot. Make one promise to yourself each day and keep it. Continue to make that daily commitment. When that promise becomes almost automatic, then build another promise on top of it. As you fulfill promise after promise, you will see and feel your body and mind changing. The resulting feeling of accomplishment and contentment is indescribable. You will experience a whole new sense of control over your life that you've never felt before.

So how do you make this happen?

Here's a great strategy that has worked for our clients:

1. Write down your Power Promise and post it in at least three places where you will see it often—your bathroom mirror, laptop screen, smartphone, workplace, or even your refrigerator.
2. Declare your promise to someone and ask for that person's support. In addition, send an email, a text, a post on Facebook—any form of communication or announcement that works for you. See our FB page to give you more suggestions on how to boost your motivation and get the most from your Transformation Team!
3. Prepare what you need to keep this commitment to yourself. For instance, if your Power Promise is to walk instead of drive, what does that entail? Do you have to leave for work earlier? Do you need to take a different kind of bag to work—a backpack to hold your meals, instead of a shoulder bag that will weigh you down? Think ahead and make adjustments as necessary to ensure you can keep your promise.

By the end of a week, go through these three steps and see how you feel. If you were able to keep that promise for one day or seven, acknowledge your victory!

## Reality Check

You will likely find yourself tempted to take on multiple promises again. If you can keep them, more power to you! Enjoy your rapid results! However, if you can't keep all of the promises, know that the consequences are disastrous. If you need to, shrink your list of promises so that you are committed to only the ones that you *know* you can keep.

Heads up: You are likely going to break your Power Promise sometime along the journey. See Lesson 16: Fall Without Failing for the formula to get back on your feet. With this formula, you can never fail!

## DAY 4

### Day 4: High-Carb Day

Meal 1: Breakfast
 Recipe: Egg and Cheddar Sandwich

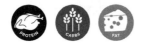

Meal 2: High-Carb Meal
 Recipe: Spiced Banana Shake

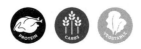

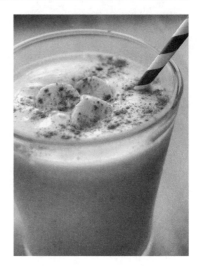

Meal 3: High-Carb Meal
 Recipe: BBQ Baked Sweet Potato, Loaded with Grilled Chicken, Corn, and Black Beans

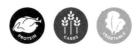

Meal 4: High-Carb Meal
 Recipe: Triple Berry Treat

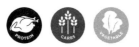

Meal 5: Low-Carb Meal
 Recipe: Zucchini and Turkey "Lasagna Roll-Ups"

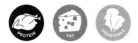

### Day 4: Metabolic Mission: Phoenix Rising (AMRAP)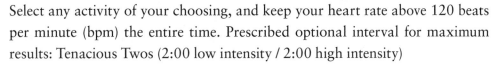

Set a running clock and perform as many rounds of the following circuit as you can in 15 minutes. Record your rounds in your Daily Tracker!

5 Push-Ups
10 Sit-Ups
15 Squats

### Day 4: Accelerator: 5 minutes (minimum)

Select any activity of your choosing, and keep your heart rate above 120 beats per minute (bpm) the entire time. Prescribed optional interval for maximum results: Tenacious Twos (2:00 low intensity / 2:00 high intensity)

## LESSON 4
## PREPARE FOR SUCCESS

*By failing to prepare, you are preparing to fail.*

—Benjamin Franklin

Success doesn't just happen. You must create it. Now that you understand and "see" the true path to transformation, it's time to get down to the nitty-gritty. With SMART goals set, your why in place, and the arsenal of all your other empowering steps under your belt, this lesson is simple, practical, and super critical to your ultimate success!

Proper nutrition will account for the majority of your weight loss success. Because of this, we have designed 21 days of delicious recipes for you. But let's get real here: Some recipes you will love, and some you may not. We designed these 21 days for you to try all kinds of different food combinations and possibilities for two reasons:

1. To help you find the recipes that you love and stick with them.
2. To give you some awesome ideas to get creative with your own food combinations and recipes.

If you love the recipes and have the time to create them, then use them to cycle away to your goal weight! But if you are limited on time or have specific tastes when it comes to your food, this lesson is for you.

## Create Your Own Meals

If you have specific tastes, or if you want to get creative with your own Extreme Cycle meal combinations, the formula is simple:

1. Create your daily menus by selecting your favorite foods (Protein, Carbs, Fats, and Veggies) from the Acceptable Foods list.
2. Follow the prescribed Extreme Cycle meal combinations (High-Carb Day, Low-Carb Day, etc.).
3. Use the 100-calorie portion reference chart (see Appendix D) to determine your portions for each meal:

|  | Breakfast | High-Carb Meal | Low-Carb Meal |
|---|---|---|---|
| **MEN** |  |  |  |
| **Protein** | 200 calories | 150 calories | 200 calories |
| **Carbs** | 150 calories | 250 calories | <30 calories |
| **Fats** | 150 calories | <30 calories | 150 calories |
| **WOMEN** |  |  |  |
| **Protein** | 150 calories | 100 calories | 150 calories |
| **Carbs** | 100 calories | 200 calories | <30 calories |
| **Fats** | 100 calories | <30 calories | 100 calories |

It's that simple. Follow these guidelines for your own custom meals, and Cycle away to a new you.

Whether you follow our recipes or make your own meal combinations, here's the unfortunate catch: If you don't have the right food with you, the usual options are fast food, convenience stores, and vending machines—none of which will likely lead you to your goal. If you want results, you'll need to establish consistency. To make a change in your body, you need to give your body repetition and time. The key to this consistency? Preparing your meals in advance. When you prepare your meals in advance, you guarantee days of nutrition consistency. Day after day, the pounds will be released. Week after week, your clothes will start falling off you and you'll start seeing muscle definition you've never seen before. Month after month, jaws will drop when your family and friends see you! Want this kind of guaranteed success? Meal prep!

### Shop, Prep, Store, and Pack

Why is it that nearly everyone who loses a significant amount of weight swears by meal prep? Why is it that all the fittest people in the world meal prep? Why is it that all the people who have lost weight, and *kept* it off for years, preach about meal prep?

Because meal prep works. Because meal prep is the most powerful way to ensure nutrition consistency for the fastest results. Because meal prep is the least expensive and most convenient way to Extreme Cycle and find success on your journey of transformation.

Yes, meal prep takes an hour or two out of your week, but think about it: If you dedicate an hour to preparing your meals in advance, you gain seven days of nutrition success! That is priceless, not to mention the hours of time you will save not having to prepare meals every three hours!

### So How Do You Shop?

1. Don't go shopping when you are hungry.
2. Purchase a week of food at a time. Use the shopping lists we provide for the weekly recipes or create your own grocery list.
3. When shopping, stay along the perimeter of the store for most of your groceries, and only go down the aisles that have foods and flavors from the list!

### *Your Good Food Grocery List*

We've organized the grocery lists by food group so that you get accustomed to thinking about all that you eat as either a protein, carbohydrate, vegetable, fat, drink, or flavoring. When you get used to these food groups, making good choices gets easier, and creating delicious dishes is simple! See Appendix B for detailed meal prep instructions for the Extreme Cycle recipes in this book.

### *How Do You Meal Prep?*

Meal prep always seems like a daunting task until you do it—and realize how easy and convenient it really is!

1. Decide which day you are going to shop and meal prep. We usually prep on Sunday. We suggest you prep your foods on your weigh-in/Reset day, or midweek if necessary.
2. Bake, grill, barbecue, and boil all meats and eggs. Flavor using seasonings you choose or sauces from the recipes.
3. Peel, chop, cut, and shred all veggies.
4. Steam, bake, or boil all starches and flavor however you choose.
5. Next, when you're done cooking, allow the dishes to cool, and then portion them out into containers to refrigerate or freeze. Refrigerate foods for meals needed in the next three or four days. Freeze foods for meals after that. And remember to label your containers with the date.
6. Get a cooler, and pack your food for each day to carry with you!

A major component to long-term meal prep is making it easy and convenient. These tools require a onetime purchase, but they will set you up for lifelong success!

- Set of pots and pans
- Set of cutlery
- Blender
- Rice cooker/steamer
- Tabletop grill
- Toaster oven
- Crock-Pot

# Reality Check

The reality is that you are going to find yourself in a bind every now and then when you didn't prep when you should have. For those times, you have to make good choices.

If you're in a convenience store, choose nuts, fruit, or a low-sugar protein bar.

If you're in a restaurant, ask your server if they can adapt a dish so that it's clean.

Keep nuts, protein bars, and other healthy snacks in your car or at your desk. If you are on the go or short on time, the following foods require little to no preparation, so they can be ready to go anywhere and anytime. They're also great when traveling—just swing by a grocery store as soon as you reach your destination and stock up!

## Proteins

Powdered proteins
Cottage cheese
Plain Greek yogurt
Canned meats
Turkey, chicken, or roast beef deli meat

## Carbohydrates

Fruit
Low-fat bran cereals and low-fat granola
Multigrain breads
Beans/lentils
Microwave-ready yams and potatoes

## Vegetables

Mixed salads
Frozen veggies in ready-to-microwave
bags

## Fats

String and sliced cheese
Peanut butter and almond butter
Pecans, almonds, and walnuts
Avocado
Salad dressing

# DAY 5

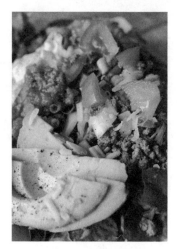

## Day 5: Low-Carb Day

Meal 1: Breakfast
   Recipe: Green Machine Pancakes

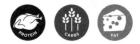

Meal 2: Low-Carb Meal
   Recipe: Stuffed Avocado

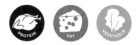

Meal 3: Low-Carb Meal
   Recipe: Citrus Salmon Slaw

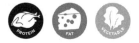

Meal 4: Low-Carb Meal
   Recipe: Greek Yogurt Parfait with Nuts

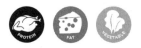

Meal 5: Low-Carb Meal
   Recipe: Taco Salad

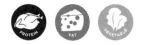

## Day 5: Metabolic Mission: A Lotta Tabata (Tabata)

For each exercise, do as many reps as you can in 20 seconds. Rest for 10 seconds, then do as many reps as you can in 20 seconds again. Repeat for 8 total rounds (for a total of 4 minutes) per exercise. The lowest number of reps you get in any round is your score. You'll get one score per exercise. Add up all three scores, and record it in your Daily Tracker!

Air Squats (lowest reps per round)
Sit-Ups
Push-Ups (lowest reps per round)
Accelerator

## Day 5: Accelerator: 5 minutes (minimum)

Select any activity of your choosing, and keep your heart rate above 120 beats per minute (bpm) the entire time. Prescribed optional interval for maximum results: Nasty Nineties (:90 low intensity / :90 high intensity)

## LESSON 5
## RALLY YOUR TEAM

*No man is an island, entire of itself; every man is a piece of the continent.*

—John Donne

Team. Support. Comrades. Unity. Something powerful happens when humans come together and cooperate toward a shared vision. They don't become twice as strong; they become exponentially stronger. You might have figured out by now that making this transformation journey alone is a daunting task, and those who have succeeded have done so because they consciously and carefully created a powerful team of supporters. This is not a solo journey: Your path to transformation *requires* interaction with others.

This is where your Transformation Team comes in. Who is this team? They are the people you declare your goals and commitments to. They are the people who hold you accountable. They are the ones who encourage you to keep your promises to yourself—even when you don't want to. They are the ones you lean on when you need to confess and unload emotional baggage. They are your trusted support network. These are people who notice you, care about you, and genuinely support your transformation.

Now, here's the catch: It may or may not be who you think it is. It might be your family and friends. It might be some of your colleagues at work. Or it might be people you don't even know yet.

Your Transformation Team can be anyone from whom you receive love and support.

Bob's Transformation Team is his church. As a devout Christian, Bob relies on his faith to fuel his commitment and keep himself feeling supported and loved. "I have to live authentically," Bob explains. "And for me that means serving others as a way to stay close to my higher power."

Jami formed her own Transformation Team. As she explains, "I started a group called BIG. It's a body image group. As a coach and mentor, I want to support other girls and women around developing a healthy, realistic body image.

Bruce's Transformation Team is—guess who? Us! He not only stays in close contact with us but also "pays it forward," as a mentor to other people who are struggling to lose weight. In turn, these "newbies" have also become Bruce's Transformation Team.

A team member might be a member of your family, church, other support groups, or maybe even people you have met online! We have hundreds of thousands of people on the journey who reach out to us and stay connected through our website, our blog, and our social networks. We invite you to "use us" as your support team. In fact, many of our peeps have connected with one another, creating ever-growing support networks among themselves. Who better to have on your team than someone who understands what the journey is all about?

Yes—these best friends in the world are waiting to meet you! They are friendly, unconditionally supportive, and want you to be healthy and happy!

## Reality Check

This may come as a shock, but it is possible that your closest family and friends may not be your biggest supporters. Or maybe they are? When creating your Transformation Team, it is important not to set high expectations of your loved ones, because it can often lead to disappointment. Understand that your goals may not resonate with their goals and aspirations. Your desire to change may threaten them and their lifestyle. It is not uncommon for spouses to be terrified of being abandoned, and best friends afraid of losing their "drinking buddy" or "drive-thru pal." Granted, your wife, brother, or best friend may turn out to be your greatest backer on your journey, but it is best to wipe the slate clean and build your team from scratch—if your family and friends want a spot on your team, let them prove to you that they belong there!

### Picking Your Team

Time to play detective: It's time to identify the people who are on your Transformation Team, and weed out the people who aren't.

On a separate sheet of paper, list the 10 people closest to you, who may deserve a spot on your Transformation Team. Then make two column headings: On My Team and Not on My Team.

Now, for each individual, answer these questions:

1. Does this person create unnecessary drama or distractions to pull you away from your transformation commitments?
2. Does this person tempt you with triggers from your past?
3. Does this person make comments or make you feel guilty for wanting to change?
4. Does this person refuse to make small changes in their lifestyle to help you reach your goals?

If your answer was no to all of the above questions, place a checkmark in the column On My Team. If your answer was yes to any of the questions, place a checkmark in the column Not on My Team.

People will come in and out of your life for as long as you live. Begin to ask yourself these questions with the people you meet, and determine if they are on your Transformation Team or if they aren't.

Note: Beware the mole! This is the person who pretends to support you on the surface, but as you move closer to your goals, he or she may begin to sabotage you and pull you off course.

If you are having difficulty identifying people to be on your Transformation Team, ask these questions to help guide your search. Your team may be closer than you think!

1. Where might I meet other people who share my goals and attitude toward success?
2. What websites or online communities might connect me with these like-minded people?

And don't forget us and our community of amazing people!

Within your Transformation Team you may find an individual who goes above and beyond motivating and supporting you. They want to see you succeed, and will go the extra mile to help you make it happen. They are there for you to vent, to confess, to open up about your struggles. They also call you out when you are making excuses or trying to rationalize bad behavior. This is your superfriend. Your superfriend tells you what you *need* to hear to better your life, not what you *want* to hear. You may not like what they have to say sometimes (because deep down, you know that they are right). Your superfriend is essential to your success, so it's important to pick this person carefully. Here are some guiding questions to help you:

1. Do I trust this person completely?
2. Do I feel comfortable being totally honest with this person, no matter what I've done?
3. Am I sure that this person will not judge me or get angry with me if I confess a setback?

You and your superfriend must make an agreement between the two of you. Why? Because being a superfriend is not easy. It is a lot easier and much less time consuming to just go along with everything *you* want. Being a superfriend is hard work. Nobody wants to hurt your feelings or for you to be upset with them...but your superfriend cares so much about you, they are willing to tell you the truth even when it might hurt—for *your* success. So take some time to let them know how much you appreciate their sacrifice for you—and that you will stay as open as possible, even when they are calling you out and you are feeling defensive!

If a fight begins, we use a code word to put everything into perspective for both parties. Just say "Superfriend." You'll both know what is happening and remember the agreement you made.

Please share this with your superfriend:

If you are chosen as a superfriend, you must agree to the following:

1. You will call out the individual when you see they are making excuses or justifying destructive behavior.
2. You will listen openly and without judgment when the other individual is confessing.
3. After their confession, the first two words out of your mouth should always be "Thank you."
4. You will be there for support (and maybe even jump into a workout or two) every chance you get.

Creating your Transformation Team is one of the crucial parts of sustaining your motivation, accountability, and perseverance on your transformation journey! Making big changes to how we think and go about our daily routines is very hard. And your Transformation Team is one of the single most important factors in holding you accountable so that you can keep your promises... and create your destiny!

# DAY 6

## Day 6: Low-Carb Day

Meal 1: Breakfast
    Recipe: Raspberry Almond Oatmeal

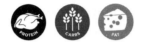

Meal 2: Low-Carb Meal
    Recipe: Chicken Slaw Dip

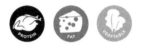

Meal 3: Low-Carb Meal
    Recipe: Vietnamese Grilled Chicken
Spring Rolls with Sweet Ginger Lime Sauce

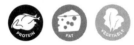

Meal 4: Low-Carb Meal
    Recipe: Vanilla Pecan Pudding

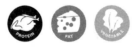

Meal 5: Low-Carb Meal
    Recipe: Citrus and Onion Fish Tacos

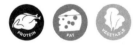

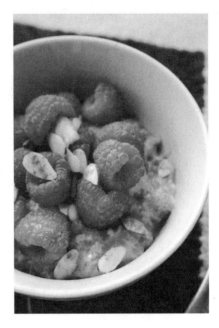

## Day 6: Metabolic Mission

No mission today!

## Day 6: Accelerator: 5 minutes (minimum)

Select any activity of your choosing, and keep your heart rate above 120 beats per minute (bpm) the entire time. Prescribed optional interval for maximum results: Mighty Minutes (1:00 low intensity / 1:00 high intensity)

### LESSON 6

# MAKE IT YOUR OWN!

*Never, ever underestimate the importance of having fun.*

—Randy Pausch

Setting SMART goals, preparing, and building a trusted Transformation Team all build the foundation for lasting transformation. But we don't want you to forget another extremely important part of your journey: having fun! It is basic common sense: If this new life isn't enjoyable, you aren't going to stick with it.

We've given you the Extreme Transformation structure and plan for success, but now it's time to make it yours—to customize the plan to fit your goals, your needs, your life. How do you do that? By customizing this new lifestyle, rewarding yourself, and trying new ways to make weight loss actually enjoyable.

We mean it: You should be excited about what you are eating and doing. If it isn't fun, then you're doing it wrong. Whether you reach your goal in three short weeks or you are on a yearlong transformation trek, it is important that this process is enjoyable for you. Keep in mind that maintenance—keeping the weight off forever—is very similar to the structure you will follow to lose the weight. So let's make this something you can do forever. Because to keep the weight off, this *is* what you're going to be doing...for life!

### The Secret of Substitutions

We mentioned earlier that we designed these 21 days of recipes to give you a plethora of new ideas and concepts for eating and enjoying food as you lose weight. When you try these recipes, we are confident that you will find ones that you absolutely love, and ones that don't suit your palate as much. That's okay! It is all part of the process.

Say you like lean ground beef over ground chicken. No problem, switch them out! Perhaps you prefer Greek yogurt to cottage cheese . . . plug it in! Maybe you prefer whole-grain pasta over potatoes. So if a recipe calls for potatoes, substitute whole-grain pasta instead! You know what to do—make the switch!

As long as you stay within the Extreme Cycle portions and calorie limits, you can substitute to your heart's content and still achieve the same phenomenal weight loss results.

### Reward Yourself!

Motivation is a tricky business. Our brains and bodies are incredibly smart and adapt to new routines easily and quickly. Which is why making changes to our behaviors is so darn hard. One of the ways we can break into our routines to make them more fun and exciting is by giving ourselves rewards. As you've seen, we have designed the Extreme Cycle to include a reward on the seventh day of every week. That means on Days 7, 14, and 21, you will be able to enjoy anything you want, in moderation of course.

The choice of when and what you reward yourself with is up to you! Of course, we wouldn't be Team Powell if we didn't also offer you a list of delicious and nutritious Clean Cheats on Reset days (see page 86 for complete list of Clean Cheats), but in reality you can choose any food you like to be your reward.

There is just one main rule to rewarding yourself: *You cannot reward yourself at or after dinner.* It must always be earlier in the day. In the evening and at night, our inhibitions are down and we are *very* likely to eat more than we should—breaking promises and starting a dangerous backslide. Because of this, any reward should be enjoyed earlier in the day, preferably at or before lunch. Dinner will always remain a sacred low-carb meal, anchoring in your commitment to this journey.

Being able to relax from a routine enables your mind to take a break and restore itself, but here's the best secret: Boosting your calorie intake also boosts your metabolism, so when you drop back into carb cycling on the next day, you will burn even more calories!

For many people, a week is still a pretty darn long time to wait to get your pizza. By the time Wednesday rolls around, it is consuming your thoughts and you can't think of anything else. That's why many people still need what we call Daily Hugs—those little treats that you reward yourself with once or twice a day…just to get you through. We get it. Here's a list of Daily Hugs that you can weave into your daily routine to keep your mind and your taste buds happy until Reset day:

- Diet soda
- Low-calorie specialty coffee
- Calorie-free (or very low-calorie) candy
- Sugar-free gum

## Two Heidi Tips

**Tip #1** I have found that when I eat such "reward" foods as potato chips or ice cream, I can't stop. It's like my body and brain crave these two foods so intensely, it's near impossible to eat just a little. So my advice is this: Know what your super-trigger foods are and stay away from them. Find a sweet or salty food that you enjoy that doesn't trigger you. Or better yet: Find another pleasurable way to reward yourself—like getting your nails done, getting a massage, or curling up on your couch to watch your favorite show. Rewards are super important, but you still need to be mindful!

**Tip #2** To get through the week without feeling any deprivation, I treat myself with one thing every day—I enjoy my own specialty coffee drink—an iced coffee with one pump of mocha and a splash of heavy cream. It has a small calorie impact (less than 100 calories), and it is the Daily Hug that I can look forward to once—or even sometimes twice—every day. It satisfies me enough so that I don't crave anything else…and just look forward to the next morning!

Reward days naturally happen on high-carb days because of their sweet and fatty content. We suggest that Sundays are great for reward days, but it's really up to you. It may make more sense for you to have your reward day (Days 7, 14, and 21 of the Extreme Cycle) on a Wednesday. It's up to you to decide, but you must declare it and commit to it in advance so that you stay clear and focused on your promises to yourself.

Rewards also help you curb your cravings for those trigger foods—sweet, salty, and fatty. But heed this word of caution: Since reward foods can be close to those comfort foods that can trigger overeating (see page 164 for more on identifying your triggers), it's wise to be mindful of your choices. By choosing from our list, you might avoid triggering those old cravings that led to your weight gain to begin with.

## Clean Cheat Recipes!

We are not kidding: These Clean Cheat snacks and meals are so delicious (and easy to make), you're going to think we are nuts! They will have your mouth watering and your bellies satisfied. You won't believe they are cleaner versions of those good ol' comfort foods! Just a heads-up, though: The Clean Cheats are cleaner, but please know that they are *still* only acceptable on Reset days, as they are higher in calories than the foods you will be eating on your high- and low-carb days. Check out the recipes in the back section of the book! And remember: Only eat these meals on Days 7, 14, and 21. Bon appétit!

### Breakfast

Hootenanny Pancakes
Chocolate Glazed Crepes
Candied Pecan Protein Waffles

### Snacks

Spinach Artichoke Dip with Pita Chips
Peanut Butter Chocolate Chip Cookie
    Dough
Muddy Buddies
Sweet Potato Nachos
Homemade Oreos
Banana Berry Ice Cream
Pigs in a Blanket
One-Minute Brownie

### Lunch/Dinner

Chunky Monkey Bowl
BLT Burger and Sweet Potato Fries
Barbecue Chicken Pita Pizza
Mac and Cheese with Bacon

If you find yourself craving some typical junk foods, try these amazing substitutions. Often we are simply seeking something that will satisfy our needs for something crunchy, sweet, and/or salty. These should do the trick!

| Instead of eating this: | Eat this: |
| --- | --- |
| Candy bar or chocolate | Protein bar or shake |
| Crackers or cookies | Flavored rice cakes |
| Potato or tortilla chips | Air-popped popcorn |
| Juice or soda | Calorie-free drink |
| Pizza | Sliced tomato with low-fat mozzarella, sprinkled with garlic, basil, and sea salt |
| Ice cream | Sugar-free Popsicle |
| High-calorie coffee beverage | Iced-coffee with sugar-free syrup |
| Candy | Sugar-free gum |

# Heidi Tip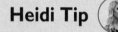

Just like a lot of folks, I get the munchies later in the day, especially after dinner when the kids are in bed and I finally unwind and relax. That's when I often find myself in the "red zone"—that high-alert place where I am craving something sweet or salty. My go-to fix? I put a bag of frozen or fresh broccoli in a bowl, sprinkle a little sea salt or ¼ cup marinara sauce on top, and microwave or steam for a few minutes. This trick not only ups my veggies for the day (always a positive) but also satisfies my cravings! Try it—my peeps have gone crazy for this treat!

### Have Fun Accelerating Your Weight Loss!

The key to long-term success is to make exercise enjoyable. If you like doing it, you're going to do it for a long time! If you don't like to do it, you will eventually stop—and go right back to your old habits. Science has found that we are programmed to play—run, jump, push, roll, pull, climb, throw, et cetera—and when we do it in a "gamified" way, the results and benefits are astounding... and fun!

Along these lines, finding the right "Accelerator" for you is a lot like dating. You've got to try them all out to find which ones you love. That's why we encourage everyone to "speed date" every aspect of sport imaginable—brisk walking, rowing, Zumba, running, soccer, basketball, CrossFit, boxing, MMA, whatever! Eventually, you will find something that you truly love to do—even if it's just watching TV while walking on the treadmill. If you enjoy it, then do it to accelerate your weight loss. There is an athlete inside all of us, and we have yet to work with anyone who hasn't found some activity they love.

Cassie rediscovered all the sports she likes. As she told us, "I'm not a gym rat. But for so long when I was overweight, I couldn't play the sports I used to love. Now I play basketball and volleyball. I do some circuit training that I set up in my house. You've just got to get out there and try different things—it's so much more fun than I ever thought."

Part of Merhbod's motivation to stick to his transformation journey was wanting to do everything he used to love—from basketball to skiing. Then he realized that doing those things he used to love was exactly how he'd get back into shape! Granted, moving up and down the court at his heaviest of 434 pounds wasn't easy at first, but he did it anyway. Day after day it got easier and easier, as he lost over 200 pounds and was running circles around his competition!

Bruce discovered CrossFit and now participates in competitions around his region.

David found MMA and trained for 60 to 90 minutes a day, losing over 200 pounds in a year.

Denise picked up tennis and now plays in a competitive doubles league.

Margaret tried Zumba and loves it!

### Variety Is the Spice of Life

When we first meet most of our peeps for the show, they seem to fall into two categories—those who love sports and think of themselves as athletes, even if they are now out of shape, and those who say they hate to exercise and would never consider themselves athletes. We are here to tell you that everyone has an athlete inside of them—you just haven't connected with the sport or exercise you love yet. Seriously. We have yet to work with anyone who didn't find something they love to do.

So now is your time! You've got to get out of your comfort zone and let yourself try something new. Take a look at the list below. We challenge you to try something new each of the three weeks of your 21-day cycle. If you don't find something that you really enjoy, keep trying. Your favorite weight-loss Accelerator is out there!

### Accelerators

#### At Home

| | | |
|---|---|---|
| Dodgeball | Stationary bike | Treadmill |
| Jump rope | Tag | |
| Rowing machine | Trampoline | |

#### At the Gym

| | | |
|---|---|---|
| Arc trainer | Rowing machine | Stationary or recumbent bike |
| Arm ergometer | Stair stepper | |
| Elliptical trainer | | Treadmill |

#### Outdoors

| | | |
|---|---|---|
| Bicycling | In-line skating | Stair running |
| Bleacher running | Jogging/running | Swimming |
| Canoeing | Kayaking | Walking |
| Cross-country skiing | Rowing | Water jogging |
| Hiking | Snow shoveling | |
| Ice skating | Snowshoeing | |

#### Sports

| | | |
|---|---|---|
| Basketball | Dodgeball | Hockey |
| Boxing | Flag football | Jiu Jitsu |

Kickball          Racquetball        Tennis
Kickboxing        Soccer             Volleyball
Lacrosse          Squash             Wrestling
Martial arts      Swimming

*Group Classes*

Aerobics          CrossFit           Step aerobics
BarSculpt         Dancing            Water aerobics
Cardio kickboxing Spinning/cycling

Pick your top five Accelerators from the list above. Choose Accelerators that you already love to do, or have always wanted to try:

Now, here are your marching orders: Do them! Pick one and have some fun with it. If or when it starts to get boring or monotonous, try the next one! Maybe even alternate and switch them up every week. However you do it, have fun!

## Become a Metabolic Master

As we described earlier, the way to boost your fat burn to lose even more weight is by including Accelerators into your daily routine. As you move through the 21-day cycles, use this chart of minimum Accelerator times to challenge yourself.

|           | Week1      | Week 2     | Week 3     |
|-----------|------------|------------|------------|
| **1st Cycle** | 5 minutes  | 10 minutes | 15 minutes |
| **2nd Cycle** | 20 minutes | 25 minutes | 30 minutes |
| **3rd Cycle** | 35 minutes | 40 minutes | 45 minutes |
| **4th Cycle** | 50 minutes | 55 minutes | 60 minutes |

# DAY 7

Congrats! You've made it to Day 7: weigh-in and reward day! We are so excited for you! You've already accomplished so much in one short week: You've begun cleaning out your body and your home; you're becoming familiar with your new routine. Now it's time to see the progress.

## Weigh In

Weigh in first thing in the morning without eating or drinking. Remove as many articles of clothing as possible to get the cleanest weight.

Your current weight: _____

At this time, feel free to take any other measurements as well and note them here: _____

## Day 7: Reset Day

It's Reset Day! Make meals easy by cooking up our Clean Cheat recipes, or simply add 1,000 extra calories of foods you love to a normal high-carb day.

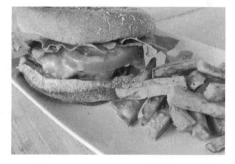

1. Meal 1: Hootenanny Pancakes
2. Meal 2: Spinach Artichoke Dip with Pita Chips
3. Meal 3: Chunky Monkey Bowl
4. Meal 4: BLT Burger and Sweet Potato Fries
5. Meal 5: Peanut Butter Chocolate Chip Cookie Dough

### Rest Day

Now relax! Take the day off and rest—no Metabolic Missions and no Accelerators!

## LESSON 7
# TROUBLESHOOT!

*Fall down seven times, get up eight.*

—Japanese proverb

As you trek through the days of this journey, you will begin to run into different challenges that can possibly derail you. Sometimes it is the frustration of not losing weight, other times it is uncontrollable cravings. Not to worry—we encounter them on a regular basis and we'll teach you all of the tips and tricks for how to get through them.

### Scale Funk

Nothing is worse than working your ass off and seeing no return on the scale. Chillax. If you did it right, you very well may have burned a lot of fat—your body just isn't showing it yet. This reaction is natural and normal. Weight loss may stall for a week or two, but then resume after that.

The body loses fat in slow motion. We recommend you weigh in once a week—the shortest amount of time to see somewhat accurate changes on the scale. We can see a much better trend for weight loss every 2 weeks, but a weekly weigh in promotes accountability and structure. While fat is gained and lost very slowly, water can be gained and lost extremely fast—sometimes we can gain or lose upwards of 10 pounds of water in a day! If you step on the scale every day, these fluctuations can cause an emotional roller coaster. Expect the scale jump up several pounds after every Reset day, then slowly drop over the course of the week. The final 2 low-carb days before the weigh-in, you should see a good drop on the scale, to reveal a clean weight for your weigh-in day.

Here are the four main physiological reasons for seeing a slow loss or even a gain on the scale, as well as some unorthodox ways to get dropping again!

## Muscle Swelling

**Reason:** It occurs to some degree after every Metabolic Mission. The amount of swelling depends upon the intensity of the workout. The higher the intensity, the greater the swelling. This lasts for one to several days, then subsides.

**Solutions:**
- Reduce the intensity of the Missions for a week; the fluid will release.
- Light massage.
- Epsom salt baths.

## Excess Water Retention

**Reason A:** When sodium intake exceeds the body's normal level, it causes excess water retention and bloat—up to 15 pounds sometimes!

**Solution:** Reduce your sodium intake and avoid processed, sugary, and salty foods. Drink *lots* of water, and your body will release the excess water over the next three days.

**Reason B:** Cortisol. This stress hormone is being released in massive amounts from physical stress (overtraining) during long bouts of exercise. The hormone causes fluid retention in the muscles and subcutaneously (under the skin).

**Solution:** Reduce your training intensity and ensure proper calorie (and carbohydrate) intake. Excess fluid will release over the week and reveal your true loss.

**Reason C:** Prior dehydration—from not drinking enough water, alcohol consumption, or some other diuretic. The body responds by retaining water.

**Solution:** Drink at least an extra quart of water daily (aim for at least a gallon daily) and give it three days to stabilize.

## Fat Gain or Plateau

**Reason:** You are consuming too many calories and not burning enough, creating a plateau or even a slow fat and/or muscle *gain*.

**Solution:** Ensure you are keeping your promises to the Extreme Cycle, Metabolic Missions, and Accelerators. Also, double-check your portions—if you have been simply eyeballing your portions, you may want to pull out the measuring cups for a week to get the portions and calories back on track.

How you can help yourself:

- Are you doing your Accelerators?
- Are you following your commitment to the Extreme Cycle?
- Have you been emotionally eating?

Now is the time to be courageous, open, and honest if you are struggling and eating more than you should. You *may* also be gaining some muscle—especially if you haven't done any form of resistance training in a long time. In the first few weeks of training, it is also common to experience a phenomenon called recomposition: It is when your body gains muscle and loses fat at the same time. This is typically most noticeable in just the first few weeks of training, but can happen subtly over the whole course of your transformation.

### Hormonal Fluctuations

**Reason A:** Women can retain fluid during their monthly cycles. This retention typically lasts no longer than a week.

**Reason B:** Thyroid, ADH, or Aldosterone fluctuations.

**Solution:** Bloodwork prescribed by a doctor can determine if this is an issue. It may require medication.

### Crush Your Cravings

Every single one of us experiences cravings—for sleep, for water, for sweets, for salty foods, you name it. Cravings are our body's way of telling us *what it thinks* we need. But we are not simple animals roaming the savannas or forests in search of immediate gratification. No. We are thinking beings and we have the power to control our cravings. Obviously, the very first step is by sticking to the Extreme Carb Cycle, exercising regularly, and getting enough sleep.

We also know enough to stay away from our trigger foods and reward ourselves so that we don't make ourselves vulnerable to cravings. But physical cravings can be overwhelming at times, so this is what we recommend:

1. Stay hydrated. Hydration is the number one way to curb cravings. Immediately do our 10-gulp water rule as soon as a craving starts. As soon as

the cup or bottle touches your lips, take 10 gulps before putting it down! It's easy to confuse thirst with hunger, so stay hydrated!

2. Chew sugar-free mint-flavored gum, eat a sugar-free breath mint, or put a dab of toothpaste on your tongue. The mint flavor overwhelms the taste buds, crushing cravings for sweet and salty foods—so you can make it to your next snack or meal.

3. Always include high-fiber foods with breakfast. Fiber-rich foods slow down digestion to keep you fuller for longer, so you will be less likely to overeat later in the day, and more likely to pay attention to your body's signals that it is full.

4. When all else fails, the last resort that is sure to nuke a craving is to use dietary fats, followed by 1 or 2 cups of liquid (water, tea). It takes about 20 minutes after eating the fats for them to close off the valve from the stomach to the intestines. Once you drink the liquid, it fills the stomach, sending an extremely strong "full" signal to the brain, and curbing the strongest of cravings. Warning: The following fats have a 100-calorie impact, so you *must* count it for your daily intake!

A small handful of almonds, then 1 to 2 cups water
1 tablespoon of peanut butter or almond butter, then 1 to 2 cups water
1 stick of string cheese, then 1 to 2 cups water
1 tablespoon of avocado, then 1 to 2 cups water

Or try one of these three delicious 100-calorie liquid treats:

Root beer float: ice-cold diet root beer + 1 tablespoon heavy cream
Coconut water: 1 cup warm water + 1 tablespoon coconut oil
Bulletproof coffee: 1 cup coffee + 1 tablespoon unsalted butter

Again, keep in mind that each of these has a 100-calorie impact, so it must be added to your daily calories. Although we recommend you use the calorie-free methods to curb cravings, if necessary these delicious treats can be used anytime on the Extreme Cycle to curb the heaviest of cravings when they hit. Limit yourself to no more than one per day and sip on it for a while—make it last!

POWELL

# LOVE IT!

So where are you now in your journey?

You're building some incredible momentum now after just seven days of Extreme Transformation! You might already be feeling better about yourself, noticing some weight loss and other positive changes in your body. You may feel lighter and cleaner. You may feel more empowered, clearheaded, and centered in yourself. You likely also feel more resolved in your new changes and commitments to yourself.

But as we cautioned you earlier in the book, the diet and exercise plan is the easy part. Just losing weight does not guarantee the deep, life-sustaining transformation we can help create for you.

So for Week Two, we share with you seven more lessons that are crucial to learning to *love* your journey of transformation. These mental and emotional tools will help you dig deep, be vulnerable, and banish the negative self-talk that can derail you. You will, once and for all, conquer your fears, unload the real weight you've been carrying around, and create a new identity that crystallizes your destiny!

# DAY 8

## Day 8: High-Carb Day

Meal 1: Breakfast
Recipe: Sweet Potato Fritters

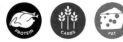

Meal 2: High-Carb Meal
Recipe: Piña Colada Dream

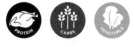

Meal 3: High-Carb Meal
Recipe: Chile Relleno, Braised Adobo Chicken, Black Bean and Quinoa Salad

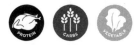

Meal 4: High-Carb Meal
Recipe: Hulk Shake

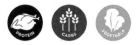

Meal 5: Low-Carb Meal
Recipe: Thai-Style Turkey Cabbage Salad

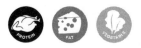

## Day 8: Metabolic Mission: The Grinder (Stepladder)

Set a running clock and, as fast as you can, do 21 reps of each exercise, then do 15 reps of each exercise, then do 9 reps of each exercise. Report your time in your Daily Tracker!

Burpees

Mountain Climbers

Back Lunges

### Day 8: Accelerator: 10 minutes (minimum)

Select any activity of your choosing, and keep your heart rate above 120 beats per minute (bpm) the entire time. Prescribed optional interval for maximum results: Dirty Two-Thirties (2:30 low intensity / 2:30 high intensity)

## LESSON 8
## BELIEVE IN YOURSELF

*Whether you think you can or whether you think you can't, you're right.*

—Henry Ford

Yes, the promises you make to yourself are concrete, convincing accomplishments. But often people feel terrified, doubtful, and just plain confused as they begin to make even the smallest of changes. In fact, beginning and sticking to this journey requires a certain "leap of faith," which often feels like moving into unknown territory. This is where you need a little faith. Faith in this process, and faith in all the people who have succeeded before you. Because if they can do it, you can do it.

But sometimes believing in yourself isn't easy, and that's where we come in.

We know you are capable of this journey. We know that it's not easy. But it is possible. As Bruce shared with us, "Chris and Heidi, I needed you. At first I didn't know if I could do it, but you helped me believe in myself again. Your support and love helped me realize that I can do this. Once I started to believe in myself, I'd say, *I'm not going to let the fat beat me today.* And you know what, it didn't. I just needed to believe!"

Our work with thousands of overweight people who have lost thousands of pounds has shown us one truth over and over again: One of the most powerful ingredients to changing your life is simply believing that you can. Seems overly simplistic, but actually getting you to *believe* in your abilities—to know in your heart of hearts that you can do this—can be a difficult task.

Belief is the magic ingredient that drives your choices and behaviors. When you believe, the light switch for transformation gets slammed into the "on" position and you excitedly put forth the effort to achieving your goals and dreams. The moment you question yourself or stop believing that you can, the switch slams off. And just as quickly, your behaviors can revert back to their old habits and patterns.

But what if you've tried and failed what seems like hundreds of times in the past?

What if you don't think that you can attain your goal?

There are a couple of ways to develop belief when you don't believe in yourself...yet.

This new commitment to transformation requires courage in the face of past experience and failures. How many diets have you tried? How many have worked for you? How many times have you gone through a dieting ordeal only to end up gaining the weight back and feeling like a failure, ashamed of your inability to succeed or stick with it?

Let us help put any doubts you have to rest. Seeing is believing. One of the most powerful sources of inspiration is seeing another person we can relate to accomplish extraordinary goals. That's why every year we select 15 to 20 new and unique individuals to embark upon the journey of transformation. As we often tell our peeps, we love working with them because they have such a long and challenging journey ahead—the literal sizes of their journeys to weight loss are daunting for almost anyone to imagine. However, time and time again they do it. They finish their yearlong journey and they just keep going. We document their journey and share it across the world so that everyone can see what we as humans are capable of. We love working with our people, because they leave no doubt on the table that anyone and everyone can change for the better.

Why are we sharing this? Because if they can do it, so can you. They not only learned to trust the process and go all in, but they came to believe in themselves.

You can trust the thousands of people who have reached their successful weight loss goals using Extreme Transformation—its eating, exercise plan, and lessons. So now it is your time. Just take a look at the before-and-after photos below.

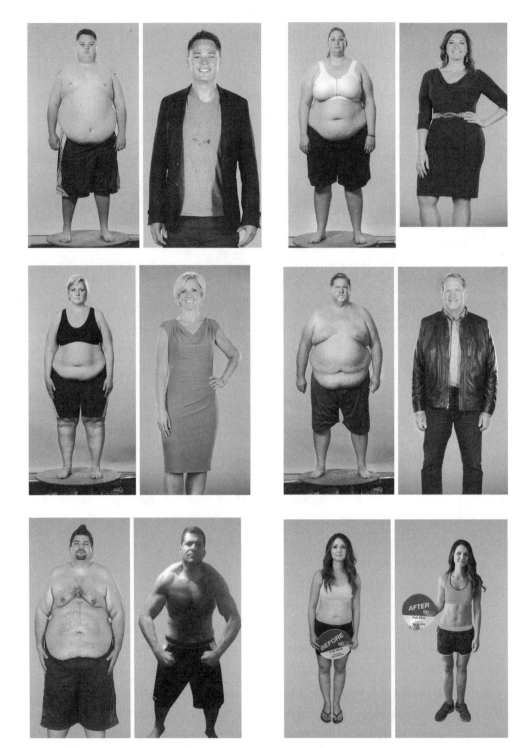

These amazing transformations are a testament to what you are also capable of.

## Call to Action: Learning How to Believe in Yourself

Begin by writing down three accomplishments that you are proud of having achieved in your life:

**1.**

**2.**

**3.**

Next, name three people whose lives you have helped:

**1.**

**2.**

**3.**

Consider these accomplishments. Reflect on them. Take pride in them. You need to remind yourself of what you have achieved.

It's possible to tap into the extraordinary—just like Bruce, Cassie, Jeff, Georgeanna, Mehrbod, and the thousands of others who have chosen to believe in themselves. We believe that though we are all ordinary humans, we all have the ability to be extraordinary. But you have to believe it's possible. Without that belief as your source, you simply will not put forward the energy and perseverance to get there.

Remember—it's okay if you don't believe in yourself yet. Turn to your Transformation Team, turn to us, turn to your online support group! Borrow their belief in you until you feel it for yourself!

Know this truth…we believe in you, we're excited for you, and we know you are going to do extraordinary things.

# DAY 9

## Day 9: High-Carb Day

Meal 1: Breakfast
Recipe: Banana Yogurt Parfait and Pumpkin Seed Granola

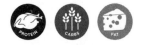

Meal 2: High-Carb Meal
Recipe: Egg Salad on Toast

Meal 3: High-Carb Meal
Recipe: Green Chili Turkey and Cilantro Rice Bowl

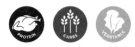

Meal 4: High-Carb Meal
Recipe: Peanut Butter Shake

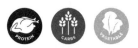

Meal 5: Low-Carb Meal
Recipe: Salmon with Pesto "Zoodles"

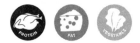

## Day 9: Metabolic Mission: Runnin' Wild (RFT)

Set a running clock and do 7 rounds of the following circuit as fast as you can. Record your time in your Daily Tracker!

10 Burpees
15 Sit-Ups
25 High Knees

## Day 9: Accelerator: 10 minutes (minimum)

Select any activity of your choosing, and keep your heart rate above 120 beats per minute (bpm) the entire time. Prescribed optional interval for maximum results: Thrilling Thirties (:30 low intensity / :30 high intensity)

## LESSON 9
# BE OPEN, HONEST, AND VULNERABLE

*Vulnerability is the greatest marker of courage.*

—Brené Brown

On Day 1 of our boot camp, we face our new group of participants and shock them to their very core. They are expecting hugs, high-fives, and for us to immediately start talking about all the weight they are going to lose. They are hoping, praying, and expecting that we give them the golden ticket of diet and exercise advice. They believe these are the true tools to changing their lives! But as you probably understand by now, true transformation actually has very little to do with diet and exercise, and everything to do with the deep, meaningful steps that truly alter your being.

So on that first day, we open the kimono. We explain that transformation has little to do with how you eat and move, and much more to do with how open, honest, and vulnerable you are willing to be. When we are vulnerable, we can grow. We can change.

Are you ready to let go and be truly vulnerable? Because that's what it's going to take. There's some tough love ahead...

### Our Need for Connection

It is human nature to seek acceptance from others—in fact, belonging is an inherent drive or need that all humans have. We all must feel loved and accepted in order to feel whole and complete. We are social animals and therefore we are "interdependent" and need help and cooperation from others for our very survival. In response to this drive, many of us—beginning when we are small children—begin to develop what we think is a "better" version of ourselves— a version that we feel is more lovable and acceptable than who we *really* are inside. This version of you strives to look its very best in front of others. This is the version that lied when you were younger so that people wouldn't think less of you. It is the version that tells everyone how well you are doing, when deep down inside you know you are struggling. It is the version that hides the donuts from the break room in its desk drawer for later—because it doesn't want to look weak in front of its co-workers. It is the version that *swears* it is doing everything right, when in reality it knows that it is breaking its promises left and right. It cannot handle embarrassment or the thought of being rejected. As we get older, that barrier becomes thicker and harder.

But this protective barrier comes at a huge cost. It is totally inauthentic, and deep down...you know it. The life you are living is a complete fraud. And even worse, because it is inauthentic, you feel like nobody could possibly love the "real you"—who you *really* are—and nobody knows how you *really* feel. You feel like you must carry on this facade, this front, forever. If you don't, you fear you will be unlovable.

Well, you're wrong. In fact, letting down this barrier is what opens your heart and mind for lifelong change—and will make you more lovable than ever!

Georgeanna, a self-described perfectionist, was unable to see herself as anything but the perfect person she thought she had to be in order to be loved. But the real Georgeanna had become over 100 pounds overweight, living two separate existences—the one in her head where she still thought she had to be a perfect mother, wife, daughter, and the one who walked around during the day, a ghost of her real self. Where was the real Georgeanna? Buried. Muted.

Georgeanna's biggest step was seeing herself naked and having the courage to say, "This is who I am right now."

Georgeanna remembers the exact moment I had her disrobe and step on the scale in front of her family and friends. She never felt more vulnerable in her entire life. She had never, ever shared how much she weighed with her husband, Scott, or anyone else in her life—let alone her whole community. She put all of her energy into doing good work for others (her "perfect" self), as if to erase the reality that she had an enormous weight problem and food addiction.

So with all the courage she could muster, Georgeanna stepped on the scale. What happened next was the exact opposite of what she thought would happen. Instead of people snickering and laughing, they began to applaud. They shouted words of encouragement and love. This first step unleashed a torrent of tears...followed by a torrent of successes. Her ability to let herself be so vulnerable paved the way for her to confront her fears, give herself permission, and ultimately declare what she wanted: weight loss, health, and a chance to change the way she was living that was making her so unhappy with herself. She realized that she could be open and honest with everyone about her mistakes and slip-ups along the way, not having to report that she was doing everything perfectly all the time—and everyone loved her *more* because of it. As she told us, "I would lie down at night and feel proud of myself and the choices I made throughout the day—instead of feeling ashamed, afraid, and filled with dread and self-loathing."

In that moment of vivid vulnerability, Georgeanna's authentic self was revealed and she was able to summon the courage to move forward into her real journey. If she hadn't allowed herself to become that open and vulnerable, she would not have succeeded.

To put our mind into a place where we are open to change, we must be truly "authentic." We must be wholly open and honest with ourselves, and with others.

To be authentic, we need to understand our ego. Our ego is the protective barrier we were speaking of earlier. It was built to protect us, but most often hinders our ability for growth and change. Embracing your ego and the role that it plays enables you to put it aside and get on with your *real* life.

So what does it take to be vulnerable? Sometimes it is a physical step like disrobing and looking in a mirror or stepping on a scale. Sometimes it's more the emotional step of being truly honest about your imperfections, and sharing openly with others about your fears, your mistakes, your dreams and aspirations. This is all part of being human that most of us hide, but being vulnerable is the only way to truly change and grow. Let yourself be truly honest about who you are. This creates the clearing for an open mind and growth. And you very well may be surprised...your vulnerability gives others around you permission to also open up for healing and growth!

## Call to Action: Step on the Scale

It doesn't matter if you're 160 pounds or 560 pounds; if you have avoided stepping on the scale earlier, it's time. It's time to be open, honest, and vulnerable with yourself. Strip down and step on the scale. Then face yourself in the mirror.

1. Write down what it feels like to see the number on the scale (for maybe the first time), what it feels like to be naked in front of the mirror, and what it feels like to face yourself in the mirror.

2. Get the feelings out. They've only been holding you back. What do you feel when you see yourself and your weight?

3. Now say good-bye to that number on the scale, and say good-bye to the old you. You have a bright, healthy, and fit future ahead, and now you are well on your way to getting there!

## Heidi Tip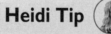

As a woman, stepping on the scale is naturally tough for me, especially having battled an eating disorder for most of my teenage years and early adulthood! But the more I do it, and the more I push myself to get comfortable with being uncomfortable, the easier it gets... and the more I love and accept myself for who I am. So don't fear the scale. Let it simply be a tool to help you stay honest and accountable.

# DAY 10

## Day 10: High-Carb Day

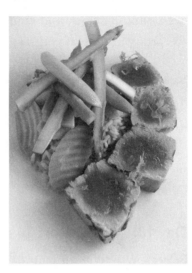

Meal 1: Breakfast
   Recipe: Huevos Rancheros

Meal 2: High-Carb Meal
   Recipe: PB & J Rice Cakes and Shake

Meal 3: High-Carb Meal
   Recipe: Grilled Ginger Lime Tuna and Steamed Vegetable Medley

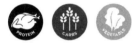

Meal 4: High-Carb Meal
   Recipe: Triple Berry Treat

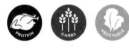

Meal 5: Low-Carb Meal
   Recipe: Pepper Jack Chicken

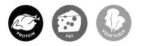

### Day 10: Metabolic Mission: Mt. Everest (Chipper)

Set a running clock and complete one round of this circuit as fast as you can. Record your time in your Daily Tracker!

20 Burpees
30 Push-Ups
40 Flutterkicks
50 Air Squats
60 Mountain Climbers
70 High Knees

### Day 10: Accelerator: 10 minutes (minimum)

Select any activity of your choosing, and keep your heart rate above 120 beats per minute (bpm) the entire time. Prescribed optional interval for maximum results: Tenacious Twos (2:00 low intensity / 2:00 high intensity)

## LESSON 10
## UNLOAD THE REAL WEIGHT

*The weak can never forgive. Forgiveness is an attribute of the strong.*
Mahatma Gandhi

Hurt. Vengeance. Sadness. Regret. Rage. We all carry emotional weight on our shoulders...some more than others. Different events in our lives when we were betrayed, hurt, abandoned—or hurt and abandoned others—can haunt us and influence the way we feel about ourselves. These emotions deeply affect our decision making every day. All of these feelings can be categorized into the two major destructive emotions: anger and shame.

Frequently we hear that people who go through massive rehabilitation, like recovery from alcohol, drug, or other addictions, often have to confront a lot of emotional pain or trauma from their past in order to finally find peace. This kind of emotional healing is critical for recovery from addiction if one wants to truly and powerfully change one's life.

However, dealing with this emotional weight is not exclusive to individuals struggling with heavy addictions. We *all* have emotional weight that we carry that is holding us back! Many times we have gone so long carrying the weight that we've almost forgotten that it is there…almost. It's like living life with the flu and forgetting what it is like to feel energetic and healthy. If we want to release this parking brake that is holding us back, we need to unload the real weight!

When Bruce first embarked on his journey of transformation he was motivated by his desire to be a more powerful, active football coach for his young players. He knew that his weight was killing him. But what he did not realize until he was knee-deep into the process is that the shame, emotions, and feelings from his past were preventing him from moving on to the future he dreamed of. He realized that in order to move on, he needed to heal from his own pain suffered at the hands of his father. During our time with Bruce, he admitted that his father had sexually and emotionally abused him for years, since he'd been a little boy. His father was now in prison on multiple counts of sexually molesting other children. But Bruce had never spoken aloud that he, too, was one of his father's victims. The shame of his silence was the real source of what was killing Bruce.

Fortunately, Bruce had an opportunity to unload the weight of his shame and anger when his father came up for parole. Afraid and shaken, Bruce summoned every bit of his courage and confronted his father in a courtroom, telling the parole hearing judge that he was also a victim and that for the safety of him and other children, his father should stay behind bars. Even in this difficult moment, Bruce told his father that he forgave him, and was ready to move on with his life—free from the control of his memories.

From that moment on, Bruce has been unstoppable. He lost weight faster than ever. He got fitter than ever. He worked himself out of debt and started dating. He unloaded the real weight—released the parking brake that had been stuck on for years—and is now living a limitless life, at half of his original body weight. Oh, and now we work side by side with him as one of our incredible transformation coaches!

Take a look at what some of our courageous people unloaded to transform:

- Cassandra chose to forgive herself for giving up her son for adoption and explained to him her wishes for his better life.
- Melissa chose to forgive her late husband for taking his life and abandoning her and her sons.
- Jeff chose to forgive himself for being an absent father and apologized to his family.
- Kenny chose to forgive himself for quitting the marines.
- David chose to forgive himself for not being there for his younger brother and sister when they needed him most.

These were all events and emotions that each of these individuals kept secret or buried for years. Whether it was hurt they endured, or the hurt they caused someone else, unable to deal with the emotions, they numbed themselves with food. It *cost* them, just like it may be costing you right now.

Sound familiar?

*What happened?* It is a powerful question we ask everyone going through transformation, because once we can identify it, we can help set you free. Here are some experiences that can create a legacy of destructive emotions that will hold you back:

- Death
- Affair
- Molestation
- Abandonment
- Bullying
- Disappointments or failures
- Sexuality
- Segregation
- Sexual assault
- Domestic violence
- Divorce
- Adoption

If you have experienced any of these, you are certainly not alone. In fact, we don't know of anyone who *hasn't* been through at least one of the traumatic events listed above. Whatever side you have been on, these major life events can cause devastating emotions of shame and anger that can, and will, prevent you from achieving your best life and body.

Keep in mind that clearing the past and unloading the weight doesn't mean that you have to forget. It doesn't mean that you are a doormat to get walked on and abused. Clearing the past is for *you* to heal and move on in *your* journey through life. That weight is not yours to carry anymore.

## Call to Action: Unloading the Weight

So how can we free ourselves from these destructive emotions and live a limitless life? There is a way...let us show you how.

1. Make amends with the past: Create a list of people you have wronged in the past, or people who have wronged *you*. Write down what happened.

2. By yourself in front of a mirror, practice forgiving those people or apologizing to them (and forgiving yourself). Notice we say to *practice* forgiveness. This is because true and authentic forgiveness can take time. It doesn't always happen immediately. Forgiveness can happen over days, weeks, months, and even years. You will likely feel the pain and hurt for a while still, but if you keep practicing, it *will* get better—we promise. Practicing forgiveness is simple: It is wish-

ing other people (or yourself) *peace*. That's it. You don't have to shower them with love and affection, you don't have to be their friend or spend time with them. Just genuinely wish them peace from what happened. It is very likely that they are dealing with their own shame or anger.

3. When you are ready, rally your superfriend or team. Let them know what happened and how you feel about it. Now is a good time to lean on them for emotional support.

4. As long as it will not do any harm to yourself or others (and only if you are truly ready), write a letter, place a phone call, text, email, what have you, to the people on your list, and practice forgiving them, or apologizing to them (and forgiving yourself). If you're not ready yet, feel free to burn the letter, or write and then delete the email.

NOTE: Remember, forgiveness is for *you,* but you will not be set free until your intentions are authentic and you genuinely *feel* it. This is not an easy process, and is one of the most difficult aspects of transformation, but this final step of unloading the weight is extremely powerful and could be the most pivotal moment in changing your life and your body!

Stay attuned to yourself, your feelings, and your triggers. Whenever you begin to experience those shameful or angry feelings, find your superfriend or someone you can confide in openly. Fear of losing connection with others fuels these emotions, so it takes the interaction with another human—to see that you are still lovable—to heal the shame.

## Reflection

Again, you may or may not be ready to confront experiences in your past that are painful and causing you shame or anger. We don't want to rush you, and we are certainly not judging you. Simply be aware of what's happened to you, what you have done to someone else, or what you might have witnessed. However, regardless of what has happened, there tends to be a moment (or a few moments) that greatly changed the way you see yourself and the world. Know that if there was no closure to this event (or events), then they will continue to weigh on your mind and hold you back from reaching your greatest potential.

You might also try to identify the source of that feeling you have that "something's wrong with me," or why you feel "different" or "all alone." These inner experiences of detachment, discomfort, and a general sense of not being good enough are common among all of us. You are not alone. When you are ready, come back to this chapter and work through it. You won't regret it.

You will know when the time is right to confront traumatic issues of the past. Being ready is a process and it's one you cannot do alone. So reach out to your team, a therapist, or a self-help group. If you're not ready right now, that's okay. Remember, this is your journey. When you are ready to move forward with no restraints, then you know what to do.

# DAY 11

## Day 11: High-Carb Day

Meal 1: Breakfast
    Recipe: Hot Quinoa Cereal with Banana

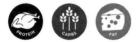

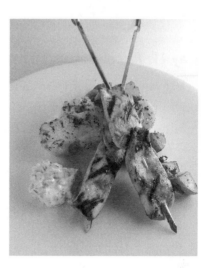

Meal 2: High-Carb Meal
    Recipe: Egg Salad on Toast

Meal 3: High-Carb Meal
    Recipe: Grilled Greek Chicken Kebabs

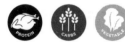

Meal 4: High-Carb Meal
    Recipe: Lemon Poppy Seed Protein Bites

Meal 5: Low-Carb Meal
    Recipe: Almond-Crusted Tilapia with Asparagus and Cauliflower Mash

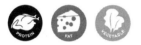

## Day 11: Metabolic Mission: Hustle Time (AMRAP)

Set a running clock and do as many rounds of the following circuit as possible in 6 minutes.

5 Burpees
7 Mountain Climbers
9 Squats

### Day 11: Accelerator: 10 minutes (minimum)

Select any activity of your choosing, and keep your heart rate above 120 beats per minute (bpm) the entire time. Prescribed optional interval for maximum results: Nasty Nineties (1:30 low intensity / 1:30 high intensity)

## LESSON 11
# BANISH THE NEGATIVE SELF-TALK

*If we talked to our friends in the same way that we talk to ourselves, we wouldn't have any friends.*

—Anonymous

You know that annoying voice in our heads that relentlessly reminds us that we could have done better or should work harder? The voice that berates us, tells us that we are not smart enough or that we are too fat? We have all, at one time or another, heard this voice of negativity of all that we aren't, all that is wrong with us, and all that is just not good enough.

Does any of this sound familiar?

"I knew I couldn't do it—I am such a loser."
"I am nothing compared with those people."
"I'm such an idiot; I can't believe I'm so stupid."
"I'm no good."
"I am bad."
"I am a failure."
"I am a terrible parent."
"I am worthless."
"Everyone else is better than me."
"I could never do that."

"I'm a monster."
"I'll never be any good at it."
"It's always my fault."
"Nobody likes me."
"I'm not popular."
"I can't cope."

We're going to shoot straight here: This kind of negative thinking brings absolutely nothing good to your life. In fact, it *costs* you joy, confidence, happiness, and ultimately the life (including the body) you want.

In this step, you are going to learn how to control that negative self-talk, to make it work for you—not against you. You are going to destroy that broken record, bury the conversation, and learn how to say affirming and empowering things to yourself. Why is this so important? Because the way we think, literally the content of our thoughts, affects how we feel and act. Behavioral researchers have shown that of the 50,000 or so thoughts we have each and every day, most are automatic, which means they pass through our minds without our realizing it. And if these thoughts are negative or self-critical, then they actually harm our confidence, our beliefs, our self-esteem, and our ability to make beneficial choices through the day.

We are asking you to make big changes to your behaviors. But before you can do that, it's critical that you first stop the barrage of negative, self-denigrating thoughts that are making you think that you can't change, that you can't succeed, and that you can't stick with it.

As humans, what we repeatedly and automatically say to ourselves becomes the foundation for our beliefs. Then it's a matter of time before these negative self-beliefs become a self-fulfilling prophecy. As the saying goes,

"Your thoughts become words, your words become actions, your actions become character, your character becomes your destiny."

In other words, when you find yourself saying negative things about yourself—in your head or out loud—you will begin to act in ways that seem to make such beliefs true.

### Letting Go of the Negative

Now is the time to deal with your mind. We are who we tell ourselves we are. Unfortunately, most of the time we are only telling ourselves how unlovable, unacceptable, inadequate, and imperfect we are. We have the hardest time seeing the good within ourselves, and tend to feel guilt when we do! Because so much of our thoughts and brain power is directed toward belittling ourselves, we do eventually become what we feel is an unlovable, unacceptable, inadequate, imperfect person. The good news is that, if we can talk ourselves into being inadequate, we can also talk ourselves into being wonderful, beautiful, powerful, and strong! We have the power to redirect our thoughts and use them to reinforce our goals. How? By replacing negative, self-sabotaging ways of thinking with positive, affirming, and dignity-inspired thoughts.

Identifying your negative thinking is the first step toward creating a positive mindset. The go-to experts in this field are cognitive behaviorists, and they have identified common types of negative thinking. There is overlap among them, but giving each type a name makes it easier to remember them. (If you do any more reading in cognitive therapy, you may come across the term *distorted thinking*. Some authors use that term instead of *negative thinking*, which we think sounds harsh. But we must say, distorted thinking feels so much more accurate because all of the negative things you are saying about yourself, simply aren't true!)

### The Big Five Types of Distorted Thinking

Just to prove to you that you are not alone, hundreds of books and thousands of articles have been written on negative thinking and how to turn it around. Why? Because as humans, we *all* do it! In fact, there are textbook categories for all of the thoughts that flow through your head on a daily basis. So to sum it up: Welcome to the club. Now, just like training a muscle, we can train our minds to turn that negative talk into something that doesn't hurt us, but actually helps us! (Source: www.cognitivetherapyguide.org.)

- **All-or-Nothing Thinking/Polarizing**—"I have to do things perfectly, because anything less than perfect is a failure." All-or-nothing thinking is the most common type of negative thinking, and leads to anxiety because you think that any mistake is a failure, which may expose you to criticism or judgment. Therefore you don't give yourself permission to even attempt many things if you don't feel you can do them perfectly. Or if you do attempt, you may tend to lie and hide any mistakes. You are terrified to be vulnerable and honest with yourself. You let your ego stand in the way of you and your authentic self.

- **Disqualifying the Positives/Filtering**—"Life feels like one disappointment after another."
- **Negative Self-Labeling**—"I feel like a failure. I'm flawed. If people knew the real me, they wouldn't like me."
- **Catastrophizing**—"If something is going to happen, it'll probably be the worst-case scenario."
- **Personalizing**—"It's always my fault." When something bad occurs, you automatically blame yourself. For example, you hear that an evening out with friends is canceled, and you assume that the change in plans is because no one wanted to be around you.

### Other Common Types of Distorted Thinking

- **Mind Reading**—"I can tell people don't like me because of the way they act around me."
- **Should Statements**—"People should be fair. If I'm nice to them, they should be nice back."
- **Excessive Need for Approval**—"I can only be happy if people like me. If someone is upset, it's probably my fault."
- **Disqualifying the Present**—"I'll relax later. But first I have to rush to finish this."
- **Dwelling on Pain**—"If I dwell on why I'm unhappy and think about what went wrong, maybe I'll feel better." Alternatively, "If I worry enough about my problem, maybe I will feel better."
- **Pessimism**—"Life is a struggle. I don't think we are meant to be happy. I don't trust people who are happy. If something good happens in my life, I usually have to pay for it with something bad."

## Call to Action

Go through the different kinds of distorted self-talk, and determine which one you use. Write it/them here: _____

### Flip the Switch: Turning the Negative into Positive

So after years of berating ourselves and beating ourselves up, how can we take this continuous conversation and change it? While we covered the power of forgiveness in the last lesson, reversing negative self-talk requires another powerful emotion: appreciation. We have seen most of our people silence these negative voices in their heads and replace them with positive, affirming, empowering voices—using appreciation. Remember, as bad as it seems life can get, there is always someone worse off. There are people in this world that are struggling through war, famine, drought, disease, severe poverty, and the list goes on. A large portion of the world's population is just trying to make it through today alive.

When you think about it, you've got a lot going for you. If you're reading this book, you're literate. And you could actually afford to buy it! You are making strides toward a better you. Let's tap into some "appreciation" and build this list even further:

- **Identify Areas to Change**—First, identify areas of your life that you typically think negatively about, whether it's work, your daily commute, or a relationship. Start small by focusing on just one of those areas to approach in a more positive way. When you say something negative, challenge yourself to think of at least one positive to go with it. Practice appreciation for what you *do* have going for you.
- **Check Yourself**—Periodically during the day, stop and evaluate what you're thinking. If you find that your thoughts are mainly negative, try to find a way to put a positive spin on them. Once again, practice appreciation for yourself and what is working in your life.
- **Be Open to Humor**—Give yourself permission to smile or laugh,

especially during difficult times. Seek humor in everyday happenings. When you can laugh at life, you feel less stressed.

- **Surround Yourself with Positive People**—Rely on your team. You created this positive, empowering network of people—surround yourself with them!
- **Practice Positive Self-Talk**—Start by following one simple rule: Don't say anything to yourself that you wouldn't say to anyone else. Be gentle and encouraging with yourself. If a negative thought enters your mind, evaluate it rationally and respond with affirmations of what is good about you.

One of the most touching and impactful experiences we've ever had with banishing negative self-talk was with Jayce. When we first met Jayce, he was a broken man. He had always been overweight, unathletic, and considered himself a worthless failure. He had recently been through an awful divorce with a verbally abusive ex-wife who berated him daily, making him feel even more worthless. When we started the process of transformation with him, he was down, depressed, and had no confidence that he could actually do it. He couldn't get out of his head the idea that he was a worthless failure—that he didn't deserve this opportunity and that he was going to fail and disappoint everyone.

The bright spot in Jayce's life was his 10-year-old son, whom he loved with all his heart. We sent Jayce home after just a few weeks of boot camp to straighten out some issues back home, and think about if he wanted to return. He chose to come back reluctantly, feeling that he had to. Jayce's mother and his son came to the airport to see him off. In the airport as he was walking toward his plane back to boot camp, his son called out his name and said, "Hey, Dad!"

When Jayce turned around, his son said to him, "You deserve this."

That moment changed everything. Jayce landed at boot camp a totally different man. His son completely flipped Jayce's negative thinking—into a positive conversation that he had with himself every single day. Jayce is now a new man. Twelve months later and 200 pounds lost is proof!!

Here are some examples (source: Mayo Clinic) of negative self-talk and how you can apply a positive twist to them:

| Negative Self-Talk | Positive Thinking |
|---|---|
| I've never done it before. | I love learning new things. |
| It's too complicated. | I'm creative. I'll tackle it from a different angle. |
| I don't have the resources. | I'm resourceful. I can find a way to make it happen. |
| I'm too lazy to get this done. | I'm committed. I wasn't able to fit it into my schedule, but I can reexamine some priorities. |
| There's no way it will work. | I can make it work. I'll just stay flexible in my approach. |
| It's too radical a change. | Let's have some fun. Let's take a chance. |
| No one bothers to communicate with me. | I'll see if I can open the channels of communication. |
| I'm not going to get any better at this. | I persevere. I'll keep trying until I get it done. Or at least I'll get a helluva lot stronger in the process! |

## Call to Action: Make Your Own List!

Make two columns. In one, write down all the negative phrases you've used in the past; in the next, write down all the same thoughts but using positive terminology. Follow the example above. Become conscious and aware of your negative feelings and thoughts about yourself and then read aloud the positive affirmations. If you do this regularly, every day for a few weeks, your thinking will begin to shift from negative to positive. You will begin to hear the true inner voice that speaks of your accomplishments, achievements, and love.

| Negative | Positive |
|---|---|
|  |  |
|  |  |
|  |  |
|  |  |
|  |  |

# DAY 12

## Day 12: Low-Carb Day

Meal 1: Breakfast
   Recipe: Apple Cinnamon Muesli

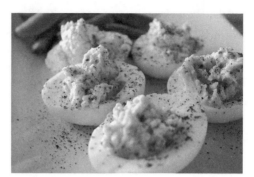

Meal 2: Low-Carb Meal
   Recipe: Deviled Eggs

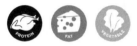

Meal 3: Low-Carb Meal
   Recipe: Chicken Basil Spaghetti

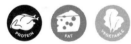

Meal 4: Low-Carb Meal
   Recipe: Chocolate Chip Almond Coconut Bites and Shake

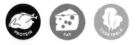

Meal 5: Low-Carb Meal
   Recipe: Cajun Salmon with Cabbage Salad and Steamed Broccoli

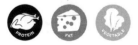

### Day 12: Metabolic Mission: Breakthrough (Tabata)

For each exercise, do as many reps as you can in 20 seconds. Rest for 10 seconds, then do as many reps as you can in 20 seconds again. Repeat for 8 total rounds (for a total of 4 minutes) per exercise. The lowest number of reps you get in any round is your score. You'll get one score per exercise. Add up all three scores, and record it in your Daily Tracker!

Burpees
Back Lunges
Hollow Rocks

### Day 12: Accelerator: 10 minutes (minimum)

Select any activity of your choosing, and keep your heart rate above 120 beats per minute (bpm) the entire time. Prescribed optional interval for maximum results: Mighty Minutes (1:00 low intensity / 1:00 high intensity)

## LESSON 12
## CREATE YOUR NEW IDENTITY

*First say to yourself what you would be; and then do what you have to do.*

—Epictetus

Who are you?

It's not a trick question, but the way you answer it will most likely have a lasting impact on your future.

Our identity says a lot about us. Our identity is defined as "the character, qualities, beliefs, etcetera, that make a particular person or group different from another." Character, qualities, beliefs. These are the components of our transformation mind-set! These are what control your choices now and the choices you make in the future. Which is why the way you think about yourself *right now* is critical to your long-term success.

As you move through these steps of transformation, your body will begin to change significantly. As it does so, however, the way you view yourself must change, too—if this transformation is going to last.

The purpose of this lesson is to help you identify the new you. The *real* you. Sometimes this new identity is tied to an aspiration, and sometimes it is linked to a younger self. Either way, it is a brand-new way of defining who you are from the inside out—from the way you act toward others, to the choices you make, to the clothes you wear. In fact, many of our peeps literally change their careers! This lesson is all about realizing who you can *be*, then becoming that person now!

Think about it.

Here's some quick and hard-hitting common sense to put things into perspective for you: If you see yourself as a loser, a disappointment, or a failure, then when faced with everyday decisions in life, you will make the choices of a loser, a disappointment, or failure. We're going out on a limb here, but chances are that those choices will not benefit your health, fitness, and long-term weight loss goals. In short, if you believe this *identity* is you, you will unintentionally choose actions that support that belief.

The same applies for the reciprocal: When you see yourself *now* as a winner, an inspiration, an achiever, a hard worker, and an athlete, that is *exactly* who you'll become.

Two people sit down at a restaurant to order a meal. One is a fat slob, and the other is a world-class athlete. What do they order?

Your meal choices for each would likely differ, wouldn't they? You may think that the fat slob would order something like a cheeseburger and fries, or maybe pizza, right? And the world-class athlete would order chicken and rice, or maybe fish and a baked potato, right?

Here's the trick to the scenario—if that's what you think they'll eat, then that's what they'll eat. So which one are you?

However you see yourself, your actions will support and you will further anchor yourself into that identity! See yourself as a fat slob, and you will become more of a fat slob. See yourself as a world-class athlete and you will become more and more of a world-class athlete!

In this process, we are *being* with the end in mind. We declare who it is that we want to be, then we become that person *now*! Every successive day we live into that new inevitable future—of being a winner, an inspiration, an achiever, a hard worker, and an athlete!

When we immediately become who it is we want to be, negative talk disappears, and positive thinking begins...because the new you, the *real* you, would *never* talk to yourself that way! When faced with decisions, you make choices that positively affect your long-term future, because that is who you are and what you do!

Bruce explains his new identity this way: "My whole life is different now. It took me a while before I understood that I'm not a loser who failed at life. I'm a role model. I'm a coach. I'm an inspiration, and I'm the hardest worker in the room. That's who I chose to be at the beginning of my journey, and that's exactly who I became. I want to help others now. I want to pay it forward."

For Melissa, her new identity emerged more subtly. As she told us, "I wasn't used to being successful in my life." Melissa's new identity was more an internal shift as she became used to feeling differently in her body—more confident and more comfortable. For years, Jami believed she was a monster. When she realized that she is a talented, beautiful inspiration...everything changed.

## How Some of Our Peeps Created New Identities

- Bruce left "fat boy" behind and became a CrossFit athlete.
- Melissa abandoned her identity as a fat and lonely widow, and became an inspirational mom to her community.
- Julianna said good-bye to the troubled, tentative teenager and became a fierce role model for her peers.

- Kenny left his discharge from the military behind and once again became a proud U.S. Marine.
- Mike left the sick old man in his past and became the superhero to his kids that he'd always dreamed of being.

What about you?

# Call to Action: Who Do You Want to Be?

Go through this quick exercise here or in your journal:

1. Identify your goal.
2. What are the emotional, physical, and lifestyle characteristics of a person who has achieved this goal?
3. What do you need to change about yourself or your life to become this person?
4. Who do you know who has achieved this goal or shares your goal?

Now, it's time to declare your new identity. Describe your new detailed character traits.

_____

_____

_____

_____

_____

_____

Now go back and read what you wrote a few times. All you have to do now, is live *into* this new you.

This "new you" may be a difficult reality to accept, but just try it out. Creating your new identity can be an amazing and powerful experience. For some it clicks right away and they never look back. Others need to practice being that person for a while until the new sense of self sinks in. Just like training muscles, many people need to train their minds to accept positive, empowering images of the self.

Begin right now and try believing it for the next 30 seconds...

Now, while you are this person, write it down:

I am_____

_____.

Great job. Now try it again for 30 more seconds.

As you face life's daily decisions of what to eat, whether or not to exercise, and what to do in certain circumstances, try out your new identity for just a few seconds at a time and see how it feels. Over time, the seconds will become minutes, which will become hours, and then days. You will realize that this new person is exactly who you will become and who you are.

## DAY 13

### Day 13: Low-Carb Day

Meal 1: Breakfast
    Recipe: "Loaded" Breakfast Potato

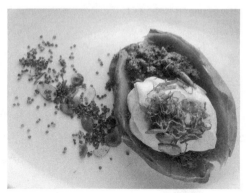

Meal 2: Low-Carb Meal
    Recipe: Edamame and Pistachio Hummus with Cucumbers and Chicken

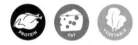

Meal 3: Low-Carb Meal
    Recipe: Grilled Wild Salmon with Quinoa and Edamame Salad

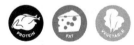

Meal 4: Low-Carb Meal
    Recipe: Chocolate Peanut Butter Shake

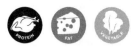

Meal 5: Low-Carb Meal
    Recipe: Cauli Mash and Meatballs

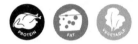

**No Metabolic Mission: Day off!**

**Day 13: Accelerator: 10 minutes (minimum)**

Select any activity of your choosing, and keep your heart rate above 120 beats per minute (bpm) the entire time. Prescribed optional interval for maximum results: Dirty Two-Thirties (2:30 low intensity / 2:30 high intensity)

## LESSON 13
## TAKE RESPONSIBILITY

*He that is good for making excuses is seldom good for anything else.*
—Benjamin Franklin

WARNING: We're going to be your superfriends and give you some tough love here. However, it is only because we care and want the best for you.

The number one red flag we look for when determining when someone is ready for transformation is acting and thinking like a victim. We know that people who blame others for their current condition, pain, suffering, and disappointment are people who have not yet accepted responsibility for their own choices. When we detect that kind of thinking, we do not choose those people for the journey of transformation…because we simply cannot help them. A victim mentality is not capable of change.

If someone cannot take responsibility for their actions, it is impossible for them to reach a goal.

You can decide whether you want to be a victim or not. But know this at the outset: Once someone chooses to take responsibility for their actions, then they *can* change! Taking responsibility is huge and scary and makes you extremely vulnerable. It takes a ton of courage, but courage is what it takes to change your life! It means you are responsible for your failures, your bad days, and all those times that you lost weight and gained it back again.

We're not saying that you haven't suffered in the past. We're not saying that awful things didn't happen to you. We're not saying that you aren't struggling, or that you don't have a chaotic and unpredictable life right now. What we *are* saying is that the only way you can change your life forever is to take full responsibility for your actions.

Here is your wake-up call: You are in the driver's seat! You always have been. You aren't struggling with your weight because someone held a gun to your head and forced you to consume 5,000 calories a day. You CHOSE to eat what you ate…when you ate it! Don't feel bad about it—heck, we've made a lot of poor choices, too, that cost us! However, take responsibility for it, and you can take your life wherever you wish. You can declare your dreams and make them a reality. You can write down your goals and achieve them. But first you need to take responsibility and stop blaming others for what has or has not happened for you.

This concept is pretty simple. Life is unexpected and unfair. Anything and everything can and will happen. You will break bones, you will throw out your back, you will have marital issues or career problems. You will be put on a different medication that causes unwanted side effects. But one thing is for sure: Life won't shove 5,000 calories down your throat. Only you can choose to do that. If you don't take responsibility and call yourself out for doing it, you're only protecting your destructive behavior…and you will never, ever change. But once you own it and admit it, you take full control of your actions and destiny!

We're not singling you out here. Heck, we *all* fall into the victim mind-set. In fact, we both struggle with this on a daily basis. It is *hard* to take responsibility for your actions. It sucks to feel like you messed up sometimes. But we're all human, and we mess up. However, it requires a ton of courage to take responsibility. Everyone around you will likely recognize your bravery.

### Jeff's Terrible, Wonderful Tuesday

Jeff and his daughter Juliana had returned home after the 90-day boot camp feeling confident and resolute about their eating and exercise routines. Michelle, Jeff's wife, was 100 percent on board and made changes to how she shopped, cooked, and prepared meals for the entire family. But when Jeff began reporting back his results to us, something was off. The numbers just didn't add up. When we asked Jeff if he was following through on his promises to meet his goals, he assured us he was. So what was happening? We decided to take things into our own hands by running some light surveillance on Jeff. We wanted to believe that he was telling us the truth, but we also knew that when people are in their old, comfortable home environments, it can be difficult to resist their triggers and old habits.

After a few days of checking up on Jeff, we found that he was not doing what he said he was going to do. Jeff was eating well, in large part thanks to Michelle's efforts. But he was barely exercising at all. He wouldn't show at the gym, and when he did go, he would only stay a few minutes then leave. If he wanted to continue to lose weight, then he had to move every day.

We confronted him. Sitting in his living room, we gently asked him how it was going for him being at home. He said everything was great. When we pressed him about the discrepancies in his numbers, he angrily insisted that he was doing everything he said he was. Clearly, he was upset that we were questioning his integrity. When we kept probing and asking him if that was true, he hesitated and then broke down.

"I was so embarrassed and felt so ashamed. Here I was, sitting in front of Chris and Heidi, who had given me so much and trusted me so much. And I was lying to them. In my mind, I had been making all sorts of excuses for why I was cutting my exercise short—I had bad knees, bad back, and I had work to do. You name it, I had an excuse for it. These excuses were all about me playing the victim—they were ways for me to deflect responsibility for my choices and my actions. Did I not want to succeed? No! I wanted to reach my goals! But it took Chris and Heidi confronting me to really understand how to take responsibility once and for all."

Who was hurt by Jeff skipping his exercise and lying about it? Jeff.

Our excuses are simply that: reflections of us not being ready to take responsibility. But in the end, this "terrible, wonderful Tuesday" was a wake-up call that worked. The confrontation with us enabled Jeff to confront not only his excuses, but the lies that lay beneath the excuses. He chose to use a "victim" excuse and say that he couldn't exercise because of his knees—when in his heart he knew that he could have easily worked around his injuries and done exercises that didn't bother his knees. Jeff saw how his not being truthful was getting in his own way. "Lying to myself was just a way of giving myself an out for not being successful. Talk about a vicious circle!"

Why was this moment such a turning point for Jeff? Because his backslide was triggered when he broke his promise one day at home, and didn't follow through on his exercise. Instead of confessing, reassessing, and recommitting (the most powerful formula for getting back on track that we will discuss in the next section), it was easier for his ego to place the blame on something else, so he didn't have to take responsibility. Once he started blaming everything and everyone else, it was hard to stop the backslide, until we stepped in and challenged him to be vulnerable and honest, and take full responsibility. That was Jeff's turning point. He changed his mind-set, which has in turn changed his life. Now Jeff will tell you that his knees and back feel absolutely amazing since he's lost the weight...and that he has never felt more proud of who he is as a father and contributor to his community. Jeff lost nearly 200 pounds in a year and is now coaching others through the journey of transformation!

## Heidi Tip

Fighting through injuries is no easy battle. I've been there! Many of you most likely have been, too—whether the result of overtraining or a freak accident, injuries even as small as a strained muscle can make us feel threatened that our fitness levels will slip away. They tend to even become excuses why we can't go to the gym, or even better yet, why we have to eat more junk food.☺ Our health and happiness have become victim to this injury. I'm not pointing fingers. I've been there, too!!! But it doesn't have to be this way—injuries are NOT excuses. There are alternative exercises around any injury.

For other people, taking responsibility is a more subtle process, but it requires the same kind of honesty and looking in the mirror. Taking responsibility isn't easy—it's the hard part. It takes vulnerability and courage, and is the true opportunity for growth and change. As we like to say, for every pointed finger, there are three pointing back! Ultimately, you didn't "end up" where you are at—your path and choices have led you to the place you are at. Life may have been rough, but you chose what you put in your mouth.

Here is the harsh reality: There are things in life we *can* control, and things in life we can't. We hear all the time, "I *have* to lose this weight or I will die."

Well, the truth is, you don't *have* to do anything. No one is holding a gun to your head…except you. If you choose to lose the weight, it is never because you *have* to. Always remember that it is because you *want* to!

## Call to Action:
## The Complain-and-Blame Exercise

1. List one to three times you attempted to lose weight and failed:

   _____
   _____
   _____
   _____
   _____
   _____

2. Now, explain why it didn't work:

   _____
   _____
   _____
   _____
   _____
   _____

3. Read over your responses and see if they contain either a complaint or a blame.

If you are placing the blame on anything or anyone other than yourself, then you are playing the victim—which will never lead to change.

What should the final response always be? The true one: "This diet didn't work because, regardless of the circumstances, I chose not to follow the program anymore."

We're not saying that something difficult or traumatic didn't happen to you. The reality of the situation is that somewhere on that time line, you *chose* not to follow the program anymore.

It's not easy to say, we know. However, this is what taking responsibility sounds like. Once you begin to think this way, you are ready for lifelong change!

Again, we say all of this out of love. Because thinking this way changed *our* lives for the better, changed our *peeps'* lives for the better, and will change *your* life for the better!

## DAY 14

### It's Time to Weigh In

Weigh in first thing in the morning without eating or drinking. Remove as many articles of clothing as possible to get the cleanest weight.

Your current weight: _____.

At this time, feel free to take any other measurements as well and note them here: _____

### Day 14: Reset Day

It's Reset Day! Make meals easy by cooking up our Clean Cheat recipes, or simply add 1,000 extra calories of foods you love to a normal high-carb day.

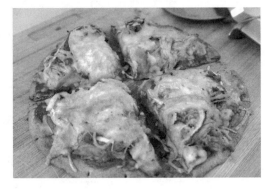

Meal 1: Chocolate Glazed Crepes

Meal 2: BBQ Chicken Pita Pizza

Meal 3: Muddy Buddies

Meal 4: Mac and Cheese with Bacon

Meal 5: Homemade Oreos

### Rest Day

Now relax! Take the day off and rest—no Metabolic Missions and no Accelerators!

## LESSON 14:
## CONQUER YOUR F.E.A.R.

*Fear does not prevent death, it prevents living.*

—Anonymous

Change is scary. We get it. Let's get it all out of the way right now:

You're scared of feeling deprived.

You're scared of the inconvenience of taking on new habits and patterns.

You're scared of feeling uncomfortable during the exercise.

You're scared of calling attention to your weight and don't want others to see or know that you're trying to do something about it.

You're scared of failing yet one more time at weight loss.

This is natural. This is normal. Fears are triggered when we explore out of our comfort zones. At the least sign of discomfort, we often automatically experience fear.

### It's Just a Mirage

But what is FEAR? It's not tangible. It's not in the present, but in the future. FEAR is something that hasn't even happened. So what are you scared of?

To break it down, fear is not real. It's a reflection of what is in our imagination. Here's how we tear it apart.

Here's the most popular acronym for FEAR, and without a doubt the most appropriate one:

F—False

E—Evidence

A—Appearing

R—Real

False Evidence Appearing Real. Basically it's something untrue; it hasn't even happened, pretending to be real. Yet, we experience a physical reaction to it as if it were real.

Sounds easy. Maybe. We all have fears. We fear heights. We fear facing traumatic moments in our life. We fear feeling uncomfortable during exercise. We fear for our children's safety. We fear for our own health. We fear for each other's health. Believe it or not, many fear success, and the responsibility that comes along with it.

There are many things we FEAR—some consciously, some subconsciously. These are some common fears we hear from our peeps:

"I'm scared I won't be able to live happily without bingeing."

"I'm scared that I'm going to fail on yet *another* diet."

"I'm scared that if I mess this up, my family and friends are going to think I'm an even bigger disappointment."

"I'm afraid that if I start to exercise I'm going to have a heart attack."

"I'm scared of hurting my knee even more if I start exercising."

"I'm scared that if I commit to this, I will never get to eat my ice cream again."

"I'm scared of having to push myself physically."

"I'm scared of losing my friends by doing this."

Right now, think what it is about these fears that *actually* scares you. You're scared of something that hasn't happened . . . and here's the punchline: Chances are, it might not!

Now, think of all the things that these FEARs have *cost* you. They have cost you your dreams and opportunities at your ideal weight. They have cost you joy. They have cost you integrity. They have cost you confidence, self-esteem, and dignity.

In this guide, we share with you all of the tips and tactics to prevent nearly every one of these scenarios. Thing is, most of what we are scared of isn't life threatening or true, yet we let it completely paralyze us. We allow fear to hold us back from our true potential and greatness. Unfortunately, until we confront this "scary monster" of false evidence in front of us, we will never fulfill our dreams.

Mitzi had been chosen to be on the show, but we didn't realize the extent of Mitzi's misery and pain. She was over 100 pounds overweight—that's what we saw. What we didn't see was hidden inside of her home: She'd become a hoarder. Her home was in shambles. She had no refrigerator, no stove, no heat, nothing. It's not that she didn't have the money to fix it. She was so terrified of a repairman coming to the house and thinking poorly of her after seeing her living situation, she couldn't bring herself to ever call for help.

She was so scared of what other people would think of her, it was costing her a better quality of life. She was living in shame and embarrassment.

Like Mitzi, when you confront your fears, something magical will happen. When we stop running away from them, and begin running toward them, they almost always disappear! Most often, what we are terrified of happening, never does. In fact, the outcome is usually more favorable than we ever expected!

For Mitzi, when she returned home from boot camp—with her Transformation Team by her side—she confronted her FEAR. She rallied her community to help clean out her house. They came out in force, acknowledging and complimenting her bravery for opening up and being vulnerable. Sure enough, that incredible day she even made new friends and some of the best supporters on her Transformation Team! Mitzi literally emptied her house and rid herself of the sad, scared person she had become. She confronted the FEAR that had kept her imprisoned for years, and now has completely liberated herself!

Mitzi's greatest fear was admitting to herself—and the world—that she was a hoarder. Georgeanna's biggest fear was that her husband and kids wouldn't need her anymore if she put herself first. Bruce's biggest fear was that he wasn't worthy of love.

You are not alone. We all have FEARs and we will all continue to have fears throughout the rest of our lives. But now you have the opportunity to resee FEAR and see each fear you harbor inside as an opportunity for growth.

When you begin to "see" FEAR as life's opportunities for growth and strength, it takes all power away from those feelings and situations that scare you, and puts you in the driver's seat.

Try this exercise.

## Call to Action: Letting Go of FEAR

1. What are you afraid of? Make a list. Most fears fall into one of four buckets:
   Fear of failure
   Fear of losing control
   Fear of losing connection/of rejection
   Fear of injury/discomfort/death

2. Now how do you respond to that fear?
   Do you sabotage your progress?
   Do you make excuses to quit or run away?
   Do you get angry or blame someone else?
   Do you withdraw into yourself so no one would know?

3. Okay. Now let's figure out what that fear is costing you.
   Have you lost love?
   Have you missed out on success?
   Have you disconnected from people you care about and who care about you?
   Have you broken a promise to yourself and lost integrity?

**4.** Next, what would it look like if you were to confront that fear? Stop with the False Evidence in your head—what is the *real* probable outcome?

The more you seek out these fears, identify what they are costing you, and then face them head-on, the more you will see them begin to shrivel and disappear.

Anytime you sense a fear cropping up, repeat the steps above.

Soon you will understand and feel that when you take on your fears and build trust in yourself, you can control them, and your life becomes limitless. Therein lies a path that is uniquely yours. Look at what you are capable of! And deep down inside, you know it. Look what FEAR has cost you. Not anymore!

## Heidi Tip
## Get Out of Your Comfort Zone!

One of my most popular blog posts from about a year ago was called "Once I Try, I'll Realize I CAN!" It was all about how hard it feels to get out of our comfort zone and try new things, which is a huge part of confronting our FEAR. Chris and I spend our lives challenging others to step outside their comfort zones to achieve a level of living that they've never before experienced. I think it's time I take my own advice and do the same. People so often think that because we help others accomplish great things, Chris and I have no fear in doing these things ourselves. I am here to correct those individuals. We *do* get scared! We *do* need people to push us to jump outside our comfort zones! Who does this for us? None other than… our show participants. ☺

When I wrote this post, I was spending time in New Zealand with one person in particular who reminds me how important it is to live my own life the way that I am teaching her to live. Melissa, because of you, I am spending this year being *UNcomfortable.* ☺ Like you have made it your mantra, I am making mine the same: I'm replacing "I can't" with "I'll try." **Once I try, I'll realize I CAN!**

POWELL

# LIVE IT!

You have bravely dug deep over the past seven days, and have begun to remove some of the major roadblocks that have kept you from achieving your lifelong goals. From this place of newfound strength and clarity, you are now ready to take all of the incredible work you accomplished in the first 14 lessons, and build upon this new foundation for transformation you are creating. In the next seven days, we will coach you through *another radical shift in thinking* so that you have the know-how to live a life of transformation forever.

These lessons show you how to make concrete changes in your behavior. We will teach you the secret to never failing, how to balance your priorities, and give you a full forecast of what to expect on the journey ahead. We are going to show you how to zero in on the bad habits that have been sabotaging your weight loss and transform them into healthy, sustainable habits that will fuel your weight loss and fitness.

These are the final seven days and lessons to live a life of transformation. Take them in, embrace them, and hang on for the ride. Here we go!

## DAY 15

### Day 15: High-Carb Day

Meal 1: Breakfast
   Recipe: Power Mocha Shake with Fruit

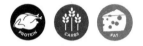

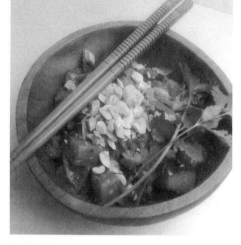

Meal 2: High-Carb Meal
   Recipe: Strawberry and Banana Quinoa Muffins

Meal 3: High-Carb Meal
   Recipe: Turkey Sliders with Sweet Potato "Bun"

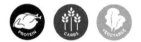

Meal 4: High-Carb Meal
   Recipe: Apple and Dip

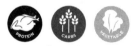

Meal 5: Low-Carb Meal
   Recipe: Eggplant Curry Stir-Fry

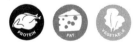

## Day 15: Metabolic Mission: The Countdown (Stepladder)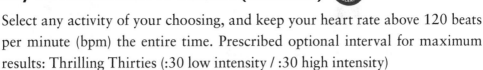

Set a running clock and, as fast as you can, do 21 reps of each exercise in the circuit, then 18 reps, then 15 reps, then 12, 9, 6, and 3.

Push-Ups
Hollow Rocks
Air Squats

## Day 15: Accelerator: 15 minutes (minimum)

Select any activity of your choosing, and keep your heart rate above 120 beats per minute (bpm) the entire time. Prescribed optional interval for maximum results: Thrilling Thirties (:30 low intensity / :30 high intensity)

## LESSON 15
# GO ALL IN

*If you always do what you've always done, you'll always get what you've always gotten.*

—Tony Robbins

When Cassie started her journey of transformation, she would never go all in. She would report following "most" of the program, but always reserved reasons why she needed to do her own portions, make her own food choices, and follow advice contrary to the advice we gave her. She would justify her behavior by saying that she was the only one who truly understood her body and how it worked—but in reality she was just protecting her food addiction and wanted the option to binge when she wanted. Most important, she was too terrified to lose control. She had always held the power, control, keys to her life. By giving them up and going all in, she would need to admit that her way didn't work. Because of this, her weight kept stalling out. By the 90-day mark she was struggling to lose a pound a week. She finally came to terms with the fact that "Cassie's way doesn't work." "When I realized that I was no longer moving toward my goal weight, I realized I had to submit to the process that Chris and Heidi laid out for me—the one that had worked for so many people."

If Cassie was going to make a lifelong change, she had to give up what we call her "ace in the pocket" and follow the program that *does* work. So she went all in. And became one of our greatest transformations of all time.

Submitting to the process is a crucial step in your transformation journey. It's not just submitting to the diet and the exercise, it is acting upon *all* the lessons of transformation! This is the step that led to Cassie's huge success and her final accomplishment: not only the loss of 176 pounds, the rejuvenation of her marriage, and being reunited with her son, but most important, loving herself for the first time in decades.

### Trust the Process

What do we mean by *trust the process*? We mean giving up that ace in your pocket, that "control card" that you hold on to, and throw down on the table to justify breaking your commitment to the plan. The mental conversation that we have is: "My body is different. I know and understand it better than anyone else, so I'll just do what works for me." Or it can also be based on a physical or emotional setback, such as "Well, they don't have a bad knee," or "They aren't dealing with the struggles that I have right now."

Trust us, we've heard it a million times before. This is the ultimate excuse, the reason of all reasons that your ego makes you feel like you are in control, because it is too afraid to show weakness or struggle. But deep down, you know you are simply protecting your bad behavior. Cassie spent so much time trying to convince herself that she knew her body better than anyone else. But she was lying to herself: Her body was *not* different. She, like all of us, abides by the laws of physics. The reality was that she did not have control over her binge eating.

Listen up: There are over 7 billion of us on this earth, and *all* of our bodies abide by the laws of physics, which dictate that if we take in less energy than we consume, we lose weight. If your body does not lose weight when at a calorie deficit, then your body defies the laws of physics. You need to put down this book and immediately check yourself in to a scientific research facility for evaluation.

Many people who struggle to lose weight and keep it off are struggling with something much larger than themselves: an unhealthy relationship with food and weight. Just take Heidi. For years as a teenager and young woman, she struggled with an eating disorder. "Although I am recovered, I still am vulnerable to the kind of thinking and behaviors that triggered my eating disorder to begin with."

And that's true for many people, Cassie included. When she was able to see that she was not in control of her food, she was able to see with clarity that she was simply a food addict. That revelation was ultimately liberating.

When you act like you don't have a problem, always justifying that your conditions in life are different, or your body is different than everyone else's, be aware that you are most likely hiding that ace in your back pocket!

## Call to Action

What have you always used as the reason to never commit fully to other programs? What's your "ace in the pocket"? _____

_____

## DAY 16

### Day 16: High-Carb Day

Meal 1: Breakfast
    Recipe: Turkey Frittata

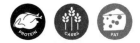

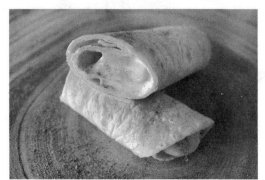

Meal 2: High-Carb Meal
    Recipe: Sweet Wrap

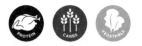

Meal 3: High-Carb Meal
    Recipe: Barbecue Chicken Salad

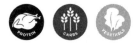

Meal 4: High-Carb Meal
    Recipe: Peanut Butter Shake

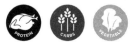

Meal 5: Low-Carb Meal
    Recipe: Curry Turkey Sliders with Cucumber and Tomato Salad

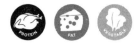

## Day 16: Metabolic Mission: Afterburner (Rounds for Time)

Set a running clock and do 5 rounds of the following exercises as fast as you can, but keeping good form!

20 Back Lunges
15 Push-Ups

## Day 16: Accelerator: 15 minutes (minimum)

Select any activity of your choosing, and keep your heart rate above 120 beats per minute (bpm) the entire time. Prescribed optional interval for maximum results: Tenacious Twos (2:00 low intensity / 2:00 high intensity)

## LESSON 16
# FALL WITHOUT FAILING

*Our greatest glory consists not in never falling, but in rising every time we fall.*

—Oliver Goldsmith

Sometimes the unexpected happens. And even though you now know how your promises are the most important thing in the world, sometimes you're just not going to keep one. This is to be expected.

Let's face it: You're human. We all make mistakes. You're going to mess up and break promises along the journey. You're going to eat what you shouldn't. You're going to skip a workout...or two. You're going to have some bad days. You're going to fall flat on your face when you least expect it.

This sounds awful, doesn't it? Because in your past, falling flat on your face meant that you'd failed yet again. Meant less self-love, less trust and belief in yourself.

Well, we have good news for you. *Falling* no longer needs to mean *failing*.

When you commit to Extreme Transformation, you are embracing a path where it's impossible to fail.

How so?

We know the secret lifeline to prevent failing.

Built into Extreme Transformation is the proven formula for getting back on your feet and continuing your journey. It is the lifeline you will *always* have the choice to grab onto when you fall. This is one of the most powerful shifts in your thinking during your journey of transformation. It is inevitable that you will mess up sometime. When you do, the backslide will begin. To stop the bleeding, and get back on your feet, you must learn and *apply* this formula:

Confess + Reassess + Recommit

These three simple actions, when done in this order, have a profound impact. This will be one of the most valuable lessons you can learn on the journey, and you will use it time and again!

## Call to Action

1. **Have the courage to confess.** If you made a mistake, fell off the wagon, or just didn't keep a promise in one way or another, you have to admit it. Trust us, this is easier said than done. If you ask *anyone* who has been through the journey of transformation, they will tell you that this is one of the most difficult parts. It takes us right back to the very first and most important step: Be vulnerable. It takes a ton of courage to admit to others our imperfections, but until you do, the weight of the broken promise will hold you back. Walk right over to the nearest mirror, look yourself in the eye, and say out loud the promise you broke to yourself. When you are ready, find someone on your trusted Transformation Team, or your superfriend, and tell them about your slip-up and that you need to confess what happened. Don't hold back and be vague—it will not be a full confession and it will hold you back. Share the details and get it *all* off of your shoulders. Confessing takes resolve and courage, but it also gives you a new sense of energy and trust in yourself. You can't look back.

   There are two dangerous reasons why most people don't confess, and eventually fail:

1. You are protecting your destructive habits and *want* to fall off the program to eat poorly again.

2. You are using negative self-talk and telling yourself that you don't want to be a burden to your Transformation Team or superfriend. This is a lie to yourself. Your team wants to see you succeed. It doesn't matter if you need to confess every week, or even every other day. Reach out to them!

2. Reassess the promise or promises that you have made and the goals that you fell short of. Ask yourself: *Why did I break that promise?* Was the commitment unattainable in your busy life and too hard to keep? Or was it a fluke day when things happened that were out of your control and you simply ran out of time? Were you feeling lonely, anxious, or stressed about something in your life? For most people, reassessing a mistake or setback reveals one of three things:

   • An emotional trigger that overpowered your promise.
   • An old excuse based upon the old you.
   • Your promise is too far out of reach of your current position and is therefore not realistic or attainable now.

Reassessing your transformation vision clarifies what's possible for you right now. You need to go back to your goals and see if they are SMART.

Ask yourself if your goal is:

• Specific
• Measurable
• Attainable
• Relevant
• Time-bound

Without our realizing it, most of our slip-ups happen because our goals become imprecise or unrealistic. Take a good look at the circumstances and decide whether to continue with the same commitment, or if you should reduce it to something that you *know* you can keep.

3. Rise up and recommit: Once you have reassessed and feel unbelievably confident that you can keep your new commitment, it is time to recommit to your promises and your goals. Contact someone on your team and declare your recommitment. Say it loud and say it clear!

   Reassessing your promise and your goals makes it possible to know exactly

where you are right now in your journey and what is realistic to expect from
yourself. When you go through the
process of establishing promises that
are truly SMART, then you will not be
afraid to move on after a setback. You
will also feel more determined and
confident that you can indeed keep that
promise and reach that goal. When you
stand up and once again declare your
promises and goals, you strengthen
your commitment to yourself!

Merhbod had lost over 100 pounds in just six months and was well on his way to his ideal weight. Then slowly but surely his weight loss slowed to a stop…and he began to gain it all back. We had no idea because he kept sending weigh-in pictures and video showing that he was continuing to lose weight, when in reality he was rigging his scale at home to make it look like he was. This went on for three months until Mehrbod finally realized that the addict had completely taken over. He was terrified to disappoint us, but he knew there was only one way to stop the backslide. He picked up the phone and called us. We met with him, and he confessed everything. We took it all in, and when he was finished he put his face in his hands and cried. We lifted his head, looked him in the eyes, and said, "Thank you. We can only imagine the courage it took to do that."

Immediately, we could see an emotional weight lifted off his shoulders. He sat back, took a deep breath, and said, "What can I do now?" We reassessed his goals and daily commitments, and when we came up with something totally attainable, he recommitted. Sure enough, he went on to break weight-loss records in the final three months of his transformation, and qualified for skin-removal surgery. When Merhbod summoned the courage to confess, reassess, and recommit, he broke free from the backslide, got back up on his feet, and surged forward with more vigor than ever before. We cannot underestimate the power of this formula.

As Lisa recalls, "I remember the first time I messed up a couple weeks into my transformation. I doubled my portions for dinner one night. Didn't seem like a big deal, but it haunted me, because deep down I knew I had broken a commitment to myself. I fell back into my old way of thinking and felt like I was a failure. Sure enough, I ended up overeating the next couple nights, until I remembered what Chris and Heidi taught me about falling without failing. I knew that if I didn't stop the bleeding, it was going to take me down, and I would fail yet again. It was so hard to pick up the phone and confess, but when I did I immediately felt control again. Together, we reassessed and recommitted. It was the lifeline I needed. I messed up a handful of times on my weight loss journey, and every time, I used this same formula—and it got me to my goal. Without a doubt, it was the greatest lesson I learned on the journey!"

As Jami described for us, "The 90-day boot camp was just the beginning of my transformation. The real work happened when I returned home. It took me a while to realize that the journey I was on was really the rest of my life. I had always lived my life in an all-or-nothing way. If I ever messed up, that was it. I was a failure and I'm done. Maybe a year later I'd try again. And that just set me up to fail—over and over again. Now I understand what Chris and Heidi mean when they say it's okay to fall—it's just an opportunity to get back up again. This way of thinking about mistakes is so much more realistic and encouraging than thinking of failure as a personal quality or source of shame. That's the old Jami. I just don't think that way anymore."

If you break a promise, will it start the downward spiral again? Will you once again give up on yourself, beat yourself up, and find yourself in a dark place?

Now you have the lifeline. You can *choose* the single most powerful and proven formula to get back on your feet, or you can *choose* to quit.

When you break a promise to yourself, it is not cause for shame or embarrassment. In fact, mistakes and setbacks are the training ground for flexing the real muscles of transformation—the muscles that get you back up on your feet and moving toward your goal. This is why during your transformation journey you will learn to fall...not fail. This is one of the key steps of your journey—learning how to clear broken promises, strategize an easier path toward your goal, and move forward with more enthusiasm than ever before.

The power is now in your hands. Any time you fall, you are always just three simple steps away from being right back on track.

### Perfectly Imperfect

Disappointment happens when expectations are not met. Simple as that. Most people make the grave mistake of setting unrealistic expectations for themselves. They create a vision of perfection that not only is impossible to fulfill but also hampers their ability to stay on their journey. When these expectations are not met, the strong emotions tied with disappointment come flooding in. In these times, most people lose the magical ingredient of *belief* and any further effort (and progression) toward the goal comes to a rapid halt.

Remember: We are all *perfectly imperfect*. That's the awesome part about being human. It is working through our setbacks and slip-ups that creates our uniqueness and character. Why place such expectations of perfection on yourself when they are simply unrealistic? Without messing up, we could never appreciate the beauty that life offers us along the way.

## Heidi Tip

I am perfect.

Perfectly imperfect, that is.

I use the word *perfect* a lot, and often people remind me that nothing is perfect. I totally disagree. I believe that everyone and everything is perfect and beautiful in its imperfect state of being. Think about that for one second—imagine that just maybe your imperfections actually make you perfect. Don't you just love the freedom that thought gives you? Well, time to realize the reality of the thought and let go of our self-judgments and negative self-talk. It's time to embrace our imperfections. Now, I'm not saying to throw caution to the wind and go indulge in a gallon of super-chunky triple chocolate fudgy goo. I'm saying that it's okay to mess up, and it's okay to have faults. For those of you who don't, I'm sorry. These faults, trials, imperfections, and stumbles are some of our greatest blessings—they're our springboards to becoming the strongest person we can possibly be!

XO Heidi

# DAY 17

## Day 17: High-Carb Day

Meal 1: Breakfast
   Recipe: Turkey and Potato Skillet Breakfast

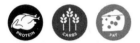

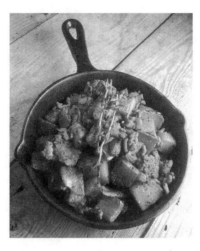

Meal 2: High-Carb Meal
   Recipe: Strawberry and Banana Quinoa Muffins

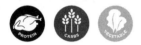

Meal 3: High-Carb Meal
   Recipe: Italian Tuna and White Bean Lettuce Wraps

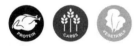

Meal 4: High-Carb Meal
   Recipe: Greek Yogurt Parfait with Fruit

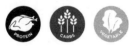

Meal 5: Low-Carb Meal
   Recipe: Barbecue Grilled Pork Tenderloin

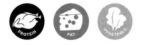

### Day 17: Metabolic Mission: Chippin' Away (Chipper)

Set a running clock and see how long it takes you to do these exercises. Record your time in your Daily Tracker!

100 Jumping Jacks
75 Air Squats
50 Push-Ups
25 Kickbacks

### Day 17: Accelerator: 15 minutes (minimum)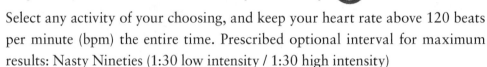

Select any activity of your choosing, and keep your heart rate above 120 beats per minute (bpm) the entire time. Prescribed optional interval for maximum results: Nasty Nineties (1:30 low intensity / 1:30 high intensity)

## LESSON 17

# BE BENEFICIALLY SELFISH

*Make your own recovery the first priority in your life.*

—Robin Norwood

The journey of transformation requires that you put yourself first. Plain and simple. If you don't put your needs, your promises, your goals first, then you will not succeed. For many (especially us parents), this can seem totally selfish. We are programmed to put our families first. However, this programming is actually a bit faulty. While our family may be the most important people in the world to us, if something happens to you that affects your ability to be a good parent, the family suffers in the long run. Nobody captured the importance of our own health better than the FAA and their safety guidelines for airplane emergency situations in the cabin.

We are ordered to put an oxygen mask over our own mouth before we turn to help a child or another person. For good reason: If you can't breathe, how can you help your child, your neighbor, and everyone else around you?

The same rule applies for your health.

If it isn't a "life-or-death" situation; Other people and their needs can wait. They can be uncomfortable for a moment while you ensure *your* health and survival—so that you can be there for them in the future.

We call this being *beneficially selfish*. Our society and culture have taught us that it is selfish to put ourselves before others. In actuality, we are taking care of ourselves first, *for the benefit of everyone around us*. Keep in mind that as you take this step and make this shift in thinking, others around you might still be programmed by society and culture, and many will likely call you "selfish" for putting yourself first. They just don't see the bigger picture. Explain it to them if you like, but either way, it is the truth.

Over time, putting everyone else's needs first pushes most people into dire health situations. Look at the position you are in right now, and what has led you here. Maybe you're frustrated with the 20 pounds that is taking forever to come off. Or perhaps you picked up this book after a triple bypass surgery. Either way, making yourself a priority in your life is of utmost importance— not just to your physical health, but to your mental and emotional health as well!

When we are fulfilling promises and taking care of ourselves, we feel better about ourselves and can bring more joy into the lives of our families and friends. How much joy did you spread when you felt like crap about yourself? Want to bring more long-term joy into the lives of everyone around you, your family, your friends, your children? Be beneficially selfish!

After years of putting her son first, Kathy declared independence so that she could finally take care of herself. David also had to learn how to put himself first. When he was working 14-hour days, he reduced his hours to 11 per day, to carve out time for his health. In fact, all the people you have met so far in this book have had to learn how to put themselves first and make their health and fitness journeys their number one priority.

.For Georgeanna this lesson, this step in her transformation journey, was one of the most difficult to actualize. "I only saw myself as a pastor's wife who was meant to serve—serve God, my husband, my children, my community. I didn't even know how to take care of myself, never mind put myself first. But I did learn. And what I realized is that when you surround yourself with loving people who really do understand what you are trying to do, then you can put yourself first without guilt or looking over your shoulder."

## Call to Action

In general we all have some predictable features of our lives, but their importance varies depending on our life and situation. Also, our priorities shift over the course of our lives. When we are young and don't yet have families to take care of, we might position education and social life over staying in touch with relatives. When we are older, education may not be as important and our health seems to shift in its importance.

When you think about your totem pole, rank these values based upon your present— where you are now, what you need now, and what your goals are now. Take a look at the following list and put these items in order, with the most important on top.

- Education
- Family
- Friends/social
- Religion
- Physical and Mental Health
- Serving others
- Work

Being beneficially selfish usually requires a sit-down meeting with your support system (and family and friends), to speak openly about your journey and priorities. Teach them what you just learned and that you are going to be putting yourself first in many situations, not because you are being generally selfish, but because you know that when you are healthy and fit, you can provide that much more to their lives. Talk openly about the journey ahead, and help them find solutions for things like transportation and meals, for when you are not available:

## Reality Check

There will always be a valid reason why you should put someone/something else first. Once again, unless the situation is truly life or death (or a health scare), you know in your heart what you *should* do—take care of yourself first.

## Chris Tip

It's necessary to have realistic expectations of life so that you are fully prepared. Here is a glimpse into your likely future. This is what you can expect from life over the course of your weight loss journey...and beyond:

- Loss and tragedy
- Family struggles
- Career struggles
- Financial struggles
- Relationship struggles
- Overall bad days

Events such as these are inevitable and unavoidable. Expect them to happen, because they will. It is our natural tendency to fall back into comforting habits, or put things on hold with our health so that we can handle such issues as those listed above. However, we are here to tell you that these are everyday occurrences in life. With many of these events ahead of you, there will never be a right time in the future to make your health and fitness a priority. The only right time...is right now.

If you play your cards right, you may have a good 75 to 100 total years here on earth. And not for one second will anyone walk in your shoes. This is *your* journey. Aggressively defend it. Do it for your health, for your happiness, and for the subsequent benefit of your family, friends, and loved ones. Let nothing get in the way of your destiny and what you deserve. Get your priorities straight!

# DAY 18

## Day 18: High-Carb Day

Meal 1: Breakfast
   Recipe: Pumpkin Spice Vanilla Protein Pancakes

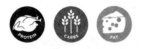

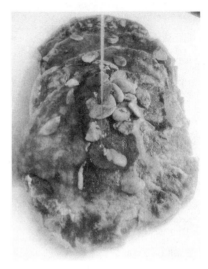

Meal 2: High-Carb Meal
   Recipe: Hulk Shake

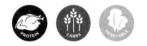

Meal 3: High-Carb Meal
   Recipe: Loaded Potato

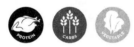

Meal 4: High-Carb Meal
   Recipe: PB & J Rice Cakes and Shake

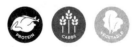

Meal 5: Low-Carb Meal
   Recipe: Fajita Chicken Roll-Ups with Roasted Squash and Avocado Puree

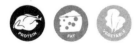

### Day 18: Metabolic Mission: "Go Time" (AMRAP)

Set a running clock and do as many rounds of the following circuit as you can in 11 minutes.

7 Push-Ups
9 Leg Levers
11 High Knees

### Day 18: Accelerator: 15 minutes (minimum)

Select any activity of your choosing, and keep your heart rate above 120 beats per minute (bpm) the entire time. Prescribed optional interval for maximum results: Mighty Minutes (1:00 low intensity / 1:00 high intensity)

## LESSON 18
## HAVE REALISTIC EXPECTATIONS OF OTHERS

*You're in the midst of a war: a battle between the limits of a crowd seeking the surrender of your dreams, and the power of your true vision to create and contribute. It is a fight between those who will tell you what you cannot do, and that part of you that knows, and has always known, that we are more than our environment; and that a dream, backed by an unrelenting will to attain it, is truly a reality with an imminent arrival.*

—Tony Robbins

You may not want to hear this, but we are determined to be honest and up front with you: Your family and friends may not be your best supporters. As you begin to make changes in your life, the people around you may very well feel uncomfortable. Your changes affect their status quo. They may claim that they want to support you and that they want you to succeed at your goals. But often, they are really, really uncomfortable with how *your* changes make *them* feel.

We are by no means saying that your family and friends are bad or malicious, but chances are that your goals and new life may not work well with what they are used to. In fact, your new lifestyle can be downright threatening. Unless they understand and embrace change, most people wince with discomfort if asked to move out of their comfort zone. So as innocent humans not yet on their own journey of transformation, some of the people in your life might react negatively to your new choices and newfound confidence.

- When you start to eat healthy, stop drinking, and spend more time at the gym, your boyfriend or wife may feel abandoned.
- When you stop indulging in pizza and wings, and instead choose healthier options every three hours, your buddy might feel angry that you've ditched him and your shared Friday-night routine.
- When you make your health a priority, your children or spouse might feel jealous of lost time and express resentment.

Everyone has a reaction. But it's up to you to surround yourself with those who understand and truly support your journey and perhaps distance yourself from those, including family, who might be trying to impede your success. Now, we are not saying that you should distance yourself from your friends, family, and loved ones simply because they may express some frustration with the process.

But by having realistic expectations of their responses to you, you will not get distracted or disappointed. You can separate your goals from *their* desires and practice patience and perseverance (and compassion for them) even in the face of adversity! There is a very good chance that your friends and family *do* love and support you…chances are, they are just terrified of losing you in their life. it's just nearly impossible for them to understand what you are going through since they are not walking in your shoes.

What's the best response? *Love!* Even if friends or family try to pull you from the process or get upset with your new routines that might be causing them an inconvenience, you can think and respond to them in love—*as long as* doing so doesn't compromise your own goals.

Part of this loving response is learning how to communicate effectively with those you care about. If the way your friend/family is being is pulling you away from your goals, you should feel confident enough to pull them aside and have a loving, open communication about what your goals are, and what you need from them (support) to get there. Express to them that you know they love you, and that is why you feel safe having this conversation.

For instance, you might say, "I know you don't think you are hurting me when you try to get me to eat dessert with the family, but it triggers an impulse in me to binge that I can't control. Please don't take it personally when I decline your homemade ice cream . . . I love you no less, but need to focus on my health."

As you make changes in how you eat, how you live, and the choices you make, you will likely trigger discomfort in your friends, family, and co-workers. Changing your routine, the way you eat, and when you're available impacts all those with whom you regularly come in contact. Many of our peeps tell us they seem to have "lost" their friends or even family members. You might hear words from them like "You've abandoned us" and "You think you're too good for us now."

You might also hear people begin to doubt you, question you, even criticize you. When one person changes, everyone around that person is affected. Sometimes this reaction will stem from a sort of jealousy—they are struggling with seeing your success while they are stuck in their unhappy life. The best thing to do is to love your friends and family regardless and lead by example.

But remember: If you aren't getting the love or support you need, you should expand (not replace) your circle of friends and supporters and include more people who are more aligned with your vision and goals. These people are most likely members of your gym, running group, or support team. As Dr. Holly says, "A connection to others who are living a similar lifestyle improves the odds of success." Which is why it's so important to look again at your social connections.

Mitzi felt that she didn't quite lose the people in her life, but rather that those who didn't understand or support all the changes she was making simply drifted away. "I didn't feel any ill will—it has just been a case of being in different places. And you know what? It's all right. It doesn't necessarily mean that our two roads won't ever converge again."

Mitzi points out something important: *It's all right.* It's all right if people don't seem to like the new you. It's all right to lose touch with a friend or family member. It's all right because you are learning to put yourself first. When you live your life with you as the number one priority, you will begin to feel so much more at ease with your choices. You will feel clear and confident, instead of tangled up in trying to please other people.

**1.** Be beneficially selfish. You can't help anyone else if you can't help yourself first! Expect some to be upset and withdraw. This is an example of conditional love. In this journey toward loving ourselves, we need unconditional love and support.

**2.** Schedule time for *you* to fulfill your commitments, and time for *them*. They might give you a hard time, but if you communicate what is important and necessary to you and your health, then you have done everything in your power to keep communication open in the relationship.

*There will always be reasons not to follow what you* know *in your heart is the path toward your health and happiness. Sometimes you have to go out of your way to get there. Honor your* word *over your* reasons, *and you will get there.*

*It is your time. Now go get 'em!*

*Chris & Heidi*

# DAY 19

## Day 19: Low-Carb Day

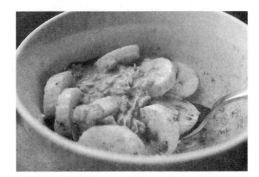

Meal 1: Breakfast
    Recipe: No-Bake Oats

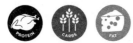

Meal 2: Low-Carb Meal
    Recipe: Quinoa Bites with
Zucchini, Tomato, and Arugula

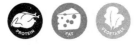

Meal 3: Low-Carb Meal
    Recipe: Citrus Salmon Slaw

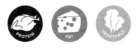

Meal 4: Low-Carb Meal
    Recipe: Popeye Shake

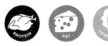

Meal 5: Low-Carb Meal
    Recipe: Chipotle Turkey Burger with House Pickles

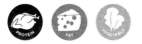

**Day 19: Metabolic Mission: Wake-Up Call (Tabata)**

For each exercise, do as many reps as you can in 20 seconds. Rest for 10 seconds, then do as many reps as you can in 20 seconds again. Repeat for 8 total rounds (for a total of 4 minutes) per exercise. The lowest number of reps you get in any round is your score. You'll get one score per exercise. Add up all three scores, and record it in your Daily Tracker!

Kickbacks
Leg Levers
Air Squats

**Day 19: Accelerator: 15 minutes (minimum)**

Select any activity of your choosing, and keep your heart rate above 120 beats per minute (bpm) the entire time. Prescribed optional interval for maximum results: Dirty Two-Thirties (2:30 low intensity / 2:30 high intensity)

## LESSON 19
## REPLACE YOUR ADDICTION

*Nothing tastes as good as being skinny feels.*

—Anonymous

In transformation, we use the word *addiction* because it is a very powerful way to describe the impact of our habits. You may be a true food addict and engage in compulsive behavior, or you may simply have a bad series of habits that led to weight gain. Either way, the fact remains that in order for a new habit to be effective, the payoff *must be* more desirable than the habit you are replacing it with. This is true of relationships with food and other addictive substances.

As you have moved through the lessons of transformation, we have pointed out places and times when it's necessary to change your behavior in order to stay committed to your new lifestyle. Essentially, what we have been asking you to do is replace your addiction to junk food or soda, with eating foods that don't create such a strong physical craving. If you don't replace the addiction, it will simply reassert its control over you. For example, we understand that junk food is both positively reinforcing and rewarding—it acts upon the reward pathways of the brain and triggers you to want to repeat the behavior—but when done repeatedly over time, it comes with a heavy cost to your appearance and health. You get fat and sick.

When it comes to the weight loss journey, we are asking you to replace the satisfaction and enjoyment of eating what you want, when you want, and living a sedentary life with little to no exercise—with eating structured meals, eating on a schedule, and moving on a daily basis.

When looking at the two lifestyles, the former is more attractive. Of course everybody wants to eat whatever they want, whenever they want! However, that lifestyle comes at a great cost. When you look at the beneficial outcome of the latter, it quickly becomes the frontrunner!

## What Is an Addiction?

Addiction is a state characterized by compulsive engagement in rewarding stimuli, despite adverse consequences. The two properties that characterize all addictive stimuli are that they are (positively) reinforcing (they increase the likelihood that a person will seek repeated exposure to them) and intrinsically rewarding (they activate the brain's "reward pathways" and are therefore perceived as being something positive or desirable).

### *The Payoff of Your New Habits*

Everything has a cost and a payoff. The major cost of your new lifestyle is no longer having the convenience of eating what you want, when you want. Instead, you eat new foods that don't have the same reward impact, but keep you full for a long period of time. You can indulge, but only when it is customized into your plan and still accommodates your weight loss. As you are on the journey of transformation, here are some of the new payoffs you are now receiving:

- You are losing weight on the scale every week—and you feel good.
- Your clothes are looser—you may just need to invest in a new wardrobe!
- You are healthier.
- You are more attractive.

- You are seeing your body develop shapely muscles.
- You are getting an endorphin rush and euphoric sense of well-being from the exercise.
- You have a sense of pride, accomplishment, and control over your life.
- You are receiving accolades and respect from others—we are certain that you are the happy recipient of compliments and well-deserved praise.

All of the above results are payoffs for your new lifestyle. These payoffs are positively reinforcing. They do not always play directly upon the reward pathways of the brain in an immediate sense, but they do offer long-term fulfillment. The question is: Are the payoffs to your transformation more rewarding than the immediate satisfaction from food?

The purpose of this lesson is to create an awareness of the trade-offs that have happened here: what you have given up with your old life, for what you are getting with your new life. Granted, your new life is much more attractive (literally), but we want you to begin thinking ahead to when you reach your goal and some of these payoffs don't occur as often. Enjoy the payoffs of the weight loss journey now, but we will explore in much more detail the process of finding another new addiction as you transition from weight loss into maintenance.

## Your *New* Addiction

When you hit your goal or are near your goal weight, some of the most powerful payoffs from the weight loss journey go away. While you once looked forward to seeing the number on the scale drop every week, it begins to remain more constant. While you beamed from the positive comments and pats on the back from your family and friends, they are all accustomed to you looking this way now, and may even become critical of your appearance again.

When the compliments stop coming, we begin to look for payoffs again. Our old habits and food addictions can creep back in. As humans we *need* something to satisfy our reward pathways. We need something to look forward to daily. When this weight loss phase is over, if you don't have a *new* addiction, you will quickly turn back to food, and begin to gain weight again.

So what will your new addiction be? See chapter 4.

# DAY 20

## Day 20: Low-Carb Day

Meal 1: Breakfast
 Recipe: Breakfast Frittata Veggie "Muffins"

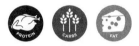

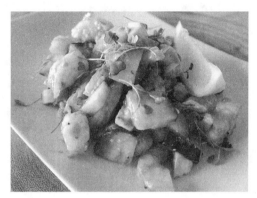

Meal 2: Low-Carb Meal
 Recipe: Protein Punch Wraps

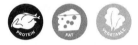

Meal 3: Low-Carb Meal
 Recipe: Grilled Lamb Kebabs

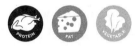

Meal 4: Low-Carb Meal
 Recipe: Shrimp Cocktail Salad

Meal 5: Low-Carb Meal
 Recipe: Creamy Cauliflower Soup

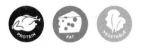

**No Metabolic Mission: Day Off!**

**Day 20: Accelerator: 15 minutes (minimum)**

Select any activity of your choosing, and keep your heart rate above 120 beats per minute (bpm) the entire time. Prescribed optional interval for maximum results: Thrilling Thirties (:30 low intensity / :30 high intensity)

LESSON 20

## TRIGGERS AND TACTICS

*God, grant me the serenity to accept the things I cannot change,*
*the courage to change the things I can, and the wisdom to know the*
*difference.*

—Serenity Prayer

We are surrounded by triggers all day, every day. The people in our lives, the places we pass through, the rituals of our daily routines. These triggers can evoke an emotional response in us. Some can be stronger than others, but either way any reaction can influence our decision-making ability.

When we encounter strong triggers, powerful emotions surface—so strong that we feel the need to soothe or numb ourselves when the emotion is negative, or to heighten the euphoria when the emotion is positive. We look outside ourselves for an instant comfort or way to make the high last longer. Unfortunately what we reach for can often set off a domino effect of old habits and behaviors, such as eating a pint of ice cream or racing over to the nearest convenience store for a package of donuts or a case of beer.

This lesson is all about being clear on your triggers—those situations, behaviors, and surroundings that tempt you to go back to your old ways. The beauty is this: Once you identify your *triggers*, you can see them more clearly. You can also train yourself to avoid them and resist them by using *tactics* that support you and your journey.

Just like habits, triggers can take time to dissipate. The purpose of a tactic is not to make the trigger go away, but to distract or empower the mind to prevent the emotional response. Most triggers can last for 5 to 15 minutes, so rest assured that if you employ these tactics to keep your mind and emotions occupied, you *can* navigate easily around or through any trigger!

### People Triggers

Oddly enough, people triggers don't have as much to do with the actual person triggering you; people triggers are more about ourselves. People triggers usually stem from a deep emotional need that we feel is not being met. For example, our parent, teacher, boss, or partner might trigger within us:

- The need to feel loved
- The need to feel trusted
- The need to feel valued
- The need to feel desired
- The need to be respected
- The need to be right
- The need to be understood
- The need for freedom
- The need to be in control

This list just scratches the surface. We have many more emotional needs that might trigger us. We become reliant on one or more of these needs because at some point in our life, that basic emotional need worked to benefit us in some way. So we learned that when that emotional need is fulfilled, the results are typically positive. However, when we feel that the need is not being met, the reaction is usually one of anger or fear—both powerful triggers that turn many of us to junk food to numb and cope.

### Tactics for People Triggers

1. Write down one to three emotional needs that you have:

   1. _____
   2. _____
   3. _____

2. Do your own reality check: Is this person really denying you of your emotional need, or preventing you from getting it? Does this person have enough relevance in your life that they have this power over you?

3. If they do hold enough relevance in your life, and you feel it is important that you receive the emotional need from this person, try communicating it with them. Let them know how you feel and how important it is to be trusted, valued, et cetera.

4. If you find yourself emotionally charged and it is clear that this individual will not help satisfy your emotional need, then it is time to separate yourself from this situation:

   • Relax and shift your focus to your breathing.

   • Choose one word that describes how you want to be in this moment: calm, relaxed, powerful, centered, or the like.

   • Reach out to a member of your Transformation Team to help you sort through your reaction to the person or situation that is triggering you.

### Food Triggers

As humans, we are programmed from infancy for food to be soothing and comforting for us. We develop an emotional connection with sweet and savory comfort foods, overloaded with sugar, salt, and fat. These "hyperpalatables" release the feel-good endorphins in our brains. Because of this, such food helps to calm and relax us when we experience feelings of anger, sadness, anxiety, or loneliness. It will even heighten feelings of happiness. It's no surprise that these hyperpalatables have become one of the biggest addictions in the United States and abroad. Because they act on many of the same systems of the brain as many drugs, these comfort foods have become an emotional "painkiller" for the masses.

It doesn't help that we are also bombarded by junk food advertisements on TV, online, in newspapers, magazines—all over our media.

### Tactics for Food Triggers

If you find that certain foods trigger binge behavior, use these tactics to beat the binge:

1. Use teamwork. Call or text someone on your Transformation Team to talk about how you are feeling. Simply talking about the issue is one of the most powerful steps in creating awareness and taking control of the trigger.

2. Clean out your environment of any trigger foods (you should have done that in Lesson 4!).

3. Avoid places, restaurants, or situations where you might find your trigger foods (the break room at work, drive-thru row, your friend's house that's loaded with junk food). Those who've successfully transformed themselves sometimes actually found alternative routes to get where they needed to go, just to avoid these dangerous pitfalls.

4. Have healthy options available at any moment: fruit, nuts, protein bars, protein shakes, gum, flavored water, and so on. Whatever you need to satisfy a sweet or salty craving, there are hundreds of amazing healthy alternatives available!

5. Stay on track with your five meals a day. Skipping a meal or snack will put you in low blood sugar, a vulnerable place for a trigger!

### Event Triggers

Some of the main triggers we experience on a regular basis are event triggers. These powerful triggers are made up of a multitude of situational events such as going to a restaurant, social gathering, party, or family reunion. Even going to work can be a trigger for some people. The drive to and from work, walking by the break room or cafeteria, finally getting the kids to bed and sitting down on the couch—these regular daily events can trigger responses in us that make us want to reach for food.

Boredom is actually one of the biggest event triggers we can experience. You know, those moments in the middle of the day when the kids are at school and the spouse is at work...and you find yourself wandering aimlessly around the kitchen pantry. Or when you have hours to kill doing xyz...

Believe it or not, another huge event trigger for some can be finishing a long workout. Many people feel the need to reward themselves after a good sweat session and then develop a food reward habit that negates all of their hard work!

Whatever habits have been formed during these daily events can be difficult to break. One of our peeps confessed to us that the simple click of his seat belt always triggered a craving for fast food because for years, nearly every time he got into a car he would hit a drive-thru wherever he was going.

Certain times of the year are loaded with powerful triggers—our birthdays, the holidays, the anniversary of a breakup. When we are reminded of certain powerful events in our lives, our triggers can be summoned.

We have created a list of tactics that can help guide you through the toughest of event triggers. Find the triggers and tactics that best apply to your life!

### Tactics for Going to a Restaurant

1. Eat something healthy before you go out and just order something extremely light when you are there.
2. Order an appetizer or side order instead of an entrée.
3. Order an entrée and cut it in half as soon as it is served. Eat half, and take the rest to go.
4. Ask your server to remove or not serve any trigger food items beforehand (say, chips, bread, soup or salad before the meal).
5. Choose a dish that has been steamed, baked, or grilled instead of fried or sautéed.

### Tactics for the Drive to and from Work

1. Avoidance. Choose a different route to and from work so you don't pass by your drive-thru trigger.
2. Be prepared. Eat something before you leave home and before you leave work. If you are hungry on your drive, your inner voice will create any excuse it can to rationalize your destructive habit. *Do not break your promise!*
3. Keep your "why" in front of you. Keep a picture on your dashboard in the car. Never forget why you are doing this and how much better your life is going to be!

### Tactics for Social Gatherings

1. Eat before you arrive.
2. Avoid the areas with food.
3. Chew gum.

4. Get a glass of water, soda water, or diet soda and keep it in your hands the whole time. We call this "glassing." It keeps your hands occupied and prevents you from feeling out of place.

### Tactics for Workplace Triggers

1. Avoid the trigger areas as much as possible. If necessary, find alternative routes around the break room, cafeteria, vending machine, and so on.
2. Keep your desk well stocked with healthy options at all times.
3. Rally your co-workers to join the health and fitness bandwagon. This has become extremely popular these days, with thousands of businesses now offering only healthy options in their break rooms, cafeterias, and vending machines.

### Tactics for End-of-Day Triggers

Typically after a long and stressful day, we feel the deep-rooted need to reward ourselves. Walking in the door from work, getting the kids to bed, or typing up those final emails can trigger some monster cravings for something that will derail you. Here's what to do:

1. Keep your hands and taste buds busy. Chew gum. Have your flavored water or low-calorie beverage in hand.
2. Grab the chopped veggies. They will give you a nice crunchy snack and fill you up.
3. Go to bed. We call the time from around 7:00 p.m. until you go to bed the "red zone." This is typically the time of the day when people are most likely to succumb to triggers and cravings. Ben Franklin said it best: "Early to bed, early to rise, makes a man healthy, wealthy, and wise."

### Tactics for Boredom

1. Call or text someone on your team and figure out something fun or relaxing to do.
2. Give yourself a project or hobby: Play a video game, build something, start a collection, clean out the closet, whatever you need to do to keep your mind busy.

3. Chew gum and drink water.

4. Volunteer for a service event in your area.

### Tactics for Holidays and Events

1. For anniversaries and birthdays, eat ahead of time and come with a full stomach. Just like social gatherings, keep a glass of water, soda water, or diet soda in hand. Chew gum. Avoid the food as much as possible.

2. Also see tactics for social gatherings and people triggers.

## Call to Action

On the left side, write your top 3 event triggers, and on the right side, write the tactics you will use to navigate around it or through it!

| Top 3 event triggers | Top 5 tactics you can use |
|---|---|
| 1. | 1.<br>2.<br>3.<br>4.<br>5. |
| 2. | 1.<br>2.<br>3.<br>4.<br>5. |
| 3. | 1.<br>2.<br>3.<br>4.<br>5. |

### Why Am I Always Hungry?

Do you ever consume thousands of calories in a sitting, and then feel hungry again within just minutes or hours? It can be so frustrating and depressing feeling like your body is an out-of-control eating machine. Many people have lost touch with their true hunger and become slaves to their emotional hunger.

There is a huge difference between the feeling of physical fullness and feeling emotionally satisfied. However, the wiring in our brains often gets crossed so that it is difficult to distinguish between the two. Through years of poor eating habits in response to emotional triggers, yo-yo dieting, and bouts of binge eating we can confuse the brain to think that loneliness and depression are hunger, and the act of eating is comfort.

This can lead to the endless consumption of thousands of calories. While your body may be full and satisfied, your emotions are not...so you continue to mindlessly eat, searching for a comfort of fullness that may never come... until you are ready to stop, take a moment, and pay attention to what is *really* going on.

It is easy to get stuck on autopilot and find yourself "blind bingeing" on junk foods. However, you need to:

- Relearn what true hunger feels like.
- Before you eat anything, stop and ask yourself, *"Am I really hungry?"*
- Log your foods.

## Reality Check

Your triggers aren't going anywhere. They are a part of life, and will be present to test you every day. However, the more aware and prepared you are, the greater the chance you will overcome them.

## DAY 21

### It's Time to Weigh In

Your End-of-Cycle Weight: _____

At this time, feel free to take any other measurements as well and note them here: _____.

### Day 21: Reset Day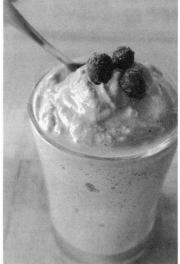

It's Reset Day! Make meals easy by cooking up our Clean Cheat recipes (see suggested menu below), or simply add 1,000 extra calories of foods you love to a normal high-carb day.

Meal 1: Candied Pecan Protein Waffles

Meal 2: Sweet Potato Nachos

Meal 3: Banana Berry Ice Cream

Meal 4: Pigs in a Blanket

Meal 5: One-Minute Brownie

### Rest Day

Now relax! Take the day off and rest—no Metabolic Missions and no Accelerators!

## LESSON 21

# LIVE WITH PURPOSE

*Man is a goal seeking animal. His life only has meaning if he is reaching out and striving for his goals.*

—Aristotle

Right now, you may be solely driven by your own personal goals, wants, and needs—which is totally awesome. Remember, in order to change you must be beneficially selfish! Setting *your* goals and declaring *your* dream has given you a direction and a purpose. And now, 21 days or more into your journey, you are seeing and feeling the difference in your life. However, to make this "difference" lifelong, we want to ask you to open up your mind to something that may seem a bit counterintuitive...

We want to ask you to begin to open your mind to the value that you can bring to others' lives. In his *7 Habits of Highly Effective People*, the great Stephen Covey wrote about the distinctions among dependence, independence, and interdependence.

We are programmed to be interdependent with others—to contribute to our family, community, and society—and when we make this connection real, we not only help others but also maximize our sense of value and belonging. When we have a contributing purpose in life, it satisfies and fulfills us on a whole new level.

In many ways, this process of transformation is akin to the process of rehabilitation, and one of the most powerful steps in true recovery is when a person becomes a sponsor to help others through their journeys. That's what we have in mind here.

So what if you could make a positive impact in someone else's life? Or many people's lives? You can. Transformation is not just about changing your life, but also about being the catalyst for change in others. In the most beneficially selfish way, reaching out to others—to help, guide, or inspire—helps keep you living a life of transformation without sliding back into your old destructive habits, and so keeps you from gaining the weight back.

# Call to Action:
# Become a Weight Loss Superstar

Start thinking about the impact that you are going to make in the world. Whether you have reached your goal in just one 21-day phase or several phases, there are millions of people out there who want to do what you have just done. You can be their motivation! Want to know where everyone is? Online. Hundreds of millions of people want to hear from you! Here are some other ideas for reaching out to others:

- Build a social media following: Start an Instagram, Facebook, and Twitter account. Follow and "like" other weight loss accounts and amazing success stories.
- Post your before and weekly pics to chart your progress for everyone.
- Post motivational quotes that resonate with you throughout your journey.
- Share the lessons of transformation that resonate most with you. Be real and vulnerable—talk about struggles you encountered during the process and struggles you currently deal with today.
- Post recipes and exercises that you love.
- Post tips and tricks that work for you on the journey.

This isn't a ploy to get free social media. In fact, we don't care for any credit. All we want for you is to live a healthier and happier life. If you have changed your life, or are in the process of change, all we ask is that you help others through the journey. Whether it is your closest friends and family, or your online community, teaching and guiding others will engrain the lessons of transformation into your life.

This is why we have dedicated our lives to helping others. It enriches our lives beyond measure. But don't take our word for it—you just have to experience it for yourself!

# PHASE ONE'S DONE: NOW WHAT?

Congratulations on completing a 21-day phase of Extreme Transformation!

If you have reached your weight loss goal, we are so darn proud of you! Very well done! ☺

If you are still on your weight loss journey, then let's get fired up to do this again!

If you are losing weight consistently and comfortably on the Extreme Cycle, then keep everything going exactly as you have been doing it. As they say, "If it ain't broke, don't fix it!"

However, if your weight loss begins to slow at any time, there are two powerful cycles that we use to jump-start your weight loss again:

## Turbocharge the Extreme Cycle

If after a full 21 days of the Extreme Cycle you aren't dropping as fast as you should or want to, we turbocharge the cycle. Replace two of the high-carb days with low-carb days. We call this the "Turbo Cycle." This is what it looks like:

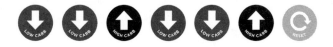

After your first 21-day phase, feel free to drop into the Turbo Cycle if you really want to speed things up.

### *The Slingshot*

If you have completed several 21-day Extreme Cycle phases, have already dropped down to the Turbo Cycle, and your weight loss has still significantly slowed or stopped, it is time for the ultimate Reset. This approach we call the Slingshot seems totally unorthodox but works like a charm to trick your body into losing weight again. Your body has likely adapted to the calorie deficit and increased activity. We have written extensively about this process in our previous books, *Choose to Lose* and *Choose More, Lose More for Life*.

Essentially, the Slingshot is a week of consecutive high-carb days—each day with double the carbs! A week doing the Slingshot looks like this:

Day 1: High-Carb Day (double your carb portion every meal)

Day 2: High-Carb Day (double your carb portion every meal)

Day 3: High-Carb Day (double your carb portion every meal)

Day 4: High-Carb Day (double your carb portion every meal)

Day 5: High-Carb Day (double your carb portion every meal)

Day 6: High-Carb Day (double your carb portion every meal)

Day 7: High-Carb Day (double your carb portion every meal)

After the Slingshot, drop back into the Extreme Cycle or Turbo Cycle and watch your weight drop like a rock again!

# Your New Life

# EMBRACING THE NEW YOU: MASTERING MAINTENANCE

**A** *huge* congratulations! Completing your Extreme Transformation is an incredible feat. It is physically, mentally, and emotionally challenging—yet unbelievably empowering in every aspect of your life. Along the way, you've lost the weight, you've come to feel more energetic, and most importantly you have created love and belief in yourself! You now know that you can do anything you set your mind to...and that you've been worth it all along. We are so proud of you.

You've been working the lessons like a warrior and we know that you feel accomplished and alive. But just like all things in life that are of value, this incredible sense of self-esteem, confidence, and love will not last forever—unless you work at it. That's what real maintenance is all about.

First, let's define what maintenance means: It's "an active process of ensuring that the necessities for a new or current state continue." Just as it takes nourishment and maintenance to keep your lawn green and your flowers in bloom, it also takes nourishment and maintenance to keep this new state of awesomeness you are now living. You must actively eat and exercise to stay at the weight you have achieved. You must also practice the lessons of transformation daily. Maintenance doesn't have to be a time-consuming process—it takes just minutes a day—but the fact remains that you still need to be beneficially selfish and spend some time and energy on yourself and your well-being every day.

In this chapter, we will lay out for you the pitfalls ahead, tell you what to expect, and help you create a bulletproof strategy to keep the weight off for years to come.

## Reality Check

If you now feel like you've completed your Extreme Transformation and believe that the process is over so you can "go back to normal"—you are very wrong. Let's not forget where living a so-called "normal" life got you last time. The majority of people who allow that mind-set to persist will spiral right back to where they started.

Remember: Transformation is a new lifestyle, not a diet that begins and ends. In other words, there is no end to your new life—it will continue forever, if you let it. Our goal is to help you find a new normal within these pages—a way to remain committed to bettering yourself and constantly striving for optimal health and happiness.

So here we are at a proverbial fork in the road. If you go in one direction, it will lead you right back to where you were. The frustration, the depression, the weight.

If you go in the other direction, it will lead you to a life of new food and physical experiences, new opportunities, and new possibilities at your ideal weight. Ten, twenty, thirty years from now, you'll still be living life at a lean and healthy weight. It is totally possible.

If you choose to continue in the direction that will lead to a fit and healthy life, we say this: Welcome to your new normal! Let's explore this new journey—to sustain your weight loss, live a happy, balanced life, and integrate some of our best tricks of the trade to handle the inevitable obstacles and challenges that lie ahead.

Read closely. This is how we do it.

## ACTIONS FOR MAINTENANCE

These **8 Actions** will help you maintain your weight loss and feel great!

## Declare Your New Goal

All of us need direction. We constantly need something to work toward. Without a goal, a purpose, it's easy to slip into a state of despair. And in despair we quickly find ourselves grasping for the comforts we once relied on to feel good and back in the grips of our vice—food.

To avoid this situation, immediately upon reaching your weight loss goal you need to have the next goal in place. Our brain needs something to strive for and a new goal or purpose to keep us happy. Think of it like that scene in *Raiders of the Lost Ark*, when Indiana Jones has to quickly switch out the gold statue with a sandbag—we've got to quickly trade your addiction again into something your brain likes for maintenance.

Over your weight loss journey, you have felt the thrill of seeing the numbers drop on the scale and squeezing into new clothes. You received accolades from your family, friends, and co-workers on a regular basis. These are payoffs you experience on a regular basis—and your brain processes these payoffs as rewards. As Bruce recalls, "Losing weight was awesome because it was always high fives and hugs from everyone. Now, nobody ever comes up to me and says, 'Bro! You're killing it in maintenance!' Or, 'Great job. You look the same!'" Now it's time to maintain because the compliments will most likely dwindle or even stop. Your clothing size will probably regulate. And the number on the scale will more or less remain the same. The satisfaction that you gained from these changes will begin to peter out and the reality of maintenance will set in.

For many, the thought of regular daily workouts for the rest of their lives can feel daunting—like an endless cycle. Let's be honest, working out just to work out can often seem more like torture. But *training* for something is totally different! We train for a payoff. Everyone we coach through maintenance continues to train for *something* to keep it fun and exciting—they regularly sign up for community events like 5Ks, triathlons, marathons, mud runs—any kind of activity to keep them getting fitter, feeling better, and thriving in their fitness community...but most important to keep them training toward another goal.

So what do you want to do?

Increase your strength? Get six-pack abs? Run a marathon? Enter a body-building contest or a CrossFit competition? Rock a slammin' body for spring break or your upcoming vacay? Your goals are limitless, and the best part is that once you reach one goal, you will always have another within reach! What-ever you choose, declare a new goal *now*, and make it SMART!

What are you going to accomplish next?

What does it look like? (Describe what it will take to achieve this goal and how you will feel when you reach it.)

When are you going to accomplish it?

Once again, surround yourself with reminders of what you will achieve next and let everyone know your new commitment. Place pictures, clothes, whatever around your house, car, workplace...everywhere!

If it's an event, sign up weeks or months in advance. Heck, sign up for several!

## Chris Tip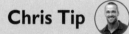

Aside from physical fitness goals, there are other incredibly powerful motivators to help engrain the maintenance lifestyle:

- Date other fitness-minded people.
- Start a weight loss website or blog.
- Begin a new career that supports your new lifestyle.
- Get involved with your community, charity, or church.

As dedicated foodies, Hannah and her husband had to replace almost all of their social activities involving food. Instead of chasing the best new restaurant, they joined a basketball league and play sand volleyball Wednesday nights. They also joined an online culinary course to learn healthy new recipes that fit into their new lifestyle!

The more you can submerge yourself in the fitness community, the greater your chances for lifelong success...oh, and you'll also meet the nicest, friendli-est, most caring people in the world!

## Review Your Support System

You've had at least 21 days to help identify who's really on your team, including your superfriend. Maybe some of your teammates have come and some have gone in that time. Whoever is on your team now will be needed just as much or more during maintenance! Sit down and communicate openly with them about your new goals and aspirations. Get them involved. They can even commit to your new maintenance activities and goals with you!

## Keep Doing the Extreme Cycle

Here's the deal. Your body still needs real, whole natural food. You still need to eat five times a day and drink plenty of water. This is for your overall health and well-being! Guys, you will need approximately 2,000 to 2,500 calories to maintain. This number can increase to 2,500 to 3,000 after about six months as your body stabilizes.

Ladies, you need approximately 1,500 calories to maintain. This number can go up to between 1,700 to 2,000 calories after six months as your body stabilizes.

The number of calories goes up or down according to how much you exercise on a daily and weekly basis, and your new physique or fitness goals.

Following the Extreme Cycle during maintenance will keep you eating five meals every day, each made up of good-quality food, and drinking plenty of water. However, there is more flexibility for introducing new foods into your lifestyle. During maintenance (and weight loss) we strongly recommend downloading a calorie tracker on your phone to monitor your daily food intake. New trackers are insanely easy to use and take literally seconds to log your food. This is what we have *all* of our participants do, and they swear by it!

And don't worry: Reset days and meals will still exist. Your body and mind will get the foods they need and crave to avoid that feeling of deprivation, even during maintenance.

## Select Your Reset Meals with Lifestyle Layers

The reset meal structure of the 21-Day Extreme Cycle may have worked perfectly for you. If rewarding yourself once a week after six days of clean eating felt good emotionally, physically, and mentally, then do not change how you reward yourself. However, if you felt deprived or restricted at all during the actual weight loss portion of the Extreme Cycle, and you feel hesitant about your ability to succeed and continue with this structure in maintenance, then it may be time to change things up a little for this next phase. Do not worry.

In this new phase of life, it is acceptable to customize your reward days, following the guidelines below, so that you feel completely physically satiated, fulfilled, and satisfied. Otherwise, maintenance will be difficult to sustain.

We call these regular rewards that are laced throughout our days "Lifestyle Layers." The layering concept relates to the idea that you will simply "lay down" more and more rewards throughout your day and week until you feel totally satisfied throughout your days, giving you the confidence to make it a long-term lifestyle.

## Choose Your Layers

Decide how many layers work for you. Here are your options:

- **Once a Week**—If you felt totally satisfied while Extreme Cycling and can maintain that pattern indefinitely, then feel free to indulge in a big reward day once a week...for life!
- **Twice a Week**—Pick two days to reward yourself. Try splitting them up, like Wednesday and Sunday.
- **Every Other Day**—If you can't have it today, you can always have it tomorrow!
- **One to Three "Daily Hugs" a Day**—First thing in the morning or later in the day, a small daily reward or two always gives us something to look forward to. Think a sugar-free candy, or low-cal specialty coffee.

Whatever you do, *do not* select to reward yourself *less* than what will satisfy you. This will lead to feelings of deprivation and inevitably going back to old destructive eating patterns. The *right* way to do maintenance is to keep laying down Lifestyle Layers until you feel satisfied, but keeping it within your calorie range!

## Heidi Tip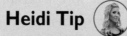

If at any time during maintenance you find the number on the scale creeping back up, simply remove one or two of your Lifestyle Layers and Extreme Cycle yourself right back down. You did it once, you can do it again!

### Plan Your Rewards

When it's time to indulge during maintenance, don't blindly wander through the days succumbing to drive-thrus and donuts that Bob from accounting brought into the office. You'll quickly find yourself pushing the parameters of maintenance.

When you plan your Lifestyle Layers, put some thought into it and treat yourself to some quality eats—because you deserve it. Maybe it's some dark chocolate, or a caramel latte from a fancy coffee shop. Think about your five favorite reward foods and list them with the portion you feel comfortable eating. Next, using the new calorie tracking app that we requested you to download, write the calorie impact of that food on the right hand side.

| Favorite Reward Food | Portion Size | Calories |
| --- | --- | --- |
|  |  |  |
|  |  |  |
|  |  |  |

Not that you have to eat from this list all of the time, but whatever you choose to indulge in, know the calorie impact and how it fits into your daily maintenance range.

### Keep Moving

For exercise, you should continue to do at least 30 minutes of moderate to intense activity daily. However, if 30 minutes is not attainable every day, then reduce your commitment to something you *know* you can do.

Maybe just start by Accelerating for 5 to 15 minutes a day again. Maybe just do one Metabolic Mission a day instead of Accelerators. As long as you keep your promises and keep moving, you will win in the long run!

## Weigh In Daily

During maintenance, weigh-ins change. It is extremely important that you weigh in at the beginning of *every* day. Start your day creating an awareness for the maintenance task at hand. While this advice may be controversial for some who worry about fixating on the scale, research has recently found that those who weigh in daily keep the weight off longer—or for life. You choose!

## The Winning Range

Research has shown that individuals who can keep their weight within a 10-pound range for over five years have a 90 percent chance of lifelong success! Give yourself an acceptable range to stay within—plus or minus 5 pounds.

My upper weight range limit for maintenance is: _____

My lower weight range limit for maintenance is: _____

Put your upper and lower range on paper and post it somewhere you will see it every day!

## Keep Taking Pictures!

Take pics of yourself weekly. Many people who have lost a significant amount of weight report still "seeing" their larger selves when they look in the mirror. Research has proven that it can take up to five years for your brain to "catch up" to the realization of your new weight. To keep a realistic view of your new body and stay motivated, take weekly pics and compare them!

# INTEGRITY IS ALWAYS THE SECRET

Building your integrity is the true secret path to dignity and ultimately losing the weight—and it is the *exact* same for maintenance. In this new chapter of your life, we set new goals, make new commitments and promises, and keep them every day. Just as keeping these promises will propel you to an extraordinary way of life and well-being, breaking these promises will do the exact opposite—they will completely derail you. Whether losing weight or keeping it off forever, your ultimate well-being will always boil down to this:

Integrity: Do what you say you're going to do, when you say you're going to do it.

## One Broken Promise Can Lead to Backslide

A lot of people lose weight. Many of them gain it back. We've all seen it— maybe it was a friend, a family member, a co-worker, or possibly even you.

We are going to teach you something very important here: Every single weight regain can be traced back to a single broken promise—a time when you didn't do what you said you were going to do, which was then followed by an internal dialogue of excuses and lies to continue to rationalize the destructive behavior. The following is a typical story of weight regain. We have dissected it so that you can see the moment integrity was broken, and how quickly the internal dialogue enabled a destructive behavior. Pay close attention; it may seem eerily familiar!

## Shari's Story

Shari lost 62 pounds over six months following the Extreme Cycle and Metabolic Missions.

Her promise: "In maintenance, I will continue to follow the Extreme Cycle and Metabolic Missions with my new added daily Lifestyle Layers to keep me satisfied and fulfilled."

Her reality: "A few weeks after hitting my goal, I felt good and on top of the world. I felt like I had weight loss and maintenance all figured out and nothing could take me down. One night, I was at a work cocktail party and kept making trips back to the bar and buffet, even though it was *way* off my maintenance plan and far beyond my Lifestyle Layers."

Her internal excuse: "I am in better shape than most of these people. I deserve to indulge here and there."

Her downslide: "A couple of days later, I was starving and stopped at a fast-food drive-thru for lunch."

Her internal excuse: "I've got this. C'mon, I've lost 62 pounds. I know what I'm doing. Plus, I worked out today."

Her further downslide: "Fast food once a day became a daily routine for me beyond my Daily Hugs and then led to more splurges in the evening. My clothes started to get tight and I was too terrified to step on the scale."

Her internal lie: "It isn't about the number on the scale anymore for me, it's about how I look and feel."

A further downslide: "Just a couple of months later I mustered up the courage to step on the scale after my clothes weren't fitting anymore, and I had gained 43 pounds back."

Reading the story, you can see numerous lessons of transformation popping out: Shari lost sight of the hidden path, she's not keeping her promises, she's not being vulnerable and authentic, she's not falling without failing to stop the downslide…the list goes on!

Whether it's eating a whole bucket of popcorn at the movies or finishing half of a pizza at your kid's party—the rules of maintenance are the same as the rules of weight loss: To get back on track and prevent sliding further downward, you must confess, reassess, and recommit. You *must* be aware of the dangerous internal conversations that follow the broken promise, full of excuses and lies. Because it always leads back to the bingeing, back to the loss of control, and back to the old you.

Nobody wants to be that cautionary tale of weight regain. We hope we've got your attention because this is the unfortunate and all-too-common reality of life after weight loss. The good news is that with your awareness, it doesn't have to happen!

# BEWARE YOUR INNER VOICE

Sometimes the first slip-up (broken promise) in maintenance is a mistake and not intentional. Sometimes it happens and we don't even realize it until later. Sometimes it seems so minuscule that you'd only be wasting someone's time to tell them about it. Doesn't matter. Once you identify the broken promise, it has to be healed. Heck, a quick phone call or three-line text to a superfriend can upright the ship in a heartbeat.

> *Messed up. Ate way too much and feel horrible about it. Recommitting now and will keep my promise to eat on plan.*

However, if the confession doesn't happen and you begin to find yourself slipping more and more…let "internal dialogue warnings" help identify when you are in a downslide situation. Here are some more dangerous internal excuses and lies that you should be aware of, and their inevitable reality. They can, and probably will, come up any day in maintenance:

Internal Dialogue: "It's finally over and I can go back to 'normal.'"

Reality: Don't forget where your old normal got you in the first place. You'll gain most, if not all, of the weight back. This way of living should be your new normal!

Internal Dialogue: "I'm going to do a muscle-bulking phase."

Reality: Addicts usually can't bulk under control. You'll be up 50 pounds before you know it. (See Lesson 20, Triggers and Tactics.)

Internal Dialogue: "I'll adjust my maintenance window 10 pounds higher because I like the way I am now."

Reality: You're only saying this because you've gained weight and don't want to put in the work to get back to your true 10-pound window. You're in a dangerous mind-set here. You're protecting your addiction, and will raise the window again as you keep gaining weight back.

Internal Dialogue: "It'll be nice to have some curves back."

Reality: Those aren't curves, it's body fat. If you want curves, lift some weight and make them *real* curves.

Internal Dialogue: "I messed up, but I'm an inspiration. I can't let them down by admitting my mistakes. They'll think less of me."

Reality: Don't get so stuck in an identity that prevents you from being great—true heroes confess, reassess, and recommit. (See Lesson 9, Be Open, Honest, and Vulnerable.) Trust us. You might be surprised at the support others give when you are authentic and share your mistakes—even coming from someone whom they consider an inspiration.

Internal Dialogue: "I saw Becky eating that junk food and she looks amazing! If she can eat that way, then I can, too, and get away with it."

Reality: You don't know *exactly* how much Becky eats or exercises during the day, so you cannot assume she's "getting away" with anything. Plus, if Becky is early in maintenance, she may be starting a slippery downward spiral. Addicts feed off other addicts to rationalize and fuel destructive behavior. Be careful.

Internal Dialogue: "I can eat this because at least I'm still smaller than Terry."

Reality: You are comparing yourself to others' weaknesses to rationalize and protect your own destructive behavior. That's not okay. You are better than that and you know it. (See Lesson 8: Believe in Yourself.)

Internal Dialogue: "I worked out extra hard today, so I've earned additional calories."

Reality: If it isn't one of your Daily Hugs, you haven't earned it. Be careful. Justification after a hard workout is a trap we can get caught in all too often. See Lesson 20: Triggers and Tactics.

What's our point here? Your inner dialogue will be around forever. Stay in touch with it and be on the lookout for negative self-talk, excuses, and other ways to rationalize breaking promises to yourself. If you're human like us, temptation will spark the voice every day. The moral of the story is that your promises *always* come first. If you end up breaking a promise, the downward spiral begins. Remember: The downward spiral doesn't have to continue. Simply confess, reassess, recommit, and get back on track to the rest of your life.

## MASTERING MAINTENANCE

As you embark upon a whole new journey of maintenance, take to heart the powerful and universal lessons you learned during your weight loss journey. We strongly advise you to *re*-learn, *re*-love, and *re*-live the 21 powerful lessons you learned during your weight loss, because they apply to your maintenance success as well! We reflect on at least one lesson every day. As Dr. Holly likes to remind our *Extreme Weight Loss* peeps, "Maintenance is a process even greater than weight loss." As her research indicates, people who not only lose weight but keep it off are those who "master" the lessons in maintenance.

Keep in mind that nobody does maintenance perfectly. However, as long as you stay connected with your support team, declare your goals, keep your promises, and stay true and vulnerable with yourself and your lifelong transformation journey, then you will always succeed. The journey of maintenance is nearly identical to the journey of weight loss. The only difference is a new goal and a few more calories. That's it.

A heartfelt welcome to the rest of your life. ☺

Chris & Heidi

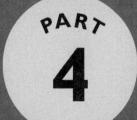

PART
4

# The Metabolic Movements

What follows is a detailed guide to all the Metabolic Movements used in the daily Missions.

## METABOLIC MISSION WARM-UP

Before your Metabolic Mission, perform this brief warm-up.

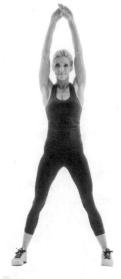

30 seconds jogging in place

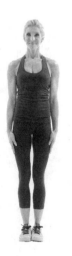
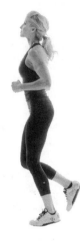
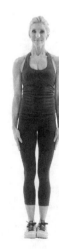

30 Jumping Jacks

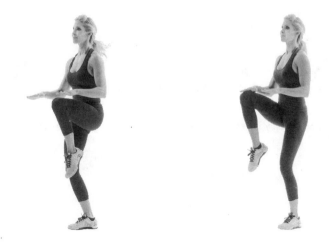

30 seconds High Knees

Then perform 10 repetitions each of the following movements. Hold each position for a brief 1–2 seconds to feel the stretch, then continue.

## Twisters

Perform 10 reps of this movement.

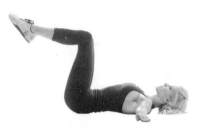 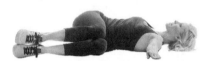 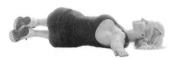

Begin lying on the floor faceup, knees and hips at a 90-degree angle as if you are sitting in a chair, arms extended to your sides.

Keeping your shoulders anchored to the floor and knees together, rotate your legs over to the left side. Touch your left knee to the floor to make a complete repetition.

Rotate your legs over to the right side and touch your right knee to the floor to make another repetition.

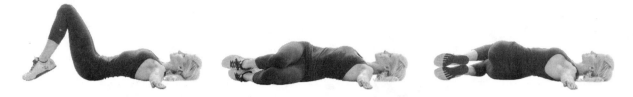

Modification: Keep your toes on the floor while rotating the knees back and forth.

## Swoops

Perform 10 reps of this movement.

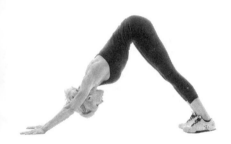 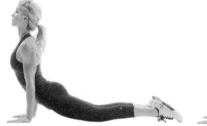 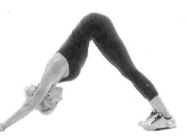

Begin in the high pike position, tucking your head between your shoulders and driving your heels into the floor.

Shift your body forward, lowering your hips to the floor. Press your shoulders down and away from your ears as you stretch your abs.

Press back into the high pike position.

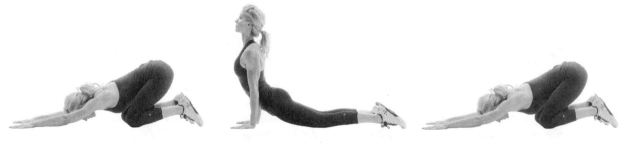

Modification: Instead of performing the movement on your feet, do it from your knees.

## Lunge Stretches

Perform 10 reps of this alternating movement.

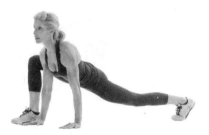 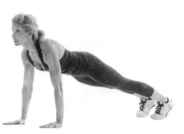 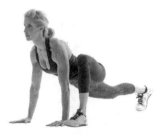

Place one foot behind you in a deep runner's lunge, keeping the back knee off the floor. Place hands on the floor inside the front knee. Shift your weight onto your front heel and feel a deep stretch in the opposition hip flexor.

Switch legs, keeping knees off the floor.

Repeat on the other side.

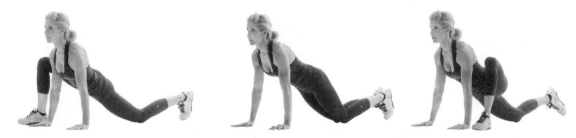

Modification: Start from your knees and alternate by placing your knees on the floor to transition into the stretch.

Here are detailed instructions for each Metabolic Movement.

## AIR SQUATS

Rules for the rep to count: At the bottom of the Air Squat, the crease of your hip must pass below the top of the kneecap. At the top of the movement, the hips and knees must be fully extended, standing upright.

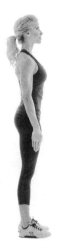
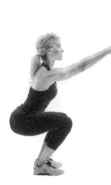
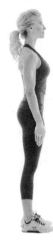

Begin in a standing position, feet shoulder width apart, toes pointed slightly out from parallel.

Keeping your weight in your heels, bend your knees and lower your buttocks down and back, as if you're being pulled backward from a belt. Reach your arms upward as the crease of your hips drops, making sure that your knees are tracking directly over your toes (not inward).

Drive upward through your heels, standing back up to the beginning position with your knees and hips extended.

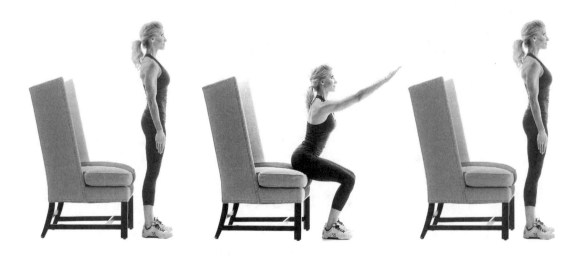

Modification: To make the exercise easier, use a chair to support the bottom of your squat. Buttocks must touch the chair.

# BACK LUNGES

Rules for the rep to count: At the bottom of the lunge, your back knee must gently "kiss" the floor. At the top of the movement, you must be standing upright with your hips and knees extended.

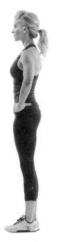
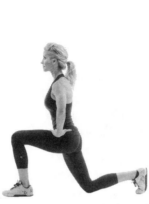
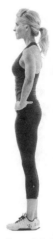

Begin in a standing position.

Take an aggressive step backward with your right foot, gently "kissing" your back knee to the floor.

Keeping your front left knee over the toe, drive the forward heel to a standing position.

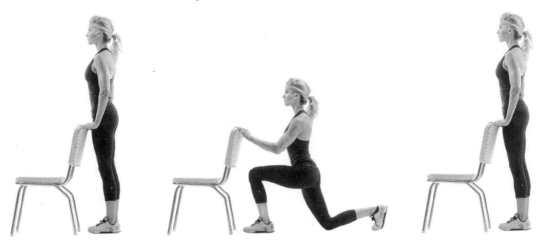

Modification: To make the exercise easier, grab onto a chair or other object for stability. When lunging, let the back knee go as low as possible, but stay in a pain-free range of motion.

# BURPEES (series)

Rules for the rep to count: You may get down to the floor however you choose, but your chest and thighs must touch the floor at the bottom of the movement, and your feet must leave the floor and hands touch overhead at the top.

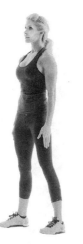

Begin standing with your feet at shoulder width.

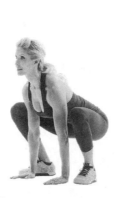

Squat down and place your hands on the floor just inside your feet.

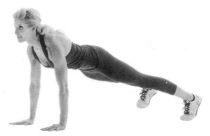

Jump back to a plank position.

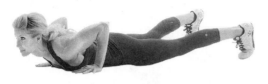

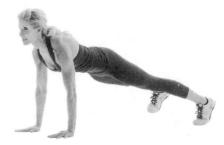

Perform a Push-Up.

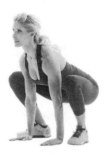

Jump forward with your feet
outside your hands.

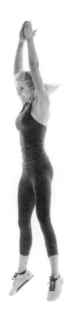

Jump up and touch your
hands overhead.

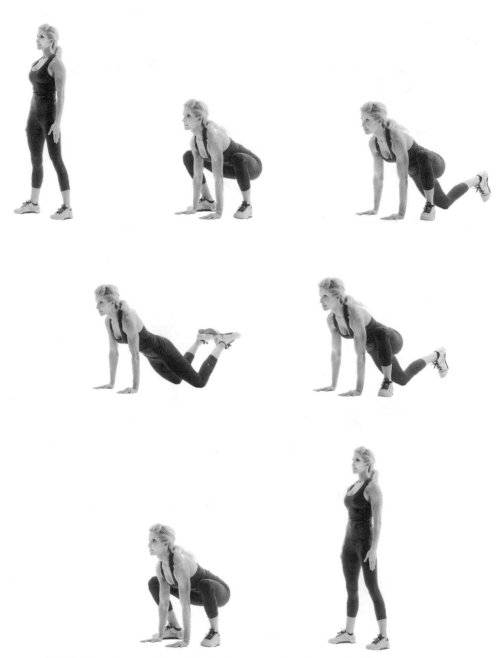

Modification: If you need to make the Burpees easier, drop to a knee or step back to the plank position. The Push-Up portion can be done from the knees or by keeping the hips on the floor. Simply stand up at the end to complete the Burpee.

## FLUTTERKICKS

Rules for the rep to count: Your knees must be extended with both feet off the floor. The heel of your top foot must rise above the toe of your bottom foot. Both legs must kick for the rep to count.

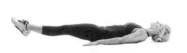 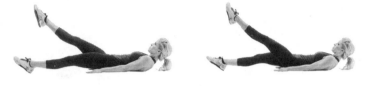

Begin lying on your back with your hands wedged under your hips. Keeping your knees extended, tighten your core and raise your feet 1 to 2 feet off the floor.

Alternate raising and lowering your legs in a "scissor kick" rhythmic motion.

Modification: Allow one heel to touch the floor while raising the other leg.

## HIGH KNEES

Rules for the rep to count: Elbows must remain at a 90-degree angle. The top of your knee must touch your hand for the rep to count.

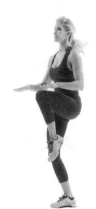 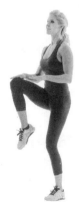 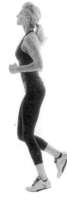

Keeping your weight on your toes, stand tall with your abs engaged. Alternate driving your knees upward toward your chest at a running tempo.

Keeping your elbows bent at 90 degrees, drive with your knees until they touch your hands.

Modification: Jog in place.

# HOLLOW ROCKS

Rules for the rep to count: At the bottom of the movement, your arms must be straight overhead and your heels must be raised at least a foot above the floor. At the top of the movement, arms must be straight overhead and your torso must be raised at least a foot off the floor.

Begin lying on your back with your arms overhead.

Lying on your back, tighten your abs and raise your arms and legs 1 to 2 feet off the floor, creating a "hollow body" position.

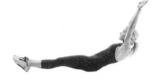

Keeping your core tight and your body rigid, allow your heels to lower back down to the floor, raising your torso off the floor.

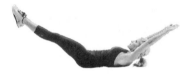

Rock back and forth in a rhythmic motion. Modification for upper body only.

Modification: Leave your heels on the floor and perform the movement using just your upper body.

# JUMPING JACKS

Rules for the rep to count: At the top of the movement you must be standing upright and hands must be touching the sides of your thighs. At the bottom of the movement, hands must touch overhead while feet land in a position wider than your shoulders.

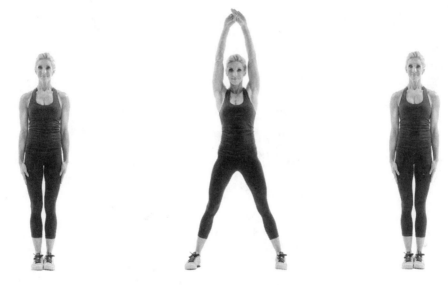

Begin in a standing position, feet together and hands at your sides.

In one motion, jump feet out to a wide stance and clap hands overhead.

Jump feet back together, bringing arms quickly back down to your sides.

Modification: Instead of jumping, step a leg out to the side.

## KICKBACKS

Rules for rep to count: At the bottom of the Kickback, your hips must be fully extended with just your hands and feet touching the floor. At the top of the movement, your hips and knees must be fully extended standing upright.

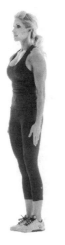
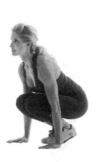
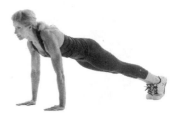

Begin standing with your feet together or at shoulder width.

Squat down and place your hands on the floor just outside your feet.

Step or jump your feet back to a Push-Up position.

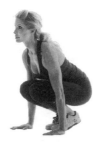
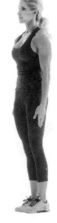

Jump forward with your feet landing outside your hands.

Stand straight up.

Modification: To make the exercise easier, step your feet back to the plank position instead of jumping.

# LEG LEVERS

Rules for the rep to count: At the bottom of the Leg Lever, the heels must touch the floor with the knees extended. At the top of the movement, with knees extended, the feet must pass through a vertical plane directly over your head.

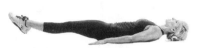 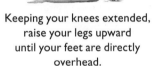 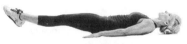

Begin lying on your back with your arms braced against the floor (or holding a chair or sofa), heels touching the floor.

Keeping your knees extended, raise your legs upward until your feet are directly overhead.

Lower your heels to the floor.

Modification: Simply alternate legs, keeping one leg on the floor and raising the other, then switch. Each leg (right and left) must raise once to count as a single rep.

## MOUNTAIN CLIMBERS (series)

Rules for rep to count: The forward foot must touch the floor at a point above the mid-shin of the back leg.

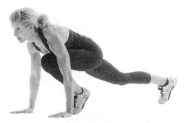

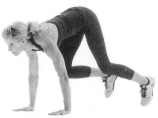

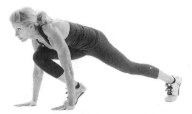

Begin in a deep runner's stance with both hands on the floor, shoulder width apart.

Keeping your abs tight, jump and switch as fast as you can.

Land gently with the opposite foot forward. As soon as your feet touch down, jump quickly and switch feet again. Switch your feet back and forth in a rhythmic motion.

Modification: To make the exercise easier, don't jump between Mountain Climbers. Just step and touch—then switch.

## PUSH-UPS

Rules for the rep to count: At the bottom of the Push-Up, your chest and thighs must touch the floor. At the top of the Push-Up, your elbows must be fully extended.

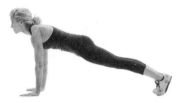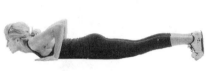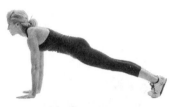

| | | |
|---|---|---|
| Begin in the plank position, hands underneath your shoulders, elbows extended and abs tight. | Bend at your elbows, lowering your body to the floor but staying rigid from your feet to your shoulders. | Immediately press upward extending your elbows, keeping your abs tight and your body rigid from your toes. |

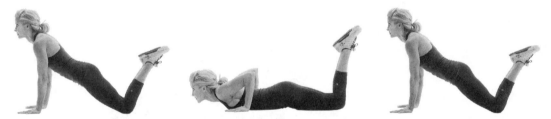

Modification 1: If you need an intermediate level Push-Up, try them from your knees.

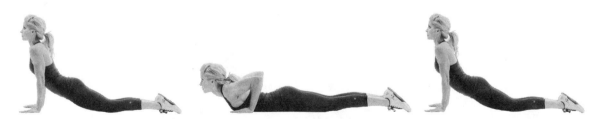

Modification 2: If you need a beginner level Push-Up, leave your hips on the floor and allow your back to extend as you press off of the floor.

# SIT-UPS

Rules for the rep to count: With legs either straight or bent, hands must touch the floor above your head at the bottom of the movement, then touch your feet at the top of the movement.

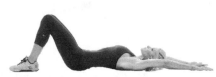
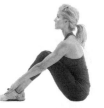
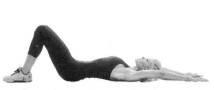

| | | |
|---|---|---|
| Begin by lying on the floor faceup, knees bent, feet flat on the floor, and arms extended overhead. | Swing your arms forward, using the momentum to raise your shoulders and torso off the floor. Touch your toes. | Extend your arms overhead as you lower your torso and shoulders back to the floor. Touch the floor overhead to complete the repetition. |

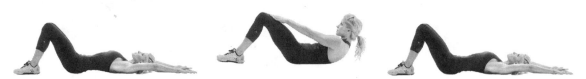

Modification 1: For a beginner Sit-Up, touch your fingers to your knees to mark the top of the rep.

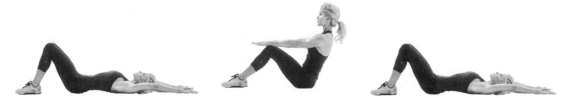

Modification 2: For an intermediate Sit-Up, touch your wrists to your knees to mark the top of the rep.

# Extreme Cycle Recipes

Although some of these recipes may seem fancy and gourmet, you don't need to be an Iron Chef to make them! If you're new to preparing your own food, don't worry—we've made it insanely simple for you. For each and every week of this program, we have created:

- A shopping list, for quick and easy grocery shopping for that week's worth of recipes.
- A meal prep guide for every three days of the program, to keep preparation for each meal to just a few minutes.
- A bulk prep cooking guide, for multiple cooking options for all of your foods.

These guides will teach you the necessary skills to conveniently prepare delicious food for the rest of your life! You'll find these step-by-step guides in the Appendices.

Note: For all recipes, 1 serving is the yield unless otherwise specified.

# BREAKFASTS

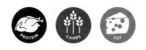

---

## Apple Cinnamon Muesli

*Breakfast*

⅓ cup rolled oats (½ cup for men)

½ cup unsweetened almond milk (¾ cup for men)

1 tablespoon fat-free plain Greek yogurt (2 tablespoons for men)

¼ cup vanilla protein powder (½ cup for men)

Dash of cinnamon

½ apple, chopped

1 tablespoon sliced almonds

Vanilla stevia drops to taste

Mix oats, almond milk, yogurt, protein powder, and cinnamon together in a bowl or in a mason jar. Top with chopped apples and sliced almonds.

Store in the fridge overnight. Eat cold. Add stevia for desired sweetness.

Women: 280 cals; 8g fat; 35g carb; 20g protein
Men: 420 cals; 11g fat; 47g carb; 37g protein

# Banana Yogurt Parfait and Pumpkin Seed Granola

*Breakfast*

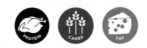

## Parfait

I cup fat-free plain Greek yogurt

I ripe banana, sliced

I tablespoon Pumpkin Seed Granola
(3 tablespoons for men)

Truvia (optional)

Top Greek yogurt and with sliced banana and Pumpkin Seed Granola (recipe follows).
Option: add some Truvia to cut the sourness of the yogurt.

## Pumpkin Seed Granola

I teaspoon extra-virgin coconut oil

¼ cup slivered almonds, raw and unsalted

¼ cup raw, unsalted pumpkin seeds

½ teaspoon Truvia sweetener

¼ teaspoon ground cinnamon or pumpkin pie spice

Pinch of ground nutmeg

Pinch of salt substitute

Heat the coconut oil in nonstick skillet over medium heat.
Toss the almonds and pumpkin seeds in coconut oil and stir to avoid burning.
Add Truvia, cinnamon, nutmeg, and salt substitute, and mix.

*Makes I serving, with leftover granola*

Women: 290 cals; 4g fat; 39g carb; 27g protein
Men: 385 cals; 12g fat; 42g carb; 30g protein

# Breakfast Frittata Veggie "Muffins"

*Breakfast*

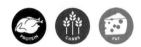

2 tablespoons extra-virgin olive oil

1 red bell pepper, small dice

3 tablespoons diced red onion

½ medium zucchini, small dice

½ medium yellow squash, small dice

6 egg whites

6 whole eggs

¼ teaspoon dried thyme

½ teaspoon salt-free onion & herb seasoning

4 ounces fat-free cheddar cheese, to be split between 12 muffins

1 cup of strawberries, sliced, on the side

Heat the olive oil over medium-high heat in a nonstick skillet.

Once oil is hot, add bell peppers, onions, zucchini, and squash. Sauté until the vegetables are soft and have a light brown color. Set aside and allow them to cool.

Meanwhile, whisk together egg whites and whole eggs along with dried thyme and onion herb seasoning.

Generously spray muffin pan with cooking spray to prevent sticking. Preheat oven to 400 degrees.

Distribute 1½ tablespoons of vegetable mixture into each muffin cup. Then evenly divide fat-free cheddar cheese between all 12 muffins.

Add egg mixture so that each cup is ¾ full.

Bake in preheated oven for approximately 20 minutes or until tops are light brown and the eggs are cooked through. Enjoy muffins with strawberries on the side.

*Makes 12 muffins*

Women (3 muffins): 285 cals; 15g fat; 17g carb; 24g protein

Men (4 muffins): 360 cals; 20g fat; 19g carb; 32g protein

## Cinnamon French Toast

*Breakfast*

1 whole egg (2 eggs for men)

1 tablespoon unsweetened almond milk

Dash of cinnamon

2 slices low-sodium Ezekiel Sprouted
   Grain Bread

¼ cup low-fat cottage cheese (½ cup for
   men) (low sodium)

Vanilla stevia drops for sweetness

¼ cup berries

2 tablespoons sugar-free syrup

Spray a pan or skillet with cooking spray and place on medium heat.

Beat the egg, almond milk, and cinnamon together in a shallow dish. Dip both slices of the bread into the mixture, coating both sides. Place on the skillet and cook until the bread is brown on both sides.

Mix together the cottage cheese and stevia drops. Top French toast with sweetened cottage cheese, berries, and syrup. Enjoy!

Women: 295 cals; 6g fat; 39g carb; 21g protein
Men: 400 cals; 11g fat; 42g carb; 33g protein

## Egg and Cheddar Sandwich

*Breakfast*

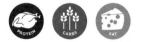

5 ounces sweet potato, cut into 4 rounds
   (6 ounces for men)

2 whole eggs (3 eggs + 1 egg white for
   men)

½ slice cheddar cheese

½ cup spinach

Preheat oven to 425 degrees. Spray baking sheet with cooking spray. Slice the sweet potato and place it on a greased baking sheet. Bake 20 minutes, then flip. Bake another 20 minutes.

Spray a frying pan with cooking spray and fry the eggs over medium-high heat until cooked through. Cut the fried eggs in half, and then fold in half.

Make 2 sandwiches by layering a sweet potato round, fried egg, ½ of the cheese and spinach, and another sweet potato round.

Women: 310 cals; 11g fat; 30g carb; 17g protein
Men: 420 cals; 15g fat; 36g carb; 27g protein

## Green Machine Pancakes

*Breakfast*

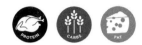

2 whole eggs (3 eggs for men)

¼ cup low-fat cottage cheese

¼ cup rolled oats (⅓ cup for men)

½ banana

½ cup of spinach (1 cup for men)

1 tablespoon sugar-free syrup

Spray skillet or griddle with cooking spray and preheat to 300 degrees.

Place all ingredients except syrup in a blender and blend until smooth.

Pour the batter slowly onto griddle. Once bubbles form on top of pancake, flip. Top with sugar-free syrup.

*Makes about 6 pancakes*

Women: 315 cals; 11g fat; 30g carb; 22g protein
Men: 411 cals; 16g fat; 35g carb; 29g protein

## Hot Quinoa Cereal with Banana

*Breakfast*

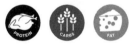

½ cup unsweetened vanilla almond milk

½ teaspoon Truvia sweetener

¼ teaspoon ground cinnamon

Pinch of ground nutmeg

½ cup cooked quinoa

½ scoop vanilla protein powder (1 scoop for men)

½ banana, sliced (1 full banana for men)

1 tablespoon Pumpkin Seed Granola (page 212)

In a small pot bring almond milk, Truvia, cinnamon, and nutmeg to a light simmer.

Add cooked quinoa and stir. Then add the scoop of protein powder and stir until protein is thoroughly dissolved.

Transfer to a bowl and top with sliced banana and granola.

Women: 300 cals; 9g fat; 37g carb; 20g protein
Men: 420 cals; 10g fat; 52g carb; 34g protein

# Huevos Rancheros

*Breakfast*

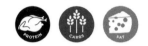

## Egg Scramble

1 teaspoon extra-virgin olive oil (2 teaspoons for men)
½ cup red bell pepper, diced
½ cup green bell pepper, diced
¼ cup red onion, diced
4 egg whites (6 egg whites for men)

Pinch of black pepper
Pinch of salt-free southwest seasoning
1 tablespoon low-fat mozzarella cheese (2 tablespoons for men)
2 tablespoons fresh salsa

In a nonstick skillet, heat the extra-virgin olive oil and lightly sauté the peppers and onions. Once the vegetables are soft, add egg whites, black pepper, and southwest seasoning.

Scramble the egg mixture until egg whites are fully cooked. Serve over tostadas. Top with cheese and fresh salsa.

## Tostadas

2 yellow corn tortillas

Lightly spray tortilla with cooking spray and bake in a 425-degree oven until golden brown and crispy.

Women: 300 cals; 8g fat; 35g carb; 21g protein
Men: 390 cals; 15g fat; 36g carb; 30g protein

## "Loaded" Breakfast Potato

*Breakfast*

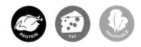

6 tablespoons fat-free plain Greek yogurt
(¾ cup for men)

Truvia sweetener

Pinch of ground cinnamon

1 tablespoon unsalted almond butter

¼ cup quinoa, cooked

4 ounces (½ cup) cooked sweet potato
(6 ounces or ¾ cup for men)

In a small dish, mix the yogurt, Truvia, and cinnamon.

In a separate dish, mix the almond butter with the quinoa.

Slice the warm potato down the middle and spread it open. Top with the almond butter mixture and then top with cinnamon yogurt.

Women: 300 cals; 10g fat; 38g carb; 15g protein
Men: 400 cals; 10g fat; 52g carb; 25g protein

## No-Bake Oats

*Breakfast*

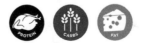

⅓ cup rolled oats

¼ cup vanilla or chocolate protein powder (½ cup for men)

2 tablespoons powdered peanut butter

2 teaspoons ground flaxseed or chia seeds

⅓ cup unsweetened almond milk

½ banana, sliced (⅔ banana for men)

Dash of cinnamon

Mix the oats, protein powder, powdered peanut butter, and flax or chia seeds. Add the almond milk. Stir. Top with banana slices and a dash of cinnamon.

Women: 300 cals; 8g fat; 40g carb; 24g protein
Men: 400 cals; 10g fat; 47g carb; 38g protein

## Power Mocha Shake with Fruit

*Breakfast*

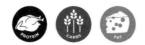

8 ounces black coffee, room temperature

1 scoop chocolate protein powder (1½ scoops for men)

¼ teaspoon ground cinnamon

½ tablespoon coconut oil

6–8 ice cubes (or 1 cup)

Blend everything in a blender until smooth. Enjoy with a side of sliced fruit: 1 banana (1½ bananas for men) or 1 cup berries (1½ cups for men).

Women: 300 cals; 10g fat; 28g carb; 28g protein
Men: 370 cals; 11g fat; 30g carb; 41g protein

## Pumpkin Spice Vanilla Protein Pancakes

*Breakfast*

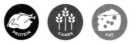

½ scoop vanilla protein powder (¾ scoop for men)

¼ cup pumpkin puree

1 teaspoon coconut oil

½ teaspoon ground cinnamon

¼ teaspoon ground nutmeg

½ teaspoon baking powder

1 large egg white

¼ cup steel-cut oats

⅓ cup water

1 teaspoon Truvia sweetener

¼ cup sugar-free pancake syrup

½ tablespoon Pumpkin Seed Granola (page 212)

½ banana, sliced (men only)

Add all ingredients except syrup, granola, and banana to the blender and blend until smooth.

Heat a nonstick griddle or skillet coated with cooking spray over medium heat. Ladle about ¼ cup of pancake batter per pancake onto griddle or skillet. Once pancake tops are covered with bubbles and edges look cooked, they are ready to flip. Cook both sides. Serve immediately. Top with syrup, granola, and banana (for men).

*Makes 4 pancakes*

Women: 310 cals; 11g fat; 34g carb; 25g protein
Men: 400 cals; 12g fat; 48g carb; 32g protein

## Raspberry Almond Oatmeal

*Breakfast*

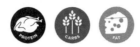

⅓ cup rolled oats (½ cup for men)

½ cup water

2 teaspoons all-natural almond butter

1 tablespoon unsweetened almond milk (2 tablespoons for men)

⅛ teaspoon pure almond extract (optional)

¼ cup vanilla protein powder (½ cup for men)

½ cup raspberries

1 teaspoon slivered almonds

Dash of cinnamon

Vanilla stevia drops for sweetness

Mix the oats and water together. Microwave 1–2 minutes.

Stir in almond butter, almond milk, and almond extract (if using). Stir in protein powder. Top with raspberries, almonds, and cinnamon. Add stevia if needed for sweetness. Eat warm.

You can also make this the night before by mixing all the ingredients together and storing in the fridge overnight without cooking. Eat cold.

Women: 285 cals; 11g fat; 30g carb; 20g protein
Men: 405 cals; 14g fat; 41g carb; 35g protein

## Scrambled Eggs and Hash

*Breakfast*

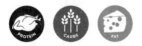

½ cup mushrooms, sliced (1 cup for men)

¼ cup yellow onions, diced

4 ounces red potatoes, grated (5 ounces for men)

1 cup spinach, chopped

2 whole eggs (3 eggs + 1 egg white for men)

2 tablespoons fresh salsa

Heat pan or skillet to medium-high heat.

Spray pan with cooking spray. Sauté the mushrooms, onions, and potatoes together for 5 minutes. Add the spinach and eggs. Cook until the eggs are cooked through. Top with salsa.

Women: 293 cals; 10g fat; 27g carb; 18g protein
Men: 414 cals; 15g fat; 33g carb; 29g protein

## Sweet Potato Fritters

*Breakfast*

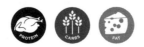

1 ounce ground beef, browned (2 ounces for men)

2 tablespoons yellow onions, browned

2 whole eggs

3 ounces sweet potatoes, grated (4 ounces for men)

Salt-free garlic & herb seasoning

Black pepper

2 tablespoons low-fat mozzarella cheese

Preheat oven to 350 degrees.

Brown the ground beef with the onions. Set aside.

Beat the eggs. Add the ground beef, sweet potatoes, and seasonings. Mix well.

Spoon mixture into 2–3 well-greased muffin cups. Bake for 20 minutes. Pull out and sprinkle with cheese. Bake an additional 5–10 minutes.

Women: 300 cals; 14g fat; 20g carb; 21g protein
Men: 400 cals; 20g fat; 22g carb; 28g protein

## Turkey and Potato Skillet Breakfast

*Breakfast*

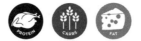

1 teaspoon extra-virgin olive oil (2 teaspoons for men)

3 ounces extra-lean ground turkey breast (4 ounces for men)

½ red bell pepper, large dice

½ green bell pepper, large dice

¼ red onion, large dice

¼ teaspoon salt-free garlic & herb seasoning

Pinch of whole fennel seed

Pinch of dried oregano

Pinch of dried basil

Pinch of salt substitute

Pinch of ground black pepper

3 small sage leaves, fresh, chopped

½ cup cooked sweet potatoes, diced (¾ cup for men)

Heat olive oil in a nonstick skillet over medium heat.

Crumble ground turkey into skillet and stir to prevent sticking.

Add bell peppers and onions and cook until soft. Add garlic and herb seasoning, fennel seed, oregano, basil, salt substitute, black pepper, and sage. Stir to mix thoroughly.

Add sweet potatoes and cook until potatoes are heated through and have slight golden color.

Women: 275 cals; 6g fat; 32g carb; 23g protein
Men: 390 cals; 11g fat; 42g carb; 31g protein

---

## Turkey Frittata

*Breakfast*

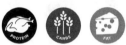

| | |
|---|---|
| 1 ounce extra-lean ground turkey | 1 tablespoon diced onion |
| ⅔ cup grated sweet potatoes (1 cup for men) | 2 small mushrooms, sliced |
| ¼ teaspoon dried oregano | 1 whole egg |
| ¼ teaspoon dried basil | 1 egg white (3 whites for men) |
| Pinch of salt substitute | 2 tablespoons shredded mozzarella cheese |
| Pinch of ground black pepper | 3 cherry tomatoes, halved |
| Pinch of whole fennel seeds | ¼ cup parsley leaves, rinsed |

Lightly spray cooking spray over the grated potatoes and microwave 2 minutes.

Heat a nonstick frying pan over medium-high heat. Spray with cooking spray and crumble in ground turkey. Once turkey has a slight brown color, add oregano, basil, salt substitute, black pepper, fennel seeds, diced onions, and sliced mushrooms.

Cook mixture until vegetables are soft and turkey is fully cooked.

Add eggs and cheese. Cover and cook until eggs are cooked through.

Toss halved cherry tomatoes and parsley and place on top.

Women: 292 cals; 8g fat; 31g carb; 24g protein
Men: 385 cals; 8g fat; 44g carb; 32g protein

# HIGH-CARB MEALS

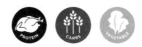

---

## Apple and Dip

*High-Carb Meal*

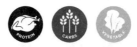

3 tablespoons fat-free plain Greek yogurt
   (6 tablespoons for men)

½ scoop vanilla protein powder
   (1 scoop for men)

2 tablespoons powdered peanut butter

Dash of cinnamon

1 medium apple (1 large apple for men)

Stevia, to taste

Mix yogurt, protein powder, peanut butter powder, stevia, and cinnamon.
Slice apple and dip!

Women: 240 cals; 3g fat; 34g carb; 24g protein
Men: 355 cals; 4g fat; 43g carb; 42g protein

---

## Barbecue Chicken Salad

*High-Carb Meal*

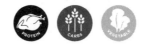

### Salad

1 ounce chicken breast, cooked and
   cubed (3 ounces for men)

1 tablespoon low-sodium barbecue sauce
   (3 tablespoons for men)

2 cups romaine lettuce, chopped

½ tomato, diced

¼ cup black beans

¼ cup fresh corn

Mix barbecue sauce with chicken, set aside.
Make salad by layering lettuce, tomatoes, beans, corn, and chicken.

## Cilantro Lime Dressing

¼ cup fat-free plain Greek yogurt
1 tablespoon Homemade Ranch Powder
   (see recipe below)

Pinch of cilantro
1 teaspoon lime juice
1 tablespoon low-sodium barbecue sauce

Make dressing by blending Greek yogurt, Ranch Powder, cilantro, and lime juice together. This recipe makes a lot of dressing; add to salad a tablespoon at a time. Top with remaining 1 tablespoon barbecue sauce.

## Homemade Ranch Powder

½ cup dried buttermilk
1 tablespoon dried parsley flakes
1 teaspoon dried dill weed
1 teaspoon dried minced onion

1 teaspoon onion powder
½ teaspoon garlic powder
¼ teaspoon ground black pepper

In a small bowl, whisk all ingredients until combined.

Women: 260 cals; 5g fat; 44g carb; 24g protein
Men: 370 cals; 7g fat; 48g carb; 41g protein

---

# BBQ Baked Sweet Potato, Loaded with Grilled Chicken, Corn, and Black Beans

*High-Carb Meal*

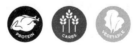

½ cup baked sweet potato (¾ cup for men)
2 ounces grilled diced chicken (3 ounces for men)
2 tablespoons frozen corn, thawed
¼ cup cooked black beans

1 tablespoon reduced-sugar barbecue sauce
Pinch of black pepper
Pinch of salt substitute
¼ cup chopped steamed broccoli

Poke holes in the sweet potato and bake it in the oven at 400 degrees for 45 minutes or for 8 minutes in the microwave.

In a mixing bowl, mix the grilled chicken, thawed corn, cooked black beans, and barbecue sauce and season with black pepper and salt substitute. Stir until all ingredients have been evenly coated with sauce. Spoon the mixture into the middle of the sweet potato. Place the broccoli on top of the chicken mixture.

Women: 290 cals; 5g fat; 44g carb; 25g protein
Men: 385 cals; 6g fat; 54g carb; 35g protein

---

# Butternut Squash Chili

### *High-Carb Meal*

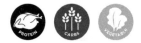

8 ounces extra-lean ground turkey

Cooking spray

2 cups peeled and cubed butternut squash

½ cup red onion, medium dice

2 tablespoons garlic, minced

½ cup red bell pepper, medium dice

½ cup green bell pepper, medium dice

½ medium jalapeño, stems and seeds removed (add more for extra heat)

2 tablespoons ground cumin

1 tablespoon light chili powder

½ tablespoon salt substitute

1 tablespoon smoked paprika

½ tablespoon ground mustard

1 quart water

1½ cups diced tomatoes in the can, no salt

4 tablespoons tomato paste

¼ cup apple cider vinegar

½ cup cooked black beans, no salt

½ cup cooked garbanzo beans, no salt

½ cup cilantro, rinsed and chopped

½ cup edamame, shelled

Brown the ground turkey and set aside. Spray a large pot with cooking spray, then over medium-high heat. Add the squash and stir until the squash has a light caramelized color.

Add the onions, garlic, red bell pepper, green bell pepper, and jalapeño. Stir and cook until the onions are translucent and the peppers are semi-soft.

Add the browned ground turkey, cumin, chili powder, salt substitute, paprika, mustard, water, canned tomatoes, tomato paste, and vinegar.

Simmer chili on medium-low for about 25 minutes or until the squash is tender.

Add the black beans, garbanzo beans, cilantro, and edamame. Stir to incorporate beans. Separate into 3 servings.

Note: This chili recipe is a Powell Pack favorite, so here's a three-serving recipe so there's enough to go around. If you're cooking for one, be sure to measure out your portion, then store and refrigerate the rest for healthy meals over the next few days.

*Makes 3 servings*

Women (1 serving): 294 cals; 3g fat; 39g carb; 29g protein
Men (1⅓ servings): 392 cals; 4g fat; 52g carb; 38g protein

## Chicken Fajita Bowl

*High-Carb Meal*

½ cup onions, chopped

½ cup bell peppers, chopped

¼ cup brown rice, cooked (⅓ cup for men)

2 ounces chicken breast, cooked and cubed (4 ounces for men)

2 tablespoons black beans (¼ cup for men)

1 tablespoon low-fat mozzarella cheese

2 tablespoons fresh salsa

1 tablespoon fat-free plain Greek yogurt

Slice the onions into rings and the peppers into thin strips. Spray a frying pan or skillet with cooking spray and sauté until peppers are tender and onions are translucent.

Layer the rice, chicken, onions, peppers, black beans, cheese, salsa, and Greek yogurt. Enjoy!

Women: 292 cals; 6g fat; 38g carb; 26g protein
Men: 394 cals; 8g fat; 49g carb; 37g protein

## Chile Relleno, Braised Adobo Chicken, Black Bean and Quinoa Salad

*High-Carb Meal*

### Adobo Chicken

½ cup fresh salsa

½ teaspoon garlic, minced

2 tablespoons red onion, diced

¼ teaspoon salt-free southwest chipotle seasoning

½ teaspoon salt-free tomato basil seasoning

½ jalapeño, stems and seeds removed and finely diced

2 ounces grilled and diced marinated chicken (3 ounces chicken for men) (Marinade recipe below)

½ teaspoon fresh lime juice

2 teaspoons cilantro, rinsed and chopped

1 medium poblano pepper, dry roasted and peeled

In a skillet over medium heat, add the salsa, garlic, onion, southwest seasoning, tomato basil seasoning, and jalapeño. Bring to a simmer; add diced grilled chicken, lime juice, and cilantro.

Heat until chicken is hot all the way through.

Cut a slit in the pepper and stuff with chicken mixture. Microwave until hot. Serve over Black Bean and Quinoa Salad.

## Marinade

3 sprigs fresh thyme or pinch of dried thyme
3 sprigs of fresh tarragon
1 tablespoon chopped garlic
1 tablespoon chopped yellow onion

2 tablespoons lemon juice
1 teaspoon salt-free chicken seasoning
½ teaspoon salt substitute
⅛ teaspoon black pepper
½ cup water

Place the thyme, tarragon, garlic, chopped onion, lemon juice, chicken seasoning, salt substitute, black pepper, and water in blender and blend until smooth.

## Black Bean and Quinoa Salad

¼ cup cooked quinoa (½ cup for men)
¼ cup thawed corn
¼ cup cooked black beans
1 teaspoon salt-free garlic & herb seasoning

½ teaspoon salt-free southwest seasoning
½ teaspoon salt-free chicken seasoning
2 tablespoons fresh lime juice
Pinch of salt substitute
1 tablespoon cilantro, chopped and rinsed

Cook the quinoa and cool, toss with corn, black beans, garlic herb seasoning, southwest seasoning, chicken seasoning, fresh lime juice, salt substitute, and cilantro.

Women: 273 cals; 2g fat; 30g carb; 19g protein
Men: 349 cals; 5g fat; 40g carb; 26g protein

# Chocolate Peanut Butter and Banana Smoothie

*High-Carb Meal*

1 frozen banana, chopped

½ scoop chocolate protein powder (1 scoop for men)

2 tablespoons chocolate peanut butter powder

1 tablespoon flax seeds

½ cup unsweetened vanilla almond milk (1 cup for men)

2 tablespoons rolled oats (men only)

6–8 ice cubes (or 1 cup)

Place all ingredients in a blender. Blend until smooth.

Women: 275 cals; 7g fat; 36g carb; 22g protein
Men: 400 cals; 11g fat; 46g carb; 37g protein

# Egg Salad on Toast

*High-Carb Meal*

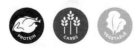

4 boiled egg whites (6 egg whites for men)

1 tablespoon low-fat mayo (2 tablespoons for men)

1 cup spinach

2 slices Ezekiel low-sodium bread, toasted

Paprika

Black pepper

½ cup blueberries (1 cup for men)

Boil eggs for 10–12 minutes. Place in ice water until cool. Peel eggs and separate yolk from white. Discard yolk.

Mash egg whites and mayo together in a bowl.

Layer ½ cup spinach on each piece of toast and top with egg salad. Sprinkle paprika and pepper over the top. Enjoy blueberries on the side.

Women: 290 cals; 3g fat; 44g carb; 24g protein
Men: 380 cals; 4g fat; 56g carb; 32g protein

# Greek Yogurt Parfait with Fruit

*High-Carb Meal*

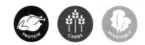

⅔ cup fat-free plain Greek yogurt
   (1¼ cups for men)
Vanilla liquid stevia drops for sweetness
   (optional)

½ cup sliced blackberries
½ cup strawberries, chopped
½ banana, sliced (1 banana for men)
Dash of cinnamon

Sweeten yogurt with stevia if desired. Top yogurt with blackberries, strawberries, bananas, and cinnamon.

Women: 290 cals; 4g fat; 36g carb; 20g protein
Men: 380 cals; 5g fat; 55g carb; 34g protein

# Green Chili Turkey and Cilantro Rice Bowl

*High-Carb Meal*

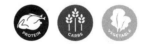

## Green Chili Turkey

3 ounces extra-lean ground turkey
   (4 ounces for men)
1 red bell pepper, diced
¼ cup red onion, chopped
1 medium poblano pepper, roasted and
   diced
1 small green tomatillo or green tomato
¼ teaspoon ground cumin

¼ teaspoon smoked paprika
¼ teaspoon dried oregano
Pinch of salt substitute
Pinch of ground black pepper
¼ cup water
Pinch of ground cayenne pepper
1 tablespoon cilantro, rinsed and chopped
Juice of ½ lime

Heat a skillet to medium-high heat. Spray with cooking spray. Crumble turkey into the skillet and stir to break up into small pieces.

Add bell peppers, red onion, roasted poblano, green tomatillo, cumin, paprika, oregano, salt substitute, black pepper, water, and cayenne. Stir and cook until turkey is cooked through.

Add cilantro and lime juice. Serve over Cilantro Rice.

## Cilantro Rice

¼ cup cooked brown rice (½ cup for
   men)
1 tablespoon chopped cilantro
½ tablespoon lime juice

Pinch of ground cumin
Pinch of salt substitute
Pinch of black pepper

Cook rice and toss with cilantro, lime juice, cumin, salt substitute, and black pepper.

## Green Beans

1 cup of green beans

Steam and toss with turkey mixture. Serve over Cilantro Rice.

Women: 305 cals; 3g fat; 44g carb; 27g protein
Men: 390 cals; 4g fat; 55g carb; 34g protein

# Grilled Ginger Lime Tuna and Steamed Vegetable Medley

*High-Carb Meal*

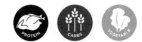

## Tuna

½ tablespoon rice vinegar, unseasoned
¾ teaspoon salt-free onion & herb
   seasoning
1 tablespoon ginger, minced
¼ teaspoon Sriracha sauce

¼ teaspoon Truvia sweetener
Pinch of salt substitute
Pinch of ground black pepper
4 ounces wild tuna (6 ounces for men)
1 lime wedge

In a medium mixing bowl, whisk together vinegar, onion and herb seasoning, minced ginger, Sriracha sauce, Truvia sweetener, salt substitute, ground black pepper, and juice from lime wedge until sweetener is dissolved. Once mixed, pour over tuna and spread evenly.
   Marinate for at least one hour, being sure to rotate after 30 minutes.
   Grill to preferred doneness, slice, and serve over rice and vegetables.

## Vegetables

¾ cup snap peas

1½ ounces carrots, cut to preference

1 ounce chopped asparagus

½ cup steamed brown rice (1 cup for men)

Steam vegetables and toss together with rice.

Women: 268 cals; 5g fat; 22g carb; 27g protein

Men: 376 cals; 6g fat; 44g carb; 32g protein

---

# Grilled Greek Chicken Kebabs

### *High-Carb Meal*

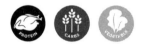

## Kebabs

2 ounces marinated chicken breast
    (4 ounces for men)

Use Marinade recipe for chicken and then weigh and skewer chicken. Grill until chicken is cooked through. Serve potatoes and cauliflower on the side, and drizzle the kebabs and vegetables with yogurt sauce. The yogurt sauce can also be used as a dipping sauce.

## Marinade

3 sprigs fresh thyme or pinch of dried thyme

3 sprigs fresh tarragon

1 tablespoon chopped garlic

1 tablespoon chopped yellow onion

2 tablespoons lemon juice

1 teaspoon salt-free chicken seasoning

½ teaspoon salt substitute

Black pepper, to taste

½ cup water

Place thyme, tarragon, garlic, chopped onion, lemon juice, chicken seasoning, salt substitute, black pepper, and water in blender and blend until smooth. Marinate chicken in mixture for 2–24 hours.

## Roasted Potatoes

1 cup red potatoes cut into wedges
   (1½ cups for men)

¼ teaspoon extra-virgin olive oil

1 sprig rosemary, chopped fine

Dash of salt substitute

Dash of ground black pepper

In a small pot, boil the potatoes in water until fork tender but not overcooked. Drain well and toss with extra-virgin olive oil.

In a skillet over high heat, lightly spray with cooking spray. Add potato wedges and stir frequently. Potatoes will get light brown in color. When this happens, add chopped rosemary, salt substitute, and ground black pepper. Stir well and remove from heat.

## Yogurt Sauce

1 tablespoon fat-free plain Greek yogurt

1 tablespoon cucumber, small dice

4 small mint leaves, chopped

½ tablespoon green onion, chopped fine

½ teaspoon fresh lemon juice

Pinch of salt substitute

Pinch of black pepper

Mix all ingredients in a small bowl and allow to sit for 30 minutes before use. This will help the flavor develop better.

## Cauliflower

4 ounces or 1 cup cauliflower "steak"—
   feel free to use florets already cut

¼ teaspoon salt-free onion & herb
   seasoning

¼ teaspoon olive oil

In a small skillet, cover cauliflower halfway with water and bring to a simmer. After 3 minutes, flip the cauliflower and let it simmer another 2 minutes. Remove from water and drain excess water.

In a small skillet, heat olive oil over medium-high heat. Season cauliflower on both sides with onion herb seasoning. Brown both sides of cauliflower, approximately 2 minutes on each side.

Women: 290 cals; 4g fat; 40g carb; 25g protein
Men: 410 cals; 5g fat; 56g carb; 36g protein

# Homemade Tortilla Chips with Tomato Salsa

*High-Carb Meal*

## *Tortilla Chips*

3 6-inch yellow corn tortillas (4 for men)
Pinch of cumin
Pinch of salt substitute

2 ounces shredded chicken (3 ounces for men)
½ cup Tomato Salsa (recipe below)

Cut the tortillas into wedges and lay them on a baking sheet lined with foil.

Preheat oven to 400 degrees. Lightly spray the tortillas with cooking spray and bake in the oven until crispy and golden brown.

Remove from the oven and sprinkle with cumin and salt substitute, then top with chicken and salsa.

## *Tomato Salsa*

1 cup chopped fresh tomatoes
½ cup chopped red onion
¼ jalapeño, stem and seeds removed
10 sprigs cilantro, rinsed
1 tablespoon chopped garlic
2 tablespoons lime juice

1 teaspoon salt-free southwest seasoning
½ teaspoon salt substitute
½ teaspoon ground cumin
½ teaspoon light chili powder
¼ teaspoon ground black pepper

Place all ingredients in a blender and pulse until a salsa-like texture has been achieved.

Women: 290 cals; 4g fat; 40g carb; 22g protein
Men: 390 cals; 6g fat; 51g carb; 32g protein

## Honey Dijon Chicken Snack Wrap

*High-Carb Meal*

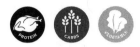

2 ounces chicken breast, cooked and
shredded (3 ounces for men)

1 Ezekiel tortilla (1½ tortillas for men)

1 cup baby spinach

½ cup sprouts

½ cup cucumbers, chopped

1 tablespoon honey Dijon mustard

Cracked pepper

Cook the chicken breast and shred it with two forks. Place it in the fridge to cool.
Pile all ingredients into the tortilla and roll up. Eat cold.

Women: 280 cals; 6g fat; 30g carb; 25g protein
Men: 400 cals; 9g fat; 42g carb; 37g protein

## Hulk Shake

*High-Carb Meal*

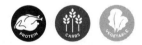

4 ounces fresh orange juice (6 ounces for
men)

2 cups power greens (spinach, chard, or
kale)

⅔ cup fat-free plain Greek yogurt

¼ cup vanilla protein powder (men only)

1 frozen banana

Vanilla stevia drops for sweetness

6–8 ice cubes (or 1 cup)

Place all ingredients in a blender. Blend until smooth. Add water if needed to blend.

Women: 270 cals; 1g fat; 49g carb; 20g protein
Men: 365 cals; 2g fat; 57g carb; 34g protein

## Italian Tuna and White Bean Lettuce Wraps

*High-Carb Meal*

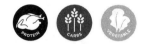

2 ounces canned light white tuna, no salt added (4 ounces for men)

⅔ cup white beans, boiled, no salt (1 cup for men)

¼ red bell pepper, diced

1 teaspoon diced red onion

½ tablespoon parsley, chopped

¼ teaspoon salt-free tomato basil seasoning

1 sprig fresh tarragon, chopped

1 medium basil leaf, chopped

1 radish, sliced thin

¼ cup diced tomatoes

1 teaspoon balsamic vinegar

Pinch of salt substitute

Pinch of black pepper

1 teaspoon fresh lemon juice

3 large lettuce leaves; Boston, Bibb, or red leaf work well (more lettuce can be used)

Drain tuna and transfer to a medium mixing bowl. Add white beans, red bell pepper, red onion, chopped parsley, tomato basil seasoning, tarragon, basil, radish, diced tomatoes, balsamic vinegar, salt substitute, black pepper, and fresh lemon juice. Toss to ensure ingredients are evenly distributed.

Distribute evenly and serve in 3 lettuce leaves.

*Makes 1 serving.*

Women: 260 cals; 2g fat; 36g carb; 27g protein
Men: 400 cals; 2g fat; 51g carb; 45g protein

## Lemon Poppy Seed Protein Bites

*High-Carb Meal*

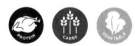

¾ cup oat flour (this can also be made by blending 1 cup of oats in a food processor)

3 scoops vanilla protein powder

½ teaspoon baking soda

2 teaspoons poppy seeds

4 egg whites

1 cup unsweetened applesauce

2 tablespoons fat-free plain Greek yogurt

¼ cup lemon juice

1½ tablespoons lemon zest

2 teaspoons vanilla extract

Preheat the oven to 350 degrees. Prepare a 9 x 9-inch tin with cooking spray. In a small bowl, mix the oat flour, protein powder, baking soda, and poppy seeds.

In a separate bowl, mix together the egg whites, applesauce, yogurt, lemon juice, lemon zest, and vanilla extract.

Slowly add the dry ingredients to the wet ingredients and stir until everything is fully incorporated.

Pour mixture into sprayed pan and bake for about 30 minutes or until a toothpick comes out clean and the sides are light brown.

Remove from oven and allow to cool completely before cutting.

Note: Freeze leftovers and save for day 11.

*Makes 12 evenly cut bars*

Women (4 bars): 245 cals; 4g fat; 27g carb; 27g protein
Men (6 bars): 370 cals; 6g fat; 40g carb; 40g protein

---

# Loaded Potato

*High-Carb Meal*

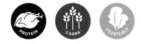

6 ounces red potato (8 ounces for men)

2 ounces extra-lean ground turkey, browned (4 ounces for men)

2 tablespoons yellow onions, browned

2 tablespoons shredded low-fat mozzarella cheese

2 tablespoons fat-free plain Greek yogurt (3 tablespoons for men)

2 teaspoons chives, chopped

½ tablespoon Homemade Ranch Powder (page 223)

Preheat oven to 400 degrees.

Poke holes in the potato with a fork. Wrap it in foil and bake for 45–60 minutes OR place in microwave-safe container and microwave for 8 minutes.

Brown turkey and onions together in a frying pan coated with cooking spray. Set aside.

Once potato is cooked, slice open and top with ground turkey and onions, cheese, yogurt, chives and Ranch Powder.

Women: 290 cals; 4g fat; 39g carb; 25g protein
Men: 400 cals; 5g fat; 49g carb; 41g protein

# PB & J Rice Cakes and Shake

*High-Carb Meal*

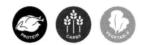

## Rice Cakes

3 tablespoons powdered peanut butter

2 tablespoons water

2 rice cakes, lightly salted (3 rice cakes for men)

Berry Puree (recipe below)

Mix powdered peanut butter and water together to reach a smooth consistency. Spread on each rice cake and top with Berry Puree. Enjoy with a protein shake.

## Berry Puree

1 cup blackberries, washed (or any berry of choice)

2 tablespoons applesauce, unsweetened

1 tablespoon Truvia sweetener

In a blender, mix all ingredients on low until fully blended.

## Shake

1 cup cold water or almond milk

½ scoop protein powder (1 scoop for men)

In a blender, mix ingredients on low until fully blended.

Women: 280 cals; 5g fat; 41g carb; 25g protein
Men: 385 cals; 6g fat; 50g carb; 39g protein

## Peanut Butter Shake

*High-Carb Meal*

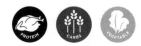

1 cup unsweetened almond milk

¼ cup vanilla protein powder (½ cup for men)

2 tablespoons powdered peanut butter (¼ cup for men)

1 frozen banana

6 ice cubes (or 1 cup)

Place all ingredients in a blender. Blend until smooth.

Women: 260 cals; 7g fat; 36g carb; 21g protein
Men: 375 cals; 9g fat; 42g carb; 39g protein

## Piña Colada Dream

*High-Carb Meal*

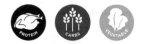

¾ cup fat-free plain Greek yogurt (1½ cups for men)

Vanilla stevia drops for sweetness

⅛ teaspoon coconut extract (optional)

1½ cups fresh pineapple chunks (2 cups for men)

2 tablespoons reduced fat, unsweetened, finely shredded coconut

Stir the Greek yogurt, stevia, and coconut extract (if using) together in a bowl. Top with pineapple and shredded coconut.

Women: 265 cals; 3g fat; 42g carb; 20g protein
Men: 410 cals; 3g fat; 60g carb; 38g protein

## Spiced Banana Shake

*High-Carb Meal*

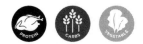

½ cup unsweetened almond milk (1 cup for men)

1 frozen banana (1⅓ banana for men)

½ cup fat-free plain Greek yogurt

¼ cup vanilla protein powder (½ cup for men)

¼ teaspoon pure vanilla extract

Dash of nutmeg

Dash of cinnamon

20 liquid stevia drops

6 ice cubes

Place all ingredients in a blender. Blend until smooth.

Women: 275 cals; 4g fat; 35g carb; 27g protein
Men: 400 cals; 7g fat; 47g carb; 42g protein

## Strawberry and Banana Quinoa Muffins

*High-Carb Meal*

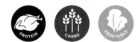

1 cup white whole-wheat flour

1 teaspoon baking powder

½ teaspoon salt substitute

2 scoops vanilla protein powder

2 large eggs, beaten

1 teaspoon vanilla extract

1 tablespoon Truvia sweetener

2 tablespoons coconut oil, melted

2 medium bananas, mashed

1 cup chopped strawberries

1 cup cooked quinoa

Preheat the oven to 375 degrees. Prepare muffin or cupcake tins with cooking spray. In a small bowl, mix the flour, baking powder, salt substitute, and protein powder.

In a separate bowl, mix together eggs, vanilla, Truvia, and coconut oil.

Slowly add the dry ingredients to the wet ingredients and stir until everything is fully incorporated.

Fold in mashed bananas, strawberries, and cooked quinoa. Stir until evenly distributed.

Divide the batter among 12 muffin cups. Bake for about 25–30 minutes or until toothpick comes out clean when tested.

Note: Freeze leftovers and save for Day 17.

*Makes 12 muffins*

Women (2 muffins): 260 cals; 8g fat; 33g carb; 16g protein
Men (3 muffins): 385 cals; 12g fat; 50g carb; 23g protein

---

# Sweet Potato Chips, Celery Sticks, and Shake

## *High-Carb Meal*

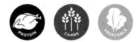

1 cup sweet potato (1½ cups for men)  
¼ teaspoon ground cumin  
¼ teaspoon smoked paprika  
¼ teaspoon garlic powder  
¼ teaspoon dried basil  

Pinch of light chili powder  
Pinch of salt substitute  
Pinch of ground black pepper  
5 celery sticks  
Cooking spray (fat-free)  

Slice the sweet potatoes about ¼ inch thick and place them in a mixing bowl.

Lightly spray the sweet potatoes with cooking spray and ensure all sides are evenly coated.

Add the spices and toss until the sweet potatoes are evenly coated with spices.

Preheat oven to 275 degrees. Lay each sweet potato slice on a baking sheet lined with aluminum foil and place in oven.

Cook sweet potato slices for 15 minutes and then flip each one. Cook another 10 minutes and flip again. Cook for another 5 minutes or until potatoes are light brown and crispy.

Enjoy with the celery sticks and protein shake (recipe follows).

## Shake

1 cup unsweetened almond milk  
1 scoop protein powder (1½ scoops for men)  

½ cup cold water (men only)  
1 cup ice (optional)  

Place all ingredients in a blender. Blend until smooth.

Women: 274 cals; 4g fat; 32g carb; 27g protein
Men: 391 cals; 4.6g fat; 47g carb; 40g protein

# Sweet Wrap

*High-Carb Meal*

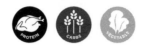

3 tablespoons fat-free plain Greek yogurt (¼ cup for men)

½ scoop vanilla protein powder (¾ scoop for men)

1 tablespoon powdered peanut butter (optional)

Vanilla stevia drops for sweetness (optional)

1 Rudi's spelt tortilla

½ banana, sliced (1 banana for men)

Dash of cinnamon

Mix Greek yogurt, powdered peanut butter, protein powder, and stevia together in a small bowl. Lay tortilla out on a plate; spread the yogurt mixture evenly down the center. Top with banana slices and cinnamon and wrap.

Women: 300 cals; 5g fat; 43g carb; 23g protein
Men: 410 cals; 6g fat; 60g carb; 32g protein

# Three-Bean Salad with Chicken and Kale

*High-Carb Meal*

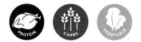

## Salad

3 ounces grilled and diced marinated chicken (see Marinade recipe for Chile Relleno, page 225)

½ cup steamed and cut green beans

¼ cup garbanzo beans, boiled, no salt (½ cup for men)

¼ cup black beans, boiled, no salt (½ cup for men)

¼ cup boiled yellow beets

1 ounce shredded carrots

1 cup kale, washed well and shredded

In a medium mixing bowl, toss the grilled chicken, steamed green beans, garbanzo beans, black beans, beets, shredded carrots, and shredded kale. Mix with dressing (recipe follows).

## *Creamy Dressing*

1 tablespoon fat-free plain Greek yogurt

1 tablespoon apple cider vinegar

Juice of ½ lemon

1 teaspoon salt-free tomato & garlic
seasoning

1 teaspoon chopped parsley

Pinch of salt substitute

Pinch of ground black pepper

In a small mixing bowl, blend the yogurt, apple cider vinegar, lemon juice, tomato and garlic seasoning, chopped parsley, salt substitute, and black pepper until all ingredients are evenly distributed.

Women: 286 cals; 4g fat; 20g carb; 27g protein
Men: 412 cals; 5g fat; 37g carb; 31g protein

# Triple Berry Treat

### *High-Carb Meal*

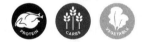

⅔ cup fat-free cottage cheese (1¼ cups
for men)

Vanilla stevia drops for sweetness

½ cup raspberries (⅔ cup for men)

½ cup blackberries (⅔ cup for men)

½ cup blueberries (⅔ cup for men)

½ cup Kashi GoLean Crisp cereal

Dash of cinnamon

Stir (or blend in a blender to make smooth) cottage cheese and stevia drops together until you reach your desired sweetness. Add berries, cereal, and cinnamon.

Women: 270 cals; 1g fat; 45g carb; 25g protein
Men: 385 cals; 2g fat; 58g carb; 40g protein

# Turkey Sliders with Sweet Potato "Bun"

*High-Carb Meal*

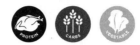

6 ounces sweet potato (8 ounces for men)

3 ounces extra-lean ground turkey (4 ounces for men)

Dash each of paprika, black pepper, garlic powder, and onion powder

2 tablespoons low-fat mozzarella cheese (3 tablespoons for men)

2 tomato slices

Spinach

1 teaspoon Dijon mustard (2 teaspoons for men)

Preheat oven to 425 degrees.

Cut the sweet potato into 4 rounds the size of a slider bun. Bake for 15 minutes. Remove from oven, flip, and then cook 15 more minutes.

Mix the ground turkey and seasonings together. Form turkey into 2 small patties. Grill or brown on a skillet. Once fully cooked, sprinkle cheese on top.

Use the sweet potato rounds for a bun and top burger with tomatoes, spinach, and mustard.

*Makes 1 slider (2 for men)*

Women: 290 cals; 3g fat; 36g carb; 25g protein
Men: 395 cals; 5g fat; 47g carb; 34g protein

# LOW-CARB MEALS

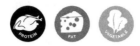

---

## Almond-Crusted Tilapia with Asparagus and Cauliflower Mash

*Low-Carb Meal*

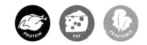

### Tilapia

½ teaspoon fat-free plain Greek yogurt

4 ounces tilapia filet (5 ounces for men)

¼ teaspoon salt-free garlic & herb seasoning

1 tablespoon Almond Crust (recipe below) (2 tablespoons for men)

¼ cup water

½ cup steamed asparagus

Spread yogurt evenly on top of tilapia. Top with garlic herb seasoning and Almond Crust. In a small nonstick skillet, add ¼ cup of water and bring to a simmer.

Carefully add the fish and simmer until the water evaporates. Once water evaporates, place the skillet in a preheated oven on high broil. Broil fish on high until crust is crispy and golden brown.

Serve with steamed asparagus, Cauliflower Mash, and Greek Yogurt Tartar Sauce.

### Almond Crust

1 cooked tostada, broken into medium pieces

¼ cup sliced raw almonds

1 teaspoon smoked paprika

Pinch salt substitute

Pinch black pepper

Place all ingredients in a blender and blend until chopped fine.

*Makes 8 servings, 1 tablespoon each*

## Cauliflower Mash

¼ head fresh cauliflower, cut into small,
  even pieces

1 tablespoon unsweetened almond milk

1 tablespoon fat-free plain Greek yogurt

2 teaspoons olive oil

Pinch of granulated garlic

Pinch of black pepper

Pinch of salt substitute

Pinch of chopped green onions

In a small pot, cover the cauliflower with water and bring to a boil. Cook for about 6 minutes or until it is fork tender.

Drain the cauliflower very well and shake off excess water.

Transfer the cooked cauliflower to a blender, food processer, or a mixing bowl with a hand masher. Add almond milk, yogurt, olive oil, garlic, pepper, salt substitute, and chopped green onions and mash well.

## Greek Yogurt Tartar Sauce

¼ cup fat-free plain Greek yogurt

¼ cup cucumber, diced fine

1 tablespoon red onion, diced fine

½ teaspoon fresh lemon juice

1 teaspoon yellow mustard

¼ teaspoon apple cider vinegar

Pinch of black pepper

Pinch of garlic powder

Pinch of paprika

Pinch of Truvia sweetener

In a mixing bowl, mix all ingredients until evenly incorporated.

*Makes 2 servings for men and 3 servings for women*

Women: 290 cals; 17.5g fat; 4g carb; 30g protein
Men: 341 cals; 22.5g fat; 6g carb; 36g protein

# Barbecue Grill Pork Tenderloin

*Low-Carb Meal*

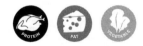

## *Pork Tenderloin*

¼ teaspoon black pepper

¼ teaspoon ground mustard powder

¼ teaspoon ground cumin

¼ teaspoon smoked paprika

¼ teaspoon garlic powder

¼ teaspoon onion powder

¼ teaspoon salt-free onion & herb seasoning

3 ounces lean pork tenderloin (5 ounces for men)

In a small bowl, mix pepper, mustard powder, cumin, paprika, garlic powder, onion powder, and onion and herb seasoning.

Rub pork generously with spice rub and marinate for 1 hour before cooking.

On a preheated grill, cook pork until it reaches 145 degrees. Let it cool for about 5 minutes before slicing. This will help keep it juicy.

## *Olive Oil Roasted Green Beans*

¼ cup water

1 cup fresh green beans, clipped and trimmed

1 tablespoon extra-virgin olive oil

¼ tablespoon fresh rosemary, chopped fine

Pinch of dried thyme

Pinch of black pepper

Pinch of salt substitute

1 tablespoon sliced raw almonds, unsalted (men only)

In a nonstick skillet over medium-high heat, bring water to a simmer.

Add green beans and cook until water evaporates.

Once water evaporates, add olive oil, rosemary, thyme, pepper, and salt substitute.

Turn heat up to high and stir until green beans have a nice golden brown color. Add sliced almonds for men's version only.

Women: 280 cals; 17g fat; 8g carb; 24g protein
Men: 400 cals; 23g fat; 9g carb; 41g protein

# Cajun Salmon with Cabbage Salad and Steamed Broccoli

*Low-Carb Meal*

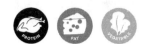

## Cajun Salmon

¼ teaspoon black pepper

¼ teaspoon ground mustard powder

¼ teaspoon ground cumin

¼ teaspoon smoked paprika

¼ teaspoon garlic powder

¼ teaspoon onion powder

Pinch of cayenne pepper

¼ teaspoon salt-free onion & herb seasoning

4 ounces wild caught salmon (5 ounces for men)

1 cup steamed broccoli

In a small bowl mix pepper, mustard, cumin, paprika, garlic powder, onion powder, cayenne pepper, and onion and herb seasoning.

Rub salmon generously with spice rub and let marinate for an hour before cooking.

Heat grill to medium heat. Lightly spray salmon with cooking spray, place on a piece of foil, and grill 5 minutes on each side. Let cool for about 5 minutes before serving. This will help keep it juicy.

Serve with steamed broccoli and Cabbage Slaw.

## Cabbage Slaw

1 cup shredded green and red cabbage

1 ounce shredded carrots

1 tablespoon parsley, rinsed and chopped

¼ teaspoon Truvia sweetener

2 teaspoons extra-virgin olive oil

Pinch of pepper

Pinch of salt substitute

1 tablespoon Pumpkin Seed Granola (page 212)

In a mixing bowl, toss the cabbage with carrots, parsley, Truvia, olive oil, pepper, salt substitute, and granola. Toss well and allow to marinate for 30 minutes before serving.

Women: 279 cals; 19g fat; 4g carb; 26g protein
Men: 312 cals; 22g fat; 5g carb; 28g protein

## Cauli Mash and Meatballs

*Low-Carb Meal*

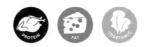

3 ounces extra-lean ground turkey, thawed (4 ounces for men)

2 tablespoons yellow onion, minced

1 tablespoon chives, chopped

1 tablespoon cilantro, chopped

¼ teaspoon garlic powder (½ teaspoon for men)

1½ cups cauliflower florets (2 cups for men)

1 tablespoon fat-free plain Greek yogurt (2 tablespoons for men)

1 tablespoon butter, unsalted (1½ tablespoons for men)

2 tablespoons low-fat mozzarella cheese

¼ teaspoon salt-free seasoning (½ teaspoon for men)

⅛ teaspoon ground pepper

Heat a skillet to medium heat.

With hands, mix together ground turkey, onion, chives, cilantro, and garlic powder.

Using a cookie scoop, form turkey into balls and place on a skillet sprayed with cooking spray. Cook 4 minutes and flip. Continue to cook and rotate until all sides are browned.

Boil cauliflower florets for 10 minutes. Drain and remove from heat. Add Greek yogurt, butter, cheese, and seasonings. Beat with hand mixer for 3–5 minutes or until smooth and creamy.

Place meatballs on mashed cauli and enjoy!

Women: 290 cals; 16g fat; 11g carb; 28g protein

Men: 390 cals; 22g fat; 14g carb; 37g protein

## Cheesy Chicken and String Beans

*Low-Carb Meal*

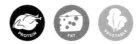

2 cups French-cut string beans

2 ounces chicken breast, chopped (4 ounces for men)

½ tablespoon coconut oil (1 tablespoon for men)

1 Laughing Cow cheese wedge

Garlic and herb salt-free seasoning

Black pepper

Cook the green beans according to the package directions. Set aside.

Brown the chicken in a skillet with coconut oil over medium heat. Add the green beans. Add the cheese and seasonings. Stir until the cheese is melted.

Women: 260 cals; 11g fat; 14g carb; 25g protein
Men: 420 cals; 20g fat; 14g carb; 43g protein

## Chicken Basil Spaghetti

*Low-Carb Meal*

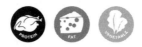

| | |
|---|---|
| 1 cup spaghetti squash | 2 tablespoons feta cheese crumbles |
| 2 ounces chicken, cooked and cubed (4 ounces for men) | ½ tablespoon olive oil |
| 2 cherry tomatoes, halved (4 for men) | 1 tablespoon fresh basil, chopped |
| 2 tablespoons black olives | 1 teaspoon dried minced onion |
| | Salt-free garlic & herb seasoning to taste |

Preheat oven to 425 degrees.

Slice the spaghetti squash into 2-inch rings. Remove seeds and place on a baking sheet sprayed with cooking spray. Bake for 20 minutes. Flip. Bake an additional 20 minutes. Squash should be tender, but not mushy. Rake with a fork into a bowl.

Layer spaghetti squash, chicken, tomatoes, olives, and cheese. Top with olive oil, basil, onion, and garlic herb seasoning.

Women: 277 cals; 15g fat; 14g carb; 22g protein
Men: 376 cals; 17g fat; 16g carb; 40g protein

## Chicken Slaw Dip

*Low-Carb Meal*

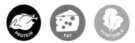

| | |
|---|---|
| 2 ounces chicken breast, cooked and shredded (4 ounces for men) | ¼ teaspoon salt-free onion & herb seasoning |
| ½ avocado, mashed | Black pepper |
| 2 tablespoons fat-free plain Greek yogurt (¼ cup for men) | 1 cup cabbage slaw |
| | 1 cup cucumbers, sliced |

Cook the chicken, shred it with two forks, and let cool in the fridge.

Combine the mashed avocado, Greek yogurt, and seasonings together. Add shredded chicken and slaw.

Dip the cucumbers in chicken slaw and eat cold.

Women: 260 cals; 13g fat; 14g carb; 23g protein
Men: 370 cals; 15g fat; 16g carb; 44g protein

# Chipotle Turkey Burger with House Pickles

*Low-Carb Meal*

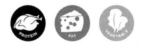

## Turkey Burger

3 ounces extra lean ground turkey
   (5 ounces for men)
Pinch of salt-free southwest seasoning
Pinch of black pepper
Pinch of dried thyme
Pinch of granulated garlic
Pinch of chili powder
Pinch of salt substitute

1 tablespoon red onion, small dice
1 small handful arugula or your preferred
   lettuce
¼ avocado, sliced (½ avocado, sliced, for
   men)
1 cup steamed broccoli
2 sliced tomatoes or cherry tomatoes
   halved

In a small bowl, mix the ground turkey, southwest seasoning, black pepper, thyme, garlic, chili powder, salt substitute, and red onion until evenly distributed. Make a patty. Lightly spray the grill with nonstick cooking spray, then cook on preheated grill until internal temperature reaches 165 degrees. Serve on top of arugula, top with avocado and serve with steamed broccoli, sliced tomatoes, and House Pickles (recipe follows).

## House Pickles

¼ sliced cucumber
2 ounces Ginger Lime Sauce (see Viet-
   namese Grilled Chicken Spring Rolls,
   page 266)

¼ teaspoon Truvia sweetener
¼ teaspoon turmeric powder

Slice cucumbers as thinly as possible.
Mix together the Ginger Lime Sauce with Truvia and turmeric.
Toss cucumbers with sauce and refrigerate for at least 24 hours.

Women: 251 cals; 10.5g fat; 6g carb; 29g protein
Men: 331 cals; 17.5g fat; 7g carb; 31g protein

---

# Chocolate Chip Almond Coconut Bites and Shake

*Low-Carb Meal*

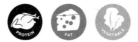

## Bites

½ cup oats

⅓ cup shredded and toasted coconut, unsweetened

¼ cup almond butter, no salt

2 tablespoons flax seeds

1 tablespoon dark chocolate chips

½ tablespoon coconut oil

½ tablespoon fat-free plain Greek yogurt

In a mixing bowl combine all ingredients until they are evenly distributed. Roll into 1-ounce balls; makes 6 bites. Store in the fridge or freezer in an airtight container. Enjoy 1 bite with a protein shake.

## Protein Shake

1 cup unsweetened almond milk

¾ scoop protein powder (1½ scoops for men)

In a blender, mix all ingredients on low until fully blended.

Women (1 bite and shake): 280 cals; 16g fat; 12g carb; 24g protein
Men (1 bite and shake): 385 cals; 18g fat; 15g carb; 44g protein

## Chocolate Peanut Butter Shake

*Low-Carb Meal*

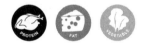

1 cup unsweetened almond milk

1 scoop chocolate protein powder (1½ scoops for men)

1 tablespoon all-natural peanut butter (1½ tablespoons for men)

6–8 ice cubes (or 1 cup)

Place all ingredients in a blender. Blend until smooth.

Women: 280 cals; 14g fat; 8g carb; 32g protein
Men: 400 cals; 19g fat; 11g carb; 47g protein

## Citrus and Onion Fish Tacos

*Low-Carb Meal*

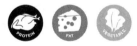

4 ounces white fish (mahi-mahi, tilapia, halibut, cod), thawed (6 ounces for men)

1 tablespoon lime juice

1 tablespoon apple cider vinegar

1 teaspoon Truvia

½ teaspoon onion powder

½ avocado, diced (¾ avocado for men)

½ Roma tomato, diced

1 tablespoon fat-free plain Greek yogurt (2 tablespoons for men)

2 tablespoons cilantro, chopped

½ lime, juiced

2 butter lettuce cups (3 for men)

Place the fish in a zip-lock bag with the tablespoon of lime juice, vinegar, Truvia, and onion powder and store in the fridge overnight.

Spray a pan with cooking spray. Pan-fry the fish with marinade over medium heat. Cook 5 minutes per side or until the fish flakes.

Layer the fish, avocado, tomatoes, Greek yogurt, cilantro, and lime juice evenly inside each butter lettuce cup. Enjoy!

Women: 265 cals; 12g fat; 18g carb; 25g protein
Men: 380 cals; 18g fat; 21g carb; 38g protein

## Citrus Salmon Slaw

*Low-Carb Meal*

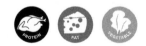

3 ounces wild caught salmon, cooked (5 ounces for men)

1 cup plain cabbage slaw (1½ cups for men)

2 asparagus spears, chopped

¼ cup sweet bell peppers

¼ avocado, sliced

2 tablespoons fat-free plain Greek yogurt (3 tablespoons for men)

2 tablespoons fresh salsa (3 tablespoons for men)

Cilantro

Lime juice

Salt-free garlic & herb seasoning, to taste

Spray a frying pan with cooking spray and pan-fry the salmon, 5 minutes on each side or until it flakes.

Layer the slaw, salmon, and veggies. Top with the yogurt, salsa, cilantro, and lime juice. Season with garlic and herb seasoning.

Women: 272 cals; 14g fat; 15g carb; 22g protein
Men: 394 cals; 20g fat; 20g carb; 34g protein

## Creamy Cauliflower Soup

*Low-Carb Meal*

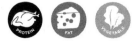

2 cups cauliflower, broken up

¼ cup yellow onion, chopped

1½ teaspoons olive oil

1 cup of low-sodium chicken broth

¼ teaspoon garlic, minced

⅓ cup fat-free plain Greek yogurt

⅓ cup low-fat mozzarella cheese

1 ounce chicken, cooked and shredded (3 ounces for men)

salt-free seasoning

Black pepper, to taste

Chives

Preheat oven to 375 degrees.

Place the cauliflower and onions in a baking dish, drizzle them with olive oil, and roast until golden, about 30 minutes.

Place the chicken, chicken broth, and garlic in a pot and bring to a boil. Add the roasted cauliflower and onions. Boil for 5 minutes. Remove from heat. Add the Greek yogurt, cheese, and seasonings. Stir.

Puree in a blender or use a hand-held emulsifier to blend in the pot until smooth. Pour into a bowl and top with chives.

Women: 280 cals; 11g fat; 16g carb; 33g protein
Men: 390 cals; 15g fat; 16g carb; 52g protein

---

# Curry Turkey Sliders with Cucumber and Tomato Salad

*Low-Carb Meal*

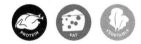

## Sliders

4 ounces extra-lean ground turkey
   (6 ounces for men)
1 teaspoon ground yellow curry powder
⅓ teaspoon turmeric powder
½ teaspoon ground ginger
½ teaspoon ground black pepper

Pinch of garam masala
Pinch of ground coriander
Pinch of cayenne pepper
1 teaspoon cilantro, rinsed and chopped
   fine

In a large mixing bowl, mix all ingredients until everything is evenly distributed.

Once turkey is mixed, separate into 1-ounce balls and lightly press into thin patties. Lightly spray each turkey slider with cooking spray and place on a preheated grill. After about 2 minutes, flip to cook the other side.

Serve with Cucumber and Tomato Salad (recipe follows).

## Cucumber and Tomato Salad

1 tablespoon fresh lime juice
½ tablespoon extra-virgin olive oil
¼ tablespoon ground ginger
¼ teaspoon ground black pepper
½ teaspoon Truvia sweetener
1 tablespoon fresh lemon juice

4 small mint leaves, chopped fine
1 medium cucumber, cubed
5 cherry tomatoes, halved
¼ avocado (½ avocado for men)
2 tablespoons red onion, minced

In a mixing bowl whisk together lime juice, olive oil, ground ginger, black pepper, Truvia, lemon juice, and mint leaves. Whisk until seasonings have been dissolved.

Add cucumbers, cherry tomatoes, avocado, and red onion.
Toss all ingredients.

Women: 285 cals; 14g fat; 15g carb; 28g protein
Men: 400 cals; 20g fat; 17g carb; 42g protein

## Deviled Eggs

*Low-Carb Meal*

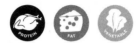

| | |
|---|---|
| 3 whole eggs (4 eggs for men) | 1 teaspoon Dijon mustard |
| ¼ cup fat-free plain Greek yogurt (men only) | Paprika |
| | Black pepper |
| 1 tablespoon low-fat mayo | 12 sugar snap peas (20 for men) |

Boil eggs for 10–12 minutes. Put in ice water until cool. Peel and cut eggs in half.
Scoop all the yolks into a bowl. Mix yolks with Greek yogurt or mayo and mustard.
Fill each egg with the yolk mixture and top with a dash of paprika and pepper. Eat snap peas on the side.

Women: 250 cals; 13g fat; 5g carb; 19g protein
Men: 355 cals; 16g fat; 8g carb; 32g protein

## Edamame and Pistachio Hummus with Cucumbers and Chicken

*Low-Carb Meal*

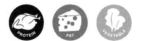

| | |
|---|---|
| ¾ cup water | 1 pinch of salt substitute |
| ½ cup raw edamame, shelled | 1 pinch of cayenne pepper |
| ½ tablespoon lemon juice | ⅛ teaspoon ground black pepper |
| ½ teaspoon garlic, chopped | 2 tablespoons extra-virgin olive oil |
| 2 tablespoons pistachios, raw and unsalted | ½ cucumber, sliced |
| ⅛ teaspoon ground cumin | 2 ounces grilled chicken (4 ounces for men) |

In a small pot, bring water to a boil and cook edamame for about 5 minutes or until fork tender. Once cooked, strain and reserve 2 tablespoons of the hot water for a later step.

Move strained edamame to a blender or food processor and add lemon juice, garlic, pistachios, cumin, salt substitute, cayenne, and black pepper. Pulsate to mix spices and coarsely blend the edamame.

With the blender going, slowly drizzle in the olive oil and then use the reserved water as needed to adjust the consistency.

Remove from blender and enjoy ½ cup hummus with sliced cucumbers and grilled chicken.

*Makes 1 cup, or 2 servings*

Women: 305 cals: 21g fat; 7g carb; 23g protein
Men: 400 cals; 23g fat; 7g carb; 41g protein

## Eggplant Curry Stir-Fry

*Low-Carb Meal*

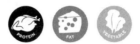

2 pieces firm tofu (4 pieces for men)
½ cup sliced yellow onions
½ medium eggplant, peeled and diced into 1-inch cubes
½ cup red bell pepper, diced
½ teaspoon cumin seed
½ teaspoon yellow mustard seed
¼ teaspoon ground turmeric
¼ teaspoon ground ginger
2 teaspoons curry powder
¼ teaspoon ground coriander
¼ teaspoon garam masala

¼ teaspoon red chili flakes
½ teaspoon salt substitute
¼ teaspoon black pepper
¼ teaspoon ground cumin
½ tablespoon Truvia sweetener
3 cups water
¼ cup lime juice
½ cup broccoli, raw and chopped
¼ cup shelled edamame
½ cup cilantro, chopped
1 tablespoon raw peanuts, unsalted, per serving

Spray a pan with cooking spray and add tofu, sliced onions, eggplant, bell peppers, cumin seed, and mustard seed. Cook this mixture until onions are golden brown, about 5–7 minutes.

Add turmeric, ginger, curry, coriander, garam masala, chili flakes, salt substitute, pepper, cumin, Truvia, and water. Bring to a simmer and cook until eggplant is tender.

Add lime juice, broccoli, edamame, and cilantro. Cook until broccoli is tender.

Serve 1 serving in a bowl with peanuts on top.

*Makes 2 servings*

Women: 285 cals; 13g fat; 25g carb; 21g protein
Men: 420 cals; 20g fat; 29g carb; 36g protein

---

# Fajita Chicken Roll-Ups with Roasted Squash and Avocado Puree

*Low-Carb Meal*

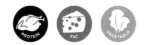

## Chicken Roll-Ups

¼ teaspoon salt-free southwest seasoning
¼ teaspoon salt-free onion & herb seasoning
¼ teaspoon salt-free chicken seasoning
Pinch of salt substitute

2 2-ounce chicken breasts, pounded thin (2 4-ounce breasts for men)
½ red bell pepper, cut into thin strips
½ red onion, cut into thin strips

In a small bowl, mix southwest seasoning, onion and herb seasoning, chicken seasoning, and salt substitute.

Lay the pounded chicken breasts out flat and evenly season with above mixture.

Mix peppers and onions and evenly distribute between the chicken breasts, ensuring the veggies are facing the same way. This will make rolling much easier.

Start by folding the closest part of the chicken over the vegetables and roll until vegetables are covered. Place seam down on a sheet tray and place in the freezer for about 20 minutes. This will help the cooking process.

Spray a nonstick skillet with cooking spray and heat over medium-high heat. Slowly add the chicken roll-ups with the open end first. Allow chicken to cook for about 4 minutes without moving. You want to create a nice seal so the roll-ups stay together. After about 4 minutes, roll the roll-ups over to cook the other side, about another 4 minutes or until internal temperature is 165 degrees. Serve with roasted squash and top with avocado puree.

*Makes 2 servings*

## Roasted Zucchini and Squash

I medium yellow squash, ½-inch dice
I medium zucchini, ½-inch dice
¼ teaspoon dried thyme

¼ teaspoon red pepper flakes
¼ teaspoon black pepper

Heat a skillet on high heat. Spray with cooking spray and add squash and zucchini; stir immediately. Keep stirring until vegetables have a light brown color and are fork tender. Add seasonings and remove from heat.

*Makes 2 servings*

## Avocado Puree

I medium ripe avocado
I tablespoon fresh lime juice
¼ teaspoon black pepper

¼ teaspoon ground cumin
Pinch of salt substitute

In a small bowl, cut avocado and smash with a spoon.
Add lime juice, pepper, cumin, and salt substitute. Mix with spoon until smooth.

*Makes 4 servings for women and 2 for men*

Women: 240 cals; 10g fat; 17g carb; 21g protein
Men: 415 cals; 19g fat; 21g carb; 39g protein

---

# Greek Yogurt Parfait with Nuts

### *Low-Carb Meal*

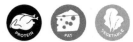

I cup fat-free plain Greek yogurt
½ scoop vanilla protein powder (men only)
Vanilla stevia drops for sweetness (optional)

2 tablespoons sliced almonds, unsalted and raw
I tablespoon chopped hazelnuts, unsalted and raw (2 tablespoons for men)

Sweeten yogurt with stevia if desired (men, stir in protein powder, too). Top with almonds and hazelnuts.

Women: 257 cals; 12g fat; 14g carb; 29g protein
Men: 360 cals; 17g fat; 16g carb; 42g protein

# Grilled Lamb Kebabs

*Low-Carb Meal*

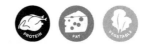

## Lamb Kebabs

3 ounces lean lamb meat, preferably shoulder (5 ounces for men)

2 ounces All-Purpose Marinade (recipe below)

Cut lean lamb into 1-inch cubes, toss with marinade, and refrigerate for up to 24 hours. On a hot grill, cook to preferred doneness.

## All-Purpose Marinade

3 sprigs fresh thyme or pinch of dried thyme

3 sprigs fresh tarragon

1 tablespoon chopped garlic

1 tablespoon chopped yellow onion

2 tablespoons lemon juice

1 teaspoon salt-free chicken seasoning

½ teaspoon salt substitute

Black pepper, to taste

½ cup water

Place thyme, tarragon, garlic, chopped onion, lemon juice, chicken seasoning, salt substitute, black pepper, and water in blender and blend until smooth.

## Vegetables

1 teaspoon extra-virgin olive oil

3 ounces yellow squash, ½-inch dice

3 ounces zucchini, ½-inch dice

Pinch of dry thyme

Pinch of red pepper flakes

Pinch of black pepper

In a skillet over high heat, add olive oil and allow it to get hot. Add squash and zucchini and stir immediately. Keep stirring until vegetables have a light brown color and are fork tender. Add seasonings and remove from heat.

Women: 275 cals; 17g fat; 6g carb; 22g protein
Men: 405 cals; 25g fat; 6g carb; 36g protein

# Grilled Wild Salmon with Quinoa and Edamame Salad

*Low-Carb Meal*

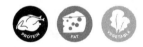

### Fish

4 ounces wild caught salmon (6 ounces for men)

1 tablespoon salt-free onion & herb seasoning

Preheat grill to medium heat. Season the salmon with salt-free seasoning. Place salmon on foil and grill about 5 minutes per side or until desired doneness.

### Salad

2 tablespoons cooked quinoa (¼ cup for men)

¼ cup edamame, shelled

2 asparagus spears, thinly chopped

½ tablespoon chopped parsley

½ teaspoon salt-free onion & herb seasoning

1 tablespoon fresh lemon juice

Dash of black pepper

Mix all ingredients together in a mixing bowl with a spatula. Serve with salmon.

Women: 280 cals; 13g fat; 12g carb; 27g protein
Men: 405 cals; 20g fat; 17g carb; 39g protein

# Pepper Jack Chicken

*Low-Carb Meal*

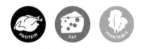

3 ounces chicken breast, thawed (4½ ounces for men)

Salt-free seasoning

2 slices pepper jack cheese

8 asparagus spears (12 spears for men)

1 tablespoon Dijon mustard

Heat a skillet to medium heat.

Pound the chicken flat in between two sheets of parchment paper. Season with your favorite salt-free seasoning.

Place cheese on one side of the flattened chicken. Place asparagus stalks on top of cheese. Fold the other half of the chicken breast over the asparagus and cheese. Place the chicken in skillet. Cover. Cook 5 minutes on each side.

Top with mustard. Enjoy!

Women: 280 cals; 12g fat; 6g carb; 32g protein
Men: 383 cals; 16g fat; 9g carb; 47g protein

---

## Popeye Shake

*Low-Carb Meal*

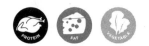

1 cup frozen spinach

1 tablespoon natural nut butter

½ cup unsweetened almond milk

1 tablespoon milled flax (2 tablespoons for men)

1 scoop protein powder (1½ scoops for men)

4–6 ice cubes (or ¾ cup)

Place all ingredients in a blender. Blend until smooth.

Women: 300 cals; 15g fat; 10g carb; 33g protein
Men: 405 cals; 19g fat; 14g carb; 48g protein

---

## Protein Punch Wraps

*Low-Carb Meal*

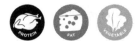

1½ ounces chicken breast, cooked and shredded (3 ounces for men)

1 piece string cheese, cut into rounds (1½ pieces for men)

½ ounce slivered almonds

Lettuce cups

Pile chicken, cheese, and almonds on top of lettuce cups. Eat cold.

Women: 235 cals; 15g fat; 6g carb; 23g protein
Men: 354 cals; 19g fat; 9g carb; 39g protein

## Quinoa Bites with Zucchini, Tomato, and Arugula

*Low-Carb Meal*

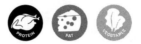

2 tablespoons extra-virgin olive oil
2 tablespoons diced red onion
½ teaspoon minced garlic
½ medium zucchini, small dice
¼ teaspoon dried thyme
¼ teaspoon dried basil

¼ teaspoon ground black pepper
½ cup diced tomatoes
¾ cup cooked quinoa
1 handful of arugula, rinsed
6 whole eggs
6 egg whites

Heat olive oil over medium-high heat in a nonstick skillet.

Once oil is hot add onions, garlic, and zucchini. Add thyme, basil, and black pepper. Sauté until the vegetables are soft and have a light brown color. Add diced tomatoes, cooked quinoa, and arugula. Cook until arugula is wilted. Set aside and allow to cool.

Meanwhile, whisk together egg whites and whole eggs.

Generously spray muffin pan with cooking spray to prevent sticking. Preheat oven to 400 degrees.

Distribute 1½ tablespoons of vegetable mixture into each muffin cup.

Add egg mixture so that each cup is ¾ full.

Bake in preheated oven for approximately 20 minutes or until tops are light brown and the eggs are cooked through.

*Makes 12 muffins*

Women (3 muffins): 234 cals; 15g fat; 5g carb; 15g protein
Men (5 muffins): 390 cals; 25g fat; 8g carb; 25g protein

## Salmon with Pesto "Zoodles"

*Low-Carb Meal*

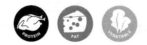

1 large zucchini squash

4 ounces wild caught salmon (6 ounces for men)

2 spears asparagus, chopped (4 spears for men)

1 tablespoon pesto sauce (1½ tablespoons for men)

Lemon juice

Spiral slice or julienne-cut the zucchini to make "zoodles." Place in a strainer and liberally salt the zucchini; let sit 20 minutes (this helps your zucchini "sweat" out all its water).

Spray a frying pan with cooking spray and heat over medium heat.

Place the thawed salmon fillet on the pan. Cook for 5 minutes on each side or until salmon begins to flake. Remove from pan and set aside.

Thoroughly rinse salt off of the zucchini and pat dry. Spray another pan with cooking spray and cook "zoodles" and asparagus over medium heat until tender. Add pesto sauce to "zoodles" and top with salmon and a squirt of lemon juice. Enjoy!

Women: 270 cals; 16g fat; 8g carb; 25g protein
Men: 390 cals; 23g fat; 10g carb; 36g protein

## Shrimp and Chicken Stir-Fry

*Low-Carb Meal*

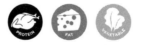

1 teaspoon coconut aminos

1 tablespoon coconut oil

½ teaspoon minced garlic

½ cup shredded carrots

½ cup sugar snap pea pods, chopped

½ cup broccoli, chopped (1 cup for men)

½ cup mushrooms, sliced

6 cocktail shrimp, thawed (10 for men)

1 ounce chicken breast, cubed (2 ounces for men)

1 tablespoon green onions, sliced (2 tablespoons for men)

⅛ teaspoon black pepper

Heat the coconut aminos, coconut oil, and garlic in a skillet over medium-high heat. Add carrots once the oil is melted. Sauté for 5 minutes.

Add the remaining veggies, shrimp, and cubed chicken. Sauté an additional 10 minutes. Garnish with green onions and black pepper. Enjoy!

Women: 260 cals; 16g fat; 12g carb; 22g protein
Men: 360 cals; 17g fat; 17g carb; 39g protein

## Shrimp Cocktail Salad

*Low-Carb Meal*

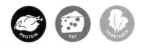

10 pieces large shrimp, halved
⅔ avocado, cubed (1 avocado for men)
1½ ounces chicken breast, cooked and
   cubed (for men only)

¼ cup cucumber, chopped
1 tablespoon cocktail sauce
1 tablespoon cilantro
Fresh lemon juice

Carefully mix shrimp, avocado, chicken (for men only), cucumber, cocktail sauce, cilantro, and lemon juice together in a small bowl. Eat cold.

Women: 240 cals; 15g fat; 13g carb; 17g protein
Men: 390 cals; 23g fat; 17g carb; 32g protein

## Stuffed Avocado

*Low-Carb Meal*

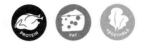

½ medium-size avocado (¾ for men)
3 ounces cooked, shredded chicken
   (4 ounces for men)
2 tablespoons fat-free plain Greek yogurt

1 tablespoon Dijon mustard
Salt-free seasoning blend blend
Ground black pepper

Slice avocado in half and remove pit. Set aside.
Mix shredded chicken, yogurt, mustard, and seasonings together. Stuff mixture into the avocado. Eat with a spoon.

Women: 285 cals; 13g fat; 7g carb; 31g protein
Men: 390 cals; 20g fat; 10g carb; 40g protein

# Taco Salad

*Low-Carb Meal*

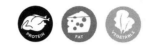

## Salad

2 ounces lean ground beef (4 ounces for men)

2 tablespoons yellow onion, chopped (¼ cup for men)

1 teaspoon homemade taco seasoning (2 teaspoons for men) (recipe below)

1½ cups romaine lettuce, chopped

½ cup chard, chopped

1 tablespoon olives, sliced

¼ avocado, sliced

1 tablespoon low-fat mozzarella cheese

1 tablespoon fat-free plain Greek yogurt

2 tablespoons fresh salsa

Chopped green onions

Heat skillet to medium-high heat.

Brown ground beef and onion together in skillet. Add taco seasoning.

To make salad, layer chopped romaine and chard, beef and onions, olives, avocado, cheese, Greek yogurt, salsa, and green onions. Enjoy!

## Taco Seasoning

1 tablespoon chili powder

1 teaspoon cumin

½ teaspoon paprika

½ teaspoon black pepper

¼ teaspoon garlic powder

¼ teaspoon onion powder

¼ teaspoon crushed red pepper flakes

¼ teaspoon dried oregano

Mix all ingredients together and store in an airtight container. Remember to label it!

Women: 260 cals; 15g fat; 13g carb; 21g protein

Men: 390 cals; 21g fat; 14g carb; 36g protein

# Thai-Style Turkey Cabbage Salad

*Low-Carb Meal*

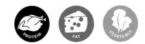

## Turkey

2 teaspoons coconut oil

3 ounces lean ground turkey (4 ounces for men)

1 teaspoon garlic, minced

1 tablespoon shallots, minced

¼ teaspoon salt substitute

¼ teaspoon black pepper

¼ teaspoon jalapeño, stems and seeds removed, minced

1 tablespoon rice vinegar, unseasoned

1 tablespoon lime juice

1 teaspoon Sriracha paste

In a nonstick skillet over high heat, melt the coconut oil and add turkey. Stir the turkey, making sure to break it up as you go.

Add the garlic, shallots, salt substitute, black pepper, jalapeños, vinegar, lime juice, and Sriracha paste.

Cook the turkey until it is cooked through all the way.

## Cabbage

1½ cups of shredded cabbage

2 teaspoons extra-virgin olive oil

3 ounces yellow squash, ½-inch dice

3 ounces zucchini, ½-inch dice

Pinch of dried thyme

Pinch of red pepper flakes

Pinch of black pepper

In a skillet over high heat, heat olive oil. Add cabbage, squash, and zucchini and stir immediately. Keep stirring until vegetables have a light brown color and are fork tender. Add seasonings and remove from heat.

Women: 278 cals; 23g fat; 3g carb; 21g protein
Men: 344 cals; 26g fat; 3g carb; 28g protein

## Vanilla Pecan Pudding

*Low-Carb Meal*

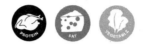

½ cup fat-free plain Greek yogurt (1 cup for men)

¼ cup vanilla protein powder

1 tablespoon all-natural almond butter

Vanilla stevia drops for sweetness

1 tablespoon chopped pecans (2 tablespoons for men)

Mix the Greek yogurt, protein powder, almond butter, and stevia together in a bowl. Top with pecans (or other nut of choice).

Women: 290 cals; 16g fat; 11g carb; 29g protein
Men: 410 cals; 21g fat; 16g carb; 41g protein

## Vietnamese Grilled Chicken Spring Rolls with Sweet Ginger Lime Sauce

*Low-Carb Meal*

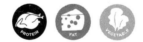

### Spring Rolls

3 sheets rice paper wrapper

1 cup cabbage slaw

¼ avocado, sliced (½ avocado for men)

¼ cup shredded carrots

3 ounces grilled chicken, cut into long, thin strips (4 ounces for men)

¼ cucumber, shredded

3 green onions, just the cut-off white stem—leave whole

Basil and mint leaves (optional)

All ingredients will be divided between three rolls.

Run rice papers under hot water until they are flexible and soft.

With the rice paper flat on the cutting board, layer cabbage slaw, avocado, carrots, grilled chicken strips, shredded cucumber, and strip of green onion.

Roll the bottom of the sheet halfway up and cover ingredients.

Roll the left side toward the middle and do the same with the right side.

Ensuring paper is kept tight, roll tightly toward the top.
Repeat for the second and third roll. Top rolls with 1 serving of sauce (recipe follows).

## Sauce

½ cup lime juice
1 teaspoon apple cider vinegar
¼ teaspoon Sriracha chili sauce
1½ tablespoons Truvia

½ teaspoon minced ginger
½ teaspoon minced garlic
Dash of salt substitute
¼ jalapeño, minced fine (optional)

*Makes 2 servings*

In a mixing bowl, whisk all ingredients together until Truvia is dissolved.

Women: 300 cals; 8g fat; 14g carb; 29g protein
Men: 400 cals; 15g fat; 17g carb; 38g protein

# Zucchini and Turkey "Lasagna Roll-Ups"

*Low-Carb Meal*

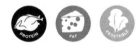

## Turkey Filling

1 tablespoon extra-virgin olive oil
1 tablespoon minced garlic
1 tablespoon yellow onion, minced
4 ounces lean ground turkey (5 ounces
    for men)
¼ teaspoon dried basil
¼ teaspoon dried oregano

¼ teaspoon dried thyme
¼ teaspoon black pepper
¼ teaspoon salt-free tomato basil
    seasoning
¼ teaspoon Truvia sweetener
½ cup diced canned tomatoes, no salt

In a nonstick skillet over medium heat, add the oil and sauté the garlic and onions until soft, stirring often. Add the ground turkey, basil, oregano, thyme, pepper, tomato basil seasoning, Truvia, and canned tomatoes. Simmer on medium until the turkey is cooked through. Set aside and allow to cool to room temperature.

## Zucchini "Noodles"

1 medium zucchini, round and long                    ¼ cup mozzarella cheese

Bring a large pot of water to boil.

Slice the zucchini lengthwise into ¼-inch strips.

Add the sliced zucchini to the boiling water and cook for about 4 minutes or until the zucchini strips are flexible without being mushy.

Remove them from the water and run under cold water until cool.

Lay the zucchini flat and divide the turkey mixture between 4 zucchini strips, placing mixture in the middle and rolling over until the end.

Place on a nonstick cookie sheet with a light spray of cooking spray.

Divide the cheese between the 4 roll-ups and broil on high until the cheese is melted and golden brown. Sprinkle with dried basil and serve.

Women: 280 cals; 16.5g fat; 4g carb; 34g protein
Men: 310 cals; 18g fat; 6g carb; 41g protein

# CLEAN CHEAT MEALS

## Banana Berry Ice Cream

*Clean Cheat*

1 cup 2% cottage cheese

½ cup berries (1 cup for men)

½ banana (1 banana for men)

2 tablespoons unsweetened almond milk

1 tablespoon nut butter

½ scoop vanilla protein powder

1 cup unsweetened almond milk

6 ice cubes (or 1 cup)

Natural sweetener of choice

The night before you intend to serve, blend cottage cheese, berries, banana, 2 tablespoons almond milk, nut butter, and protein powder. Pour into an ice cube tray and freeze overnight.

Place frozen cubes back in blender, and blend with 1 cup almond milk, ice cubes, and natural sweetener of choice, to desired sweetness. Enjoy!

Note: Make this the night before serving.

Women: 500 cals; 18g fat; 44g carb; 48g protein
Men: 607 cals; 19g fat; 70g carb; 49g protein

## Barbecue Chicken Pita Pizza

*Clean Cheat*

1 whole-wheat flatbread
(1½ for men)

2 tablespoons reduced-sugar barbecue
sauce (3 tablespoons for men) (we like
the smoky mesquite flavor)

½ cup shredded Monterey jack and
cheddar cheese

2 ounces cooked and shredded chicken

Red onion, thinly sliced

Cilantro

Preheat oven to 350 degrees.

Spread the barbecue sauce on pita, then layer ¼ cup of cheese, chicken, red onion, cilantro, and remaining ¼ cup of cheese.

Bake on a baking sheet for 15–20 minutes. Enjoy!

Women: 495 cals; 16g fat; 53g carb; 40g protein
Men: 600 cals; 17g fat; 74g carb; 43g protein

## BLT Burger and Sweet Potato Fries

*Clean Cheat*

½ cup sweet potatoes

Sea salt to taste

4 ounces beef

Dash each of salt, pepper, cumin, salt-free
seasoning blend, dried minced onion

1 slice nitrate-free turkey bacon

½ whole-grain bun (1 whole bun for men)

Lettuce

Tomato

1 tablespoon reduced-sugar barbecue
sauce

½ tablespoon olive oil mayo OR homemade mayo

Heat oven to 425 degrees. Heat grill or skillet to medium-high heat.

Slice ½ cup sweet potatoes into fries. Place a single layer of fries on a baking sheet lined with a crinkled and greased piece of tinfoil. Spray the tops with cooking spray or an olive oil misto and sprinkle with sea salt. Bake 15 minutes, flip. Bake another 15 minutes.

Mix beef and seasonings together with your hands and form a patty. Grill burger and bacon or cook on skillet to desired doneness.

Place burger patty on bun. Layer with bacon, lettuce, tomato, barbecue sauce, and mayo. (Women, leave off the top of the bun.) Eat fries on the side OR try to stack them on your burger. Enjoy!

Women: 496 cals; 22g fat; 41g carb; 31g protein
Men: 590 cals; 24g fat; 57g carb; 36g protein

---

## Candied Pecan Protein Waffles

*Clean Cheat*

4 egg whites
¼ cup 2% cottage cheese
½ scoop vanilla protein powder
¼ banana (¾ banana for men)
⅓ cup oats (½ cup for men)

1 tablespoon ground flaxseed
1 teaspoon cinnamon
Topping:
1 tablespoon chopped pecans
2 tablespoons pure maple syrup

Heat waffle iron.

Blend egg whites, cottage cheese, protein powder, banana, oats, flaxseed, and cinnamon. Pour into a waffle iron that's been sprayed with cooking spray. Cook 2 minutes. Transfer to a plate.

Toast pecans in a frying pan over medium heat for 3–5 minutes. Add syrup to pan. Stir together. Once bubbles begin to form, pour over waffle. Enjoy!

Women: 525 cals; 13g fat; 66g carb; 41g protein
Men: 600 cals; 14g fat; 82g carb; 43g protein

# Chocolate Glazed Crepes

*Clean Cheat*

## Crepes

½ banana
½ cup oats (⅔ cup for men)
¼ cup unsweetened almond milk
1 whole egg

3 egg whites
1–2 teaspoons stevia
Dash of cinnamon

## Chocolate Glaze

½ tablespoon almond butter
½ tablespoon coconut oil
1 tablespoon unsweetened almond milk
1 tablespoon raw honey

2 tablespoons chocolate protein powder
Topping (for men only):
½ banana, sliced

Spray a small frying pan with cooking spray and place over medium heat.

Blend the banana, oats, almond milk, eggs, stevia, and cinnamon for 2 minutes.

Pour ¼ of the batter into the frying pan and swirl around to cover base of the pan. Once bubbles form on the top, flip. Cook another minute, transfer to a plate and roll up. Should make 4 crepes.

For the glaze, place almond butter and coconut oil in a small bowl and heat for 20 seconds in the microwave. Stir in almond milk, honey, and protein powder. Drizzle over your crepes. Men, top with banana slices. Enjoy!

Women: 500 cals; 21g fat; 50g carb; 31g protein
Men: 603 cals; 22g fat; 72g carb; 33g protein

## Chunky Monkey Bowl

*Clean Cheat*

¼ cup plain Greek yogurt
1 tablespoon peanut butter
1 frozen banana
½ scoop chocolate or vanilla protein
    powder (1 scoop for men)
4 ice cubes (or ½ cup)

Toppings:
½ banana, sliced
2 large strawberries, sliced
2 tablespoons granola
15 extra-dark chocolate chips
1 teaspoon raw honey

Blend yogurt, peanut butter, frozen banana, protein powder, and ice cubes.
Pour in a bowl and top with all toppings. Enjoy!

Women: 492 cals; 14g fat; 72g carb; 28g protein
Men: 562 cals; 15g fat; 74g carb; 41g protein

## Homemade Oreos

*Clean Cheat*

### Cookies

6 tablespoons whole-wheat flour
2 tablespoons chocolate protein powder
1 tablespoon cocoa powder
Dash of sea salt

2 tablespoons melted coconut oil
3 tablespoons pure maple syrup
1 whole egg
¼ teaspoon pure vanilla extract

### Cream Filling

¼ cup full-fat whipped cream cheese
2 tablespoons vanilla protein powder

¼ teaspoon pure vanilla extract
½ tablespoon pure maple syrup

Preheat oven to 325 degrees. Line a baking sheet with parchment paper.

Sift together the flour, chocolate protein powder, cocoa powder, and salt. Set aside. Beat together the melted coconut oil and maple syrup. Add egg and vanilla. Mix. Add dry ingredients to wet ingredients. Mix.

Scoop into 1-inch balls and place on baking sheet; this should make 8 cookies. Bake for 7–9 minutes. Transfer to a cooling rack.

Beat together all ingredients for the cream filling. Once cookies are cooled, spoon 1 tablespoon filling onto each of 4 cookies and sandwich with the remaining 4 cookies. Enjoy!

*Makes 4 cookies*

Women (2 cookies): 445 cals; 24g fat; 49g carb; 16g protein
Men (3 cookies): 665 cals; 36g fat; 73g carb; 23g protein

---

# Hootenanny Pancakes

*Clean Cheat*

## Pancakes

½ tablespoon coconut oil

4 egg whites

1 whole egg

½ cup Kodiak Cakes pancake mix

½ cup unsweetened almond milk

¼ teaspoon sea salt

¼ teaspoon pure vanilla extract

Toppings:

¼ cup sliced strawberries (½ cup for men)

1 tablespoon heavy whipping cream (2 tablespoons for men)

½ tablespoon pure maple syrup (1 tablespoon for men)

Preheat oven to 425 degrees. Spray an 8 x 8-inch baking pan with cooking spray. Place the coconut oil in the pan and put in the oven to melt.

Place all the other ingredients except the toppings in a blender and blend for 5 minutes (do not skip this step!).

Pull the pan out of the oven and pour the blended mixture into the melted coconut oil.

Return the pan to oven and bake for 20 minutes. Top with strawberries, cream, and syrup. Enjoy!!

Women: 492 cals; 21g fat; 41g carb; 35g protein
Men: 599 cals; 27g fat; 55g carb; 36g protein

## Mac and Cheese with Bacon

*Clean Cheat*

3 ounces brown rice pasta (4 ounces for men)

2 tablespoons minced onion

½ teaspoon minced garlic

Dash of cayenne pepper

¼ cup reserved pasta water

⅓ cup 2% cheddar cheese

2 tablespoons plain Greek yogurt

1 slice turkey bacon, chopped

1 tablespoon whole-grain breadcrumbs

1 tablespoon Parmesan cheese

Preheat oven to 425 degrees. Cook the pasta a couple minutes using the package directions. Add a pinch of sea salt to the water. Once cooked, drain and save ¼ cup of the pasta water.

Sauté the onions, garlic, and cayenne pepper in a small frying pan over medium-high heat. Once the onions are soft, add ¼ cup of your pasta water to the pan and lower heat to low-medium. Then add the cheddar cheese and stir until melted. Turn to low heat.

Return pasta to its original pot without any heat. Add yogurt, bacon, melted cheese mixture from the frying pan, and salt and pepper to taste. Mix well.

Pour into a small baking dish. Top with breadcrumbs and Parmesan cheese. Bake for 10 minutes or until cheese is melted. Enjoy!!

Women: 505 cals; 17g fat; 69g carb; 25g protein
Men: 602 cals; 19g fat; 90g carb; 27g protein

## Muddy Buddies

*Clean Cheat*

1½ tablespoons peanut butter (2 tablespoons for men)

3 tablespoons honey

½ teaspoon cocoa powder

2 tablespoons chocolate protein powder

1 cup corn or rice Chex cereal (1½ cups for men)

2 tablespoons peanut butter powder

Melt peanut butter and honey together in the microwave for 20 seconds in a medium-size bowl. Stir in cocoa powder and protein powder. Add Chex and coat well.

Pour mixture into a zip-lock bag. Add peanut butter powder, seal bag, and shake until well coated. Enjoy!

Women: 500 cals; 14g fat; 89g carb; 21g protein
Men: 597 cals; 18g fat; 103g carb; 24g protein

## One-Minute Brownie

*Clean Cheat*

| | |
|---|---|
| 1 whole egg | ¼ teaspoon sea salt |
| 1 tablespoon pure maple syrup | ¼ teaspoon baking powder |
| 1 tablespoon unsweetened almond milk | 10 extra-dark chocolate chips (20 chips for men) |
| 2 tablespoons nut butter | 2 tablespoons heavy cream sweetened with stevia (3 tablespoons for men) |
| ½ scoop chocolate protein powder | |
| 1 tablespoon cocoa powder | |

Beat together the egg, maple syrup, almond milk, and nut butter. Add the protein powder, cocoa powder, sea salt, baking powder, and chocolate chips. Mix well.

Pour into a microwave-safe bowl that's been sprayed with cooking spray and microwave for 1 minute. Top with cream and enjoy!

Women: 538 cals; 36g fat; 33g carb; 25g protein
Men: 615 cals; 43g fat; 36g carb; 26g protein

## Peanut Butter Chocolate Chip Cookie Dough

*Clean Cheat*

| | |
|---|---|
| 2 tablespoons peanut butter (2½ tablespoons for men) | 2 tablespoons vanilla protein powder |
| 1 tablespoon raw honey (2 tablespoons for men) | ⅓ cup oat flour |
| ¼ teaspoon pure vanilla extract | 15 extra-dark chocolate chips |

Mix all ingredients together and eat as is OR scoop into cookie dough balls. Enjoy!

Women: 495 cals; 33g fat; 34g carb; 20g protein
Men: 599 cals; 26g fat; 73g carb; 23g protein

---

## Pigs in a Blanket

*Clean Cheat*

½ cup Kodiak Cakes pancake mix (¾ cup for men)

½ tablespoon olive oil (1 tablespoon for men)

2 tablespoons warm water (3 tablespoons for men)

1 large chicken sausage

2 tablespoons ketchup

Side salad (optional)

Preheat oven to 450 degrees. Line a baking sheet with parchment paper.
Mix together Kodiak Cakes mix, olive oil, and warm water until the mixture resembles bread dough.
Wrap dough around the chicken sausage. Place on a baking sheet and bake for 10 minutes. Dip in ketchup. Enjoy a side salad with your meal.

Women: 430 cals; 17g fat; 40g carb; 30g protein
Men: 585 cals; 25g fat; 55g carb; 37g protein

---

## Spinach Artichoke Dip with Pita Chips

*Clean Cheat*

1 cup spinach, finely chopped

5 ounces canned artichoke hearts, chopped

⅓ cup Parmesan cheese

⅓ cup mozzarella cheese

⅔ cup plain Greek yogurt

½ teaspoon minced garlic

½ teaspoon lemon juice

½ teaspoon salt-free seasoning blend

12 Stacy's pita chips (20 chips for men)

Preheat oven to 375 degrees.

Mix the spinach, artichokes, Parmesan, and mozzarella in a medium-size bowl. In a separate bowl, mix the yogurt, garlic, lemon juice, and seasonings. Add the yogurt mixture to the cheese and spinach mixture. Mix well.

Pour into a greased 8 x 8-inch baking pan that's been sprayed with cooking spray. Bake for 25 minutes or until the cheese is golden around the edges.

Sprinkle the top with Parmesan cheese when finished and enjoy with pita chips!

Women: 511 cals; 21g fat; 35g carb; 41g protein
Men: 615 cals; 25g fat; 51g carb; 43g protein

---

## Sweet Potato Nachos

*Clean Cheat*

6 ounces sweet potatoes, very thinly
    sliced (10 ounces for men)

⅓ cup Monterey jack and cheddar cheese

4 ounces lean ground turkey, cooked

1 teaspoon taco seasoning

1 tablespoon guacamole

1 tablespoon salsa

1 tablespoon plain Greek yogurt

2 tablespoons sliced olives

Jalapeño slices (optional)

Green onions (optional)

Preheat oven to 250 degrees. Line a baking sheet with parchment paper. Place the sweet potato slices in a single layer on the baking sheet. Bake for 1 hour. If they are still soft, flip and bake an additional 15 minutes.

Transfer hot sweet potato chips to a plate and top with cheese, hot ground turkey, taco seasoning, guacamole, salsa, yogurt, olives, jalapeños, and green onions. Dig in!

Women: 500 cals; 22g fat; 42g carb; 34g protein
Men: 600 cals; 23g fat; 66g carb; 36g protein

# Appendices

# APPENDIX A
## *21-Day Daily Tracker*

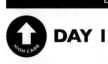 **DAY 1**

**MEALS**
Note what went well, struggles, likes, and dislikes.

 **FITNESS TEST**
Do each exercise for 1 min. Record # done.
Push-ups:
Sit-ups:
Squats:
Burpees:

 **GO THE DISTANCE**
What round did you get to?

 **MIGHTY MINUTES**
5-minute *minimum* then record progress.

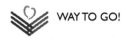 **LESSON INSIGHTS**
Find Your *What* and Your *Why*
Record your thoughts and insights below.

---

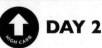 **DAY 2**

**MEALS**
Note what went well, struggles, likes, and dislikes.

 **THE WHOLE 9**
What was your time?

 **DIRTY TWO-THIRTIES**
5-minute *minimum* then record progress.

 **LESSON INSIGHTS**
Discover the True Path to Transformation
Record your thoughts and insights below.

---

WAY TO GO!

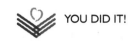 YOU DID IT!

**EXTREME TRANSFORMATION • 21-DAY TRACKER**

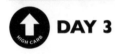 **DAY 3**

### MEALS
Note what went well, struggles, likes, and dislikes.

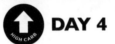 **BURPEE LOVE**
What was your time?

**THRILLING THIRTIES**
5-minute *minimum* then record progress.

**LESSON INSIGHTS**
Keep Your Promises
Record your thoughts and insights below.

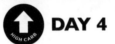 **DAY 4**

### MEALS
Note what went well, struggles, likes, and dislikes.

**PHOENIX RISING**
How many rounds did you get?

**TENACIOUS TWOS**
5-minute *minimum* then record progress.

**LESSON INSIGHTS**
Prepare for Success
Record your thoughts and insights below.

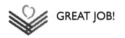 GREAT JOB!

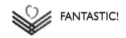 FANTASTIC!

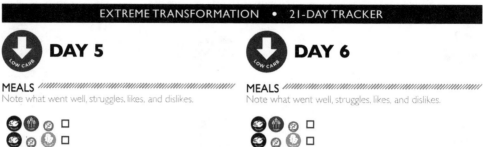

 **DAY 5**

**MEALS**
Note what went well, struggles, likes, and dislikes.

 **A LOTTA TABATA**
What was your lowest rep count per round for
each exercise?

 **NASTY NINETIES**
5-minute *minimum* then record progress.

**LESSON INSIGHTS**
Rally Your Team
Record your thoughts and insights below.

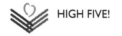 HIGH FIVE!

 **DAY 6**

**MEALS**
Note what went well, struggles, likes, and dislikes.

**MIGHTY MINUTES**
5-minute *minimum* then record progress.

 **LESSON INSIGHTS**
Make It Your Own!
Record your thoughts and insights below.

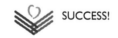 SUCCESS!

## EXTREME TRANSFORMATION • 21-DAY TRACKER

 **DAY 7**

**MEALS**
Note what went well, struggles, likes, and dislikes.

 **WEIGH IN**
Start your day by weighing in and
record your weight. How did you do?

**LESSON INSIGHTS**
Troubleshoot!
Record your thoughts and insights below.

 **DAY 8**

**MEALS**
Note what went well, struggles, likes, and dislikes.

**THE GRINDER**
What was your time?

**DIRTY TWO-THIRTIES**
10-minute *minimum* then record progress.

 **LESSON INSIGHTS**
Believe In Yourself
Record your thoughts and insights below.

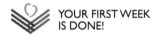 **YOUR FIRST WEEK
IS DONE!**

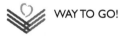 **WAY TO GO!**

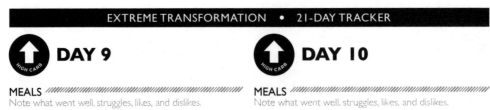

## DAY 9

**MEALS**
Note what went well, struggles, likes, and dislikes.

**RUNNIN' WILD**
What was your time?

**THRILLING THIRTIES**
10-minute *minimum* then record progress.

**LESSON INSIGHTS**
Be Open, Honest, and Vulnerable
Record your thoughts and insights below.

## DAY 10

**MEALS**
Note what went well, struggles, likes, and dislikes.

**MT. EVEREST**
What was your time?

**TENACIOUS TWOS**
10-minute *minimum* then record progress.

**LESSON INSIGHTS**
Unload the Real Weight
Record your thoughts and insights below.

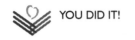 YOU DID IT!

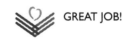 GREAT JOB!

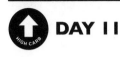 **DAY 11**

**MEALS**
Note what went well, struggles, likes, and dislikes.

**HUSTLE TIME**
How many rounds did you get?

**NASTY NINETIES**
10-minute *minimum* then record progress.

**LESSON INSIGHTS**
Banish the Negative Self-Talk
Record your thoughts and insights below.

**DAY 12**

**MEALS**
Note what went well, struggles, likes, and dislikes.

**BREAKTHROUGH**
What was your lowest rep count per round for each exercise?

**MIGHTY MINUTES**
10-minute *minimum* then record progress.

**LESSON INSIGHTS**
Create Your New Identity
Record your thoughts and insights below.

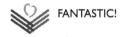 FANTASTIC!

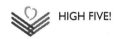 HIGH FIVE!

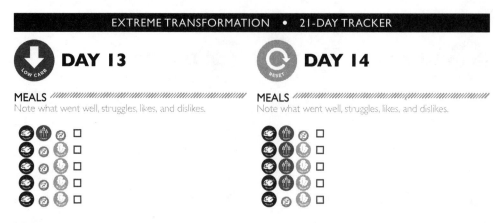

## DAY 13

**MEALS**
Note what went well, struggles, likes, and dislikes.

**DIRTY TWO-THIRTIES**
10-minute *minimum* then record progress.

**LESSON INSIGHTS**
Take Responsibility
Record your thoughts and insights below.

## DAY 14

**MEALS**
Note what went well, struggles, likes, and dislikes.

**WEIGH IN**
Start your day by weighing in and
record your weight. How did you do?

**LESSON INSIGHTS**
Conquer Your F.E.A.R.
Record your thoughts and insights below.

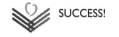 SUCCESS!

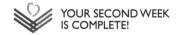 YOUR SECOND WEEK
IS COMPLETE!

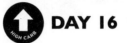

EXTREME TRANSFORMATION • 21-DAY TRACKER

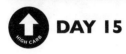 **DAY 15**

## MEALS
Note what went well, struggles, likes, and dislikes.

 ☐
☐
☐
☐
☐

 **THE COUNTDOWN**
What was your time?

 **THRILLING THIRTIES**
15-minute *minimum* then record progress.

 **LESSON INSIGHTS**
Go All In
Record your thoughts and insights below.

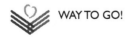 WAY TO GO!

**DAY 16**

## MEALS
Note what went well, struggles, likes, and dislikes.

☐
☐
☐
☐
☐

 **AFTERBURNER**
What was your time?

 **TENACIOUS TWOS**
15-minute *minimum* then record progress.

 **LESSON INSIGHTS**
Fall Without Failing
Record your thoughts and insights below.

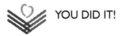 YOU DID IT!

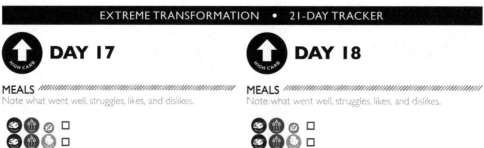

## EXTREME TRANSFORMATION • 21-DAY TRACKER

 **DAY 17**

**MEALS**
Note what went well, struggles, likes, and dislikes.

**CHIPPIN' AWAY**
What was your time?

**NASTY NINETIES**
15-minute *minimum* then record progress.

**LESSON INSIGHTS**
Be Beneficially Selfish
Record your thoughts and insights below.

**DAY 18**

**MEALS**
Note what went well, struggles, likes, and dislikes.

**GO TIME**
How many rounds did you get?

**MIGHTY MINUTES**
15-minute *minimum* then record progress.

**LESSON INSIGHTS**
Have Realistic Expectations of Others
Record your thoughts and insights below.

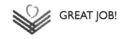 GREAT JOB!

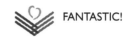 FANTASTIC!

## EXTREME TRANSFORMATION • 21-DAY TRACKER

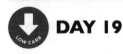 **DAY 19**

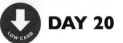 **DAY 20**

**MEALS** ////////////////////////////////////////
Note what went well, struggles, likes, and dislikes.

**MEALS** ////////////////////////////////////////
Note what went well, struggles, likes, and dislikes.

 **WAKE-UP CALL** /////////////////////////////
What was your lowest rep count per round for each exercise?

 **THRILLING THIRTIES** /////////////////////////
15-minute *minimum* then record progress.

 **DIRTY TWO-THIRTIES** /////////////////////////
15-minute *minimum* then record progress.

**LESSON INSIGHTS** /////////////////////////
Triggers and Tactics
Record your thoughts and insights below.

 **LESSON INSIGHTS** /////////////////////////
Replace Your Addiction
Record your thoughts and insights below.

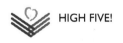 HIGH FIVE!

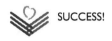 SUCCESS!

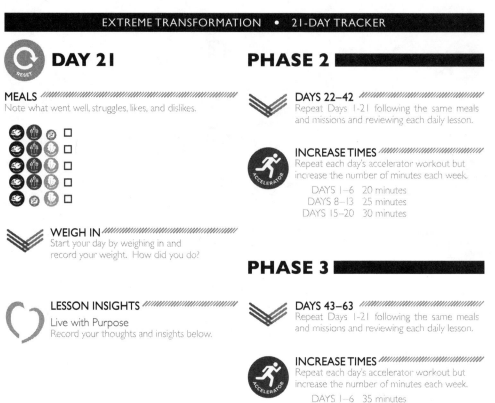

EXTREME TRANSFORMATION • 21-DAY TRACKER

## DAY 21

### MEALS
Note what went well, struggles, likes, and dislikes.

### WEIGH IN
Start your day by weighing in and
record your weight. How did you do?

### LESSON INSIGHTS
Live with Purpose
Record your thoughts and insights below.

## PHASE 2

**DAYS 22–42**
Repeat Days 1-21 following the same meals
and missions and reviewing each daily lesson.

**INCREASE TIMES**
Repeat each day's accelerator workout but
increase the number of minutes each week.

DAYS 1–6    20 minutes
DAYS 8–13   25 minutes
DAYS 15–20  30 minutes

## PHASE 3

**DAYS 43–63**
Repeat Days 1-21 following the same meals
and missions and reviewing each daily lesson.

**INCREASE TIMES**
Repeat each day's accelerator workout but
increase the number of minutes each week.

DAYS 1–6    35 minutes
DAYS 8–13   40 minutes
DAYS 15–20  45 minutes

## PHASE 4

**DAYS 64–84**
Repeat Days 1-21 following the same meals
and missions and reviewing each daily lesson.

**INCREASE TIMES**
Repeat each day's accelerator workout but
increase the number of minutes each week.

DAYS 1–6    50 minutes
DAYS 8–13   55 minutes
DAYS 15–20  60 minutes

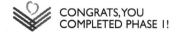
CONGRATS, YOU
COMPLETED PHASE 1!

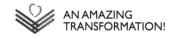
AN AMAZING
TRANSFORMATION!

# APPENDIX B
## *Shopping Lists and Meal Prep*

We've created these Shopping Lists, separated by women and men, to give you an organized week-by-week list of what foods you'll need during your Extreme Transformation, including lists for Clean Cheat days. There's a separate Meal Prep Guide as well, so that after you bring home all the delicious ingredients, you can eliminate the guesswork by planning and prepping your meals ahead of time.

# Shopping Lists

## Week 1 Shopping List

### PROTEIN

| Women | Men | Item | Women | Men | Item | Women | Men | Item |
|---|---|---|---|---|---|---|---|---|
| 8 | 12 | whole eggs | 7 | 11 | scoops protein powder | 6 | 8 | ounces organic lean ground beef |
| 8 | 10 | egg whites | 22 | 35 | ounces chicken breasts | 4 | 6 | ounces white fish |
| 12 | 16 | ounces low-sodium cottage cheese | 12 | 13 | ounces extra-lean ground turkey | 3 | 5 | ounces wild caught salmon |
| 10 | 40 | ounces fat-free plain Greek yogurt | 4 | 4 | ounces nitrate-free turkey bacon | 6 | 10 | large shrimp |

### FRUIT

| Women | Men | Item | Women | Men | Item | Women | Men | Item |
|---|---|---|---|---|---|---|---|---|
| 6 | 7 | bananas | 1 | 1 | apple | 6 | 8 | ounces blackberries |
| 3 | 1 | lemons | 6 | 14 | ounces strawberries | 4 | 6 | ounces blueberries |
| 5 | 5 | limes | 8 | 10 | ounces raspberries | | | |

### VEGGIES AND HERBS

| Women | Men | Item | Women | Men | Item | Women | Men | Item |
|---|---|---|---|---|---|---|---|---|
| 20 | 20 | ounces fresh green beans | 1 | 1 | yellow beet | 1 | 1 | bunch parsley |
| 4 | 4 | ounces shredded carrots | 1 | 1 | large yellow onion | 1 | 1 | bunch chives |
| 1 | 1 | package alfalfa sprouts | 1 | 1 | large red onion | 2 | 2 | bunches green onions |
| 1 | 1 | cup shredded kale | 1 | 1 | green bell pepper | 1 | 1 | bunch cilantro |
| 4 | 5 | cups spinach | 2 | 2 | red bell peppers | 1 | 1 | bunch fresh basil (optional) |
| 1 | 1 | 5-ounce can artichoke hearts | 4 | 4 | ounces sugar snap peas | 1 | 1 | bunch fresh mint (optional) |
| 1 | 1 | romaine lettuce heart | 8 | 12 | ounces mushrooms | 1 | 1 | small bag frozen corn |
| 1 | 1 | head chard | 1 | 1 | zucchini | 1 | 1 | small jar minced garlic |
| 1 | 1 | head butter lettuce | 2 | 2 | cucumbers | 10 | 10 | ounces fresh salsa |
| 3 | 4 | cups cabbage slaw | 1 | 1 | bunch asparagus spears | 1 | 1 | 16-ounce can diced tomatoes, no salt |
| 2 | 2 | celery stalks | 1 | 1 | tomato | | | |
| 1 | 1 | head cauliflower | 8 | 8 | ounces edamame | 1 | 1 | 6-ounce can tomato paste |
| 1 | 1 | head broccoli | 1 | 1 | jalapeño | | | |

### CARBOHYDRATES

| Women | Men | Item | Women | Men | Item | Women | Men | Item |
|---|---|---|---|---|---|---|---|---|
| 1 | 1 | loaf Ezekiel low-sodium bread (frozen section) | 3 | 4 | sweet potatoes | 1 | 2 | Ezekiel tortilla(s) |
| | | | 4 | 5 | small red potatoes | | | Kashi GoLean Crisp cereal |
| ½ | ½ | cup Kodiak Cakes pancake mix | 16 | 16 | ounces butternut squash | | | rice paper wrapper |
| 1 | 1 | whole-grain bun | 16 | 20 | ounces old-fashioned rolled oats | | | Stacy's pita chips |
| 1 | 1 | 15-ounce can garbanzo beans, no salt | 1 | 1 | small bag brown rice | | | extra-dark chocolate chips |
| 1 | 2 | 15-ounce can(s) black beans, no salt | 3 | 4 | yellow corn tortillas | | | granola (optional) |

### FAT

| Women | Men | Item | Women | Men | Item | Women | Men | Item |
|---|---|---|---|---|---|---|---|---|
| | | heavy whipping cream | 1 | 1 | 6-ounce container Laughing Cow cheese wedges | 3 | 4 | tablespoons all-natural peanut butter |
| | | extra-virgin olive oil | | | | | | |
| | | coconut oil | ½ | ½ | slice low-sodium cheddar | 1 | 1 | serving(s) all-natural almond butter (see product label) |
| | | low-fat mayonnaise | 2½ | 2½ | ounces Parmesan cheese | | | |
| 1 | 1 | 2¼-ounce can sliced olives | 2 | 2 | ounces sliced or slivered almonds | | | almond flour |
| 3 | 4 | avocados | | | | | | milled flaxseed |
| 10½ | 10½ | ounces low-fat mozzarella cheese | 1 | 2 | ounce(s) chopped pecans | 0 | 1 | ounce chopped hazelnuts |

### SEASONINGS

|  |  |  |
|---|---|---|
| salt-free seasoning blend | smoked paprika | poppy seeds |
| salt-free tomato & garlic seasoning | ground ginger | ground mustard |
| salt-free garlic & herb seasoning | garlic powder | nutmeg |
| salt-free tomato basil seasoning | dried minced onion | cinnamon |
| salt-free onion & herb seasoning | onion powder | dried basil |
| salt substitute | crushed red pepper flakes | dried oregano |
| ground black pepper | dried basil | dried thyme |
| ground cumin | chili powder | sea salt |

### MISCELLANEOUS ITEMS

| Women | Men | Item | Item | Item |
|---|---|---|---|---|
| 24 | 28 | ounces unsweetened almond milk | Sriracha chili sauce | baking soda |
| 8 | 8 | ounces low-sodium chicken broth | Dijon mustard | pure vanilla extract |
| 8 | 8 | ounces unsweetened applesauce | reduced-sugar barbecue sauce | almond extract (optional) |
| | | raw honey | peanut butter powder | Truvia |
| | | sugar-free syrup | apple cider vinegar | vanilla liquid stevia drops |
| | | pure maple syrup | coconut aminos | |

# EXTREME TRANSFORMATION MEAL PREP—WEEK I

## Days 1–3

Cook 12 ounces boneless, skinless chicken breast (20 ounces for men)

Cook 4 ounces extra-lean ground turkey

Cook ¼ cup brown rice (⅓ cup for men)

Make Lemon Poppy Seed Protein Bites (freeze extras)

Make Tomato Salsa

Thaw shrimp in fridge (see recipe for amount)

## Days 4–6

Cook 10 ounces boneless, skinless chicken breast (15 ounces for men)

Cook 4 ounces extra-lean ground turkey (5 ounces for men)

Cook 2 ounces lean ground beef (4 ounces for men)

Bake 5 ounces sweet potatoes, cut into 4 rounds (6 ounces for men)

Bake ½ cup sweet potatoes, whole (¾ cup for men)

Make Taco Seasoning

Make Sweet Ginger Lime Sauce

Place salmon in fridge to thaw (see recipe for amount)

Marinate 4 ounces white fish in fridge for Citrus and Onion Fish Tacos

# Week 2 Shopping List

Go through your cupboards and cross off anything that you may already have.

## PROTEIN

| Women | Men | Item | Women | Men | Item | Women | Men | Item |
|---|---|---|---|---|---|---|---|---|
| 7 | 8 | whole eggs | 3 | 6½ | scoops protein powder | 1 | 2 | ounce(s) organic lean ground beef |
| 15 | 21 | egg whites | 13 | 22½ | ounces chicken breast | 12 | 17 | ounces wild caught salmon |
| 33 | 37 | ounces fat-free plain Greek yogurt | 9 | 12 | ounces extra-lean ground turkey | 4 | 6 | ounces wild tuna |
| 6 | 10 | ounces low-sodium, fat-free cottage cheese | 1–2 | 1–2 | slices nitrate-free turkey bacon | 4 | 5 | ounces tilapia |

## FRUITS

| Women | Men | Item | Women | Men | Item | Women | Men | Item |
|---|---|---|---|---|---|---|---|---|
| 1 | 1 | pineapple | 1 | 2 | large orange(s) | 12 | 16 | ounces blackberries |
| 3 | 3 | limes | 5 | 6 | bananas | 4 | 8 | ounces raspberries |
| 4 | 4 | lemons | 12 | 24 | ounces blueberries | 1 | 1 | apple |

## VEGGIES AND HERBS

| Women | Men | Item | Women | Men | Item | Women | Men | Item |
|---|---|---|---|---|---|---|---|---|
| 8 | 8 | ounces fresh green beans | 1 | 1 | green bell pepper | 1 | 1 | bunch fresh basil |
| 1 | 2 | head(s) cauliflower | 2 | 2 | bunches asparagus spears | 1 | 1 | bunch fresh parsley |
| 1 | 1 | head broccoli | 12 | 16 | ounces sugar snap peas | 1 | 1 | bunch cilantro |
| 1 | 1 | head green cabbage | 1 | 1 | cucumber | 4 | 4 | small mint leaves |
| 1 | 1 | head red cabbage | 1 | 1 | spaghetti squash | 1 | 1 | bunch green onions |
| 4 | 4 | cups spinach | 2 | 2 | cherry tomatoes | 1 | 1 | bunch chives |
| 1 | 1 | yellow onion | 6 | 6 | ounces raw edamame, shelled | | | fresh ginger |
| 2 | 2 | red onions | 2 | 2 | medium poblano peppers | 1 | 1 | shallot |
| 4 | 4 | ounces frozen corn | 1 | 1 | jalapeño | | | minced garlic |
| 2 | 2 | zucchini | 1 | 1 | small green tomatillo | 4 | 4 | ounces fresh salsa |
| 1 | 1 | yellow squash | 6 | 6 | sprigs fresh tarragon | | | |
| 2 | 2 | red bell peppers | 1 | 1 | sprig rosemary | | | |

## CARBOHYDRATES

| Women | Men | Item | Women | Men | Item | Women | Men | Item |
|---|---|---|---|---|---|---|---|---|
| 7 | 10 | ounces sweet potatoes | 4 | 4 | slices Ezekiel low-sodium bread (frozen section) | 2 | 3 | rice cakes |
| 3 | 4 | small red potatoes | | | | | | Kashi GoLean Crisp cereal |
| 6 | 9 | ounces quinoa | 1 | 1 | whole-wheat pita (Papa Pita brand) | | | Corn Chex cereal |
| 6 | 12 | ounces brown rice | | | whole-grain bread crumbs | 11 | 12 | ounces old-fashioned rolled oats |
| 3 | 3 | ounces brown rice pasta | 3 | 3 | ounces whole-wheat flour | | | |
| 1 | 1 | 15-ounce can black beans | 3 | 3 | yellow corn tortillas | | | dark chocolate chips |

## FATS

| Women | Men | Item | Women | Men | Item | Women | Men | Item |
|---|---|---|---|---|---|---|---|---|
| 2 | 2 | ounces whipped cream cheese | 4 | 4 | ounces cheddar jack cheese | 1 | 1 | ounce pistachios |
| 1 | 1 | ounce reduced-fat unsweetened shredded coconut | 2 | 2 | slices pepper jack cheese | 2 | 2 | ounces raw pumpkin seeds |
| 4 | 4 | ounces low-fat mozzarella cheese | | | low-fat mayonnaise | 1 | 1 | 2¼-ounce can sliced olives |
| 1 | 1 | ounce shredded Parmesan cheese | | | pesto sauce | | | all-natural almond butter |
| 2 | 2 | tablespoons feta cheese | | | coconut oil | | | all-natural peanut butter |
| 6 | 6 | ounces cheddar cheese | | | extra-virgin olive oil | 1 | 1½ | tablespoon unsalted butter |
| | | | 5 | 5 | ounces slivered almonds | | | milled flaxseed |

## SEASONINGS

|  |  |  |
|---|---|---|
| sea salt | dried thyme | dried oregano |
| black pepper | red pepper flakes | cayenne pepper |
| salt-free garlic & herb seasoning | cocoa powder | granulated garlic |
| salt-free southwest seasoning | powdered peanut butter | garlic powder |
| salt-free tomato basil seasoning | cinnamon | ground mustard |
| salt-free chicken seasoning | nutmeg | onion powder |
| salt-free onion & herb seasoning | paprika | dried minced onion |
| salt substitute | cumin | |

## MISCELLANEOUS ITEMS

| Women | Men | Item | Women | Men | Item | Women | Men | Item |
|---|---|---|---|---|---|---|---|---|
| | | raw honey | | | rice vinegar | 8 | 8 | ounces unsweetened applesauce |
| | | pure maple syrup | | | Sriracha chili sauce | | | Dijon mustard |
| | | vanilla liquid stevia drops | 36 | 36 | ounces unsweetened almond milk | | | reduced-sugar barbecue sauce |
| | | pure vanilla extract | | | powdered peanut butter | | | apple cider vinegar |
| | | coconut extract (optional) | | | zero-calorie nonstick cooking spray | | | |
| | | Truvia | | | | | | |

# EXTREME TRANSFORMATION MEAL PREP—WEEK 2

## Days 8–10

Cook 1 ounce lean ground beef
(2 ounces for men)

Cook 2 ounces boneless, skinless
chicken breast (3 ounces for men)

Cook 6 ounces extra-lean ground
turkey (8 ounces for men)

Cook ¼ cup quinoa (½ cup for men)

Cook ¾ cup brown rice (1½ cups for
men)

Boil 4 eggs (6 eggs for men)

Make Pumpkin Seed Granola
(refrigerate extras)

Make Berry Puree

Thaw salmon in fridge (see recipe for
amount)

Thaw and marinate tuna in fridge (see
recipe for amount)

## Days 11–13

Cook 6 ounces boneless, skinless
chicken breast (12 ounces for men)

Cook 1 cup quinoa

Bake ½ cup sweet potatoes, whole
(¾ cup for men)

Boil 1 cup red potatoes (1½ cups for
men)

Boil 7 eggs (10 eggs for men)

Make Marinade for chicken

Make Yogurt Sauce

Make Greek Yogurt Tartar Sauce

Make Chocolate Chip Almond Coconut
Bites (freeze extras)

Make Hummus

Thaw 3 ounces extra-lean ground
turkey in fridge (4 ounces for men)

# Week 3 Shopping List

## Go through your cupboards and cross off anything that you may already have.

### PROTEIN

| Women | Men | Item | Women | Men | Item | Women | Men | Item |
|---|---|---|---|---|---|---|---|---|
| ☐ | 13 | 13 | whole eggs | ☐ | 26 | 34 | ounces fat-free plain Greek yogurt | ☐ | 3 | 5 | ounces lean lamb meat (shoulder) |
| ☐ | 18 | 20 | egg whites | ☐ | 1 | 1 | large chicken sausage | ☐ | 2 | 4 | pieces firm tofu |
| ☐ | 6½ | 11 | scoops protein powder | ☐ | 6½ | 16½ | ounces chicken breast | ☐ | 2 | 4 | ounces canned tuna |
| ☐ | 10 | 10 | ounces cottage cheese | ☐ | 14 | 22 | ounces extra-lean ground turkey | ☐ | 3 | 5 | ounces wild caught salmon |
| ☐ | | | protein powder | ☐ | 3 | 5 | ounces lean pork tenderloin | ☐ | 10 | 10 | large shrimp |

### FRUITS

| Women | Men | Item | Women | Men | Item | Women | Men | Item |
|---|---|---|---|---|---|---|---|---|
| ☐ | 3 | 3 | limes | ☐ | 1 | 1 | pear | ☐ | 20 | 20 | ounces strawberries |
| ☐ | 2 | 2 | lemons | ☐ | 8 | 10 | bananas | ☐ | 12 | 12 | ounces blackberries |
| ☐ | 2 | 2 | apples | ☐ | 1 | 2 | large orange(s) | ☐ | 4 | 4 | ounces berries of choice |

### VEGGIES AND HERBS

| Women | Men | Item | Women | Men | Item | Women | Men | Item |
|---|---|---|---|---|---|---|---|---|
| ☐ | 4 | 4 | tomatoes on the vine | ☐ | 2 | 2 | yellow onions | ☐ | 2 | 2 | ounces pumpkin puree |
| ☐ | 1 | 1 | head broccoli | ☐ | 2 | 2 | red onions | ☐ | | | minced garlic |
| ☐ | 1 | 1 | head cauliflower | ☐ | 4 | 4 | red bell peppers | ☐ | | | fresh salsa |
| ☐ | 1 | 1 | cup cabbage or cabbage slaw | ☐ | 1 | 1 | green bell pepper | ☐ | | | fresh rosemary |
| ☐ | 1 | 1 | romaine lettuce heart | ☐ | 1 | 1 | jalapeño (optional) | ☐ | 1 | 1 | bunch cilantro |
| ☐ | | | Boston, Bibb, or red leaf lettuce | ☐ | 1 | 1 | bunch asparagus spears | ☐ | 1 | 1 | bunch parsley |
| ☐ | 2 | 2 | cups arugula | ☐ | 8 | 8 | ounces fresh green beans | ☐ | 4 | 4 | small mint leaves |
| ☐ | 4 | 4 | cups spinach | ☐ | 1 | 1 | radish | ☐ | 1 | 1 | basil leaf |
| ☐ | 1 | 1 | eggplant | ☐ | 2 | 2 | small mushrooms | ☐ | 3 | 3 | small sage leaves |
| ☐ | 2 | 2 | cucumbers | ☐ | 10 | 10 | cherry tomatoes | ☐ | 1 | 1 | bunch green onions |
| ☐ | 3 | 3 | zucchini squash | ☐ | 2 | 2 | ounces edamame, shelled | ☐ | 1 | 1 | bunch chives |
| ☐ | 2 | 2 | yellow squash | ☐ | 2 | 2 | ounces frozen or fresh corn | ☐ | 3 | 3 | sprigs tarragon |

### CARBOHYDRATES

| Women | Men | Item | Women | Men | Item | Women | Men | Item |
|---|---|---|---|---|---|---|---|---|
| ☐ | 8 | 8 | ounces whole-wheat flour | ☐ | | | Kodiak Cakes pancake mix | ☐ | 6 | 6 | ounces old-fashioned rolled oats |
| ☐ | 14 | 14 | ounces quinoa, cooked | ☐ | 1 | 1 | spelt tortilla (Rudi's brand) | ☐ | 2 | 3 | rice cakes |
| ☐ | 16 | 22 | ounces sweet potatoes | ☐ | 2 | 2 | ounces black beans | ☐ | | | extra-dark chocolate chips |
| ☐ | 1 | 1 | small sweet potato | ☐ | 6 | 8 | ounces white beans | | | | |
| ☐ | 6 | 8 | ounces red potatoes | ☐ | 2 | 2 | ounces steel-cut oats | | | | |

### FAT

| Women | Men | Item | Women | Men | Item | Women | Men | Item |
|---|---|---|---|---|---|---|---|---|
| ☐ | | | heavy whipping cream | ☐ | 1 | 2 | piece(s) string cheese | ☐ | 3 | 4 | ounces milled flaxseed or chia seeds |
| ☐ | | | coconut oil | ☐ | 2 | 2 | ounces raw peanuts, unsalted | ☐ | | | all-natural nut butter of choice |
| ☐ | 6 | 6 | ounces low-fat mozzarella cheese | ☐ | 1 | 1 | ounce chopped pecans | ☐ | 1 | 1 | ounce sliced olives |
| ☐ | 4 | 4 | ounces fat-free cheddar cheese | ☐ | 4 | 5 | avocados | | | | |
| ☐ | 3 | 3 | ounces cheddar jack cheese | ☐ | | | extra-virgin olive oil | | | | |
| | | | | ☐ | 1½ | 2½ | ounces slivered almonds | | | | |

### SEASONINGS

| Women | Men | Item | Women | Men | Item | Women | Men | Item |
|---|---|---|---|---|---|---|---|---|
| ☐ | | | cinnamon | ☐ | | | granulated garlic | ☐ | | | red pepper flakes |
| ☐ | | | sea salt | ☐ | | | cumin seed | ☐ | | | ground cumin |
| ☐ | | | salt substitute | ☐ | | | yellow mustard seed | ☐ | | | onion powder |
| ☐ | | | salt-free garlic & herb seasoning | ☐ | | | ground mustard powder | ☐ | | | dried oregano |
| ☐ | | | salt-free tomato basil seasoning | ☐ | | | ground turmeric | ☐ | | | dried basil |
| ☐ | | | salt-free onion & herb seasoning | ☐ | | | ground ginger | ☐ | | | whole fennel seeds |
| ☐ | | | salt-free southwest seasoning | ☐ | | | yellow curry powder | ☐ | | | dried thyme |
| ☐ | | | salt-free chicken seasoning | ☐ | | | ground coriander | ☐ | | | ground nutmeg |
| ☐ | | | paprika | ☐ | | | garam masala | ☐ | | | ketchup |
| ☐ | | | black pepper | ☐ | | | chili powder | | | | |
| ☐ | | | garlic powder | ☐ | | | red chili flakes | | | | |

### MISCELLANEOUS ITEMS

| Women | Men | Item | Women | Men | Item | Women | Men | Item |
|---|---|---|---|---|---|---|---|---|
| ☐ | | | zero-calorie nonstick cooking spray | ☐ | | | powdered peanut butter | ☐ | 8 | 8 | ounces unsweetened applesauce |
| ☐ | 8 | 8 | ounces black coffee | ☐ | | | vanilla liquid stevia drops | ☐ | | | cocktail sauce |
| ☐ | | | Dijon mustard | ☐ | | | reduced-sugar barbecue sauce | ☐ | 8 | 8 | ounces low-sodium chicken broth |
| ☐ | | | pure vanilla extract | ☐ | 22 | 22 | ounces unsweetened almond milk | ☐ | | | cocoa powder |
| ☐ | | | Truvia baking powder | ☐ | | | balsamic vinegar | | | | |
| | | | | ☐ | | | sugar-free pancake syrup | | | | |

# EXTREME TRANSFORMATION MEAL PREP—WEEK 3

## Days 15–17

Cook 4 ounces extra-lean ground turkey (5 ounces for men)

Cook 1 ounce boneless, skinless chicken breast (3 ounces for men)

Bake 6 ounces sweet potatoes, 4 rounds (8 ounces for men)

Bake ½ cup sweet potatoes, diced (¾ cup for men)

Make Strawberry and Banana Quinoa Muffins (freeze extras)

Make Cilantro Lime Dressing

Thaw 3 ounces pork on Day 16 (5 ounces for men) (marinate in refrigerator overnight)

Thaw 7 ounces extra-lean ground turkey in fridge (10 ounces for men)

## Days 18–20

Cook 1½ ounces boneless, skinless chicken breast (3 ounces for men)

Cook 2 ounces extra-lean ground turkey (4 ounces for men)

Cook ¾ cup quinoa

Bake 6 ounces red potatoes (8 ounces for men)

Make Homemade Ranch Powder

Make Berry Puree

Make Avocado Puree

Make House Pickles

Make Breakfast Frittata Veggie "Muffins"

Marinate 3 ounces lamb in All-Purpose Marinade in fridge (5 ounces for men)

Thaw 3 ounces extra-lean ground turkey in fridge (5 ounces for men)

# APPENDIX C
## *Extreme Transformation Bulk Prep Cooking Guide*

## Bulk Prep Cooking Guide

## PROTEIN

### Chicken

### Grill

1. Preheat outdoor or countertop grill on high heat.
2. Lightly spray the grill with nonstick cooking spray.
3. Grill 12–15 minutes per side.
4. Chicken is done when it is no longer pink and juices run clear.
5. Add seasonings, and serve or store.

### Boil

1. Place chicken in a large pot and add enough water to cover it completely.
2. Cover the pot and bring the water to a boil.
3. Reduce heat to a simmer and gently boil for 60 minutes.
4. Remove chicken, let cool, and shred or chop the meat.
5. Add seasonings, and serve or store.

## Bake

1. Preheat oven to 400°F.
2. Spray baking sheet or dish with nonstick cooking spray, or line with foil or parchment paper.
3. Bake for 20–25 minutes or until chicken is no longer pink in the center and juices run clear.
4. Add seasonings, and serve or store.

## Broil

1. Preheat oven to broil.
2. Spray broiler pan with nonstick cooking spray.
3. Butterfly-cut the chicken.
4. Move oven rack to the top.
5. Broil for 8 minutes per side.
6. Add seasonings, serve, or store.

## Ground Turkey or Beef

### Skillet or Frying Pan

1. Lightly spray large skillet or pan with nonstick cooking spray.
2. Cook the ground turkey or beef over medium heat for 5–10 minutes.
3. While cooking, continue to chop and break chicken into smaller and smaller chunks until browned.
4. Add seasonings, serve, or store.

## Eggs

### Hard-Boil

1. Bring a large pot of water to a boil.
2. Using a large spoon, carefully place each egg in the boiling water one at a time. Bring water back to a boil and let cook 10 minutes.
3. Drain and run cold water over the eggs until cool to touch.
4. Cool in fridge. Peel when ready to eat.

# CARBS

## Brown Rice

### Cooked on the Stovetop

1. Place pot on the stove and add water and brown rice (for every 1 cup of brown rice, add 1½ cups water).
2. Bring water to a boil, cover with a lid, reduce heat, and simmer for 50 minutes.
3. Remove from heat and fluff with a fork.
4. Add seasonings, and serve or store.

### Cooked in a Grain Cooker

1. Pour brown rice and water into the grain cooker (for every 1 cup brown rice, add 1½ cups water).
2. Close the lid and press START.
3. When cooked, open lid slowly and fluff with a fork.
4. Add seasonings, serve, or store.

## Quinoa

### Cooked on the Stovetop

1. Rinse quinoa with cold running water.
2. Follow directions on package.

## Potatoes and Sweet Potatoes

### Boil

1. Chop potatoes or yams and place in a pot.
2. Fill with water so that they are just covered.
3. Bring to a boil, reduce heat, and simmer for 50–60 minutes.
4. Remove from the heat and run under cold water until cool.
5. Add seasonings. Serve (with skins or mashed) or store.

## Bake (chopped)

1. Preheat oven to 425°F.
2. Cover baking sheet with foil and spray with nonstick cooking spray.
3. Slice sweet potatoes into rounds or dice into cubes.
4. Bake 20 minutes. Flip. Bake another 15–20 minutes or until fork tender (not hard, but not mushy).

## Bake (whole)

1. Preheat oven to 350°F.
2. Stab potatoes or yams with fork 8–10 times each to penetrate the skin.
3. Wrap each potato or yam in aluminum foil (optional).
4. Bake for 60 minutes.
5. Remove from oven and allow to cool for 30 minutes before serving or storing.

# APPENDIX D

## EXTREME CYCLE ACCEPTABLE FOODS
## AND 100-CALORIE PORTIONS

### CARBS

#### Breads
| | |
|---|---|
| Breads, whole-grain | 1 slice |
| Tortillas, brown rice | ¾ tortilla |
| Tortillas, corn | 1½ tortillas |

#### Cereal
| | |
|---|---|
| All-Bran | ½ cup |
| Fiber One | 1 cup |
| Granola (low-fat) | ⅓ cup |
| Kashi cereals | ½ cup |
| Oatmeal | ¾ cup |

#### Fruits
| | |
|---|---|
| Apples | 1½ apple |
| Apricots | 5 apricots |
| Bananas | 1 banana |
| Berries | 1½ cups |
| Grapes | 1½ cups |
| Kiwi | 3 kiwi |
| Lemon juice | 8 ounces |
| Lime juice | 8 ounces |
| Melons | 2 cups |
| Monk fruit | Unlimited! |
| Oranges/Tangerines | 1 whole |
| Peaches/Nectarines | 2 whole |
| Pears | 1 pear |
| Pineapple | 1 cup |
| Plums | 3 plums |

#### Grains
| | |
|---|---|
| Amaranth | ½ cup |
| Barley | ½ cup |
| Buckwheat | ½ cup |
| Couscous | ½ cup |
| Popcorn (air-popped) | 3½ cups |
| Quinoa | ½ cup |
| Rice, brown (long-grain) | ½ cup |
| Rice, wild | ½ cup |

### Legumes
| | |
|---|---|
| Beans (low-sodium only) | ½ cup |
| Hummus | 2 tablespoons |
| Lentils (low-sodium only) | ½ cup |

#### Starchy Veggies
| | |
|---|---|
| Corn | ½ cup |
| Peas | 1 cup |
| Potatoes (medium) | 1 potato |
| Sweet potatoes/Yams (medium) | ¾ cup |

#### Pasta
| | |
|---|---|
| Pasta, brown rice | ½ cup |
| Pasta, whole-grain | ½ cup |

### CONDIMENTS/DRESSINGS/MISC

| | |
|---|---|
| Chili paste | ½ tablespoon |
| Chili sauce | 1½ tablespoons |
| Marinara sauce (Newman's Own) | ½ cup |
| Mayonnaise (fat-free) | 4 tablespoons |
| Mustard | 6 teaspoons |
| Nonstick cooking spray (butter flavor) | 10 sprays |
| Salad dressing, creamy | 1.5 tablespoons |
| Salad dressing, French (fat-free) | 4 tablespoons |
| Salad dressing, Italian (low-fat) | 2 tablespoons |
| Salsa (Newman's Own All-Natural) | 12 tablespoons |
| Soy sauce (low-sodium) | 6 teaspoons |
| Tabasco sauce | 20 teaspoons |
| Tomato paste | 4 tablespoons |
| Tomato sauce | 1 cup |
| Vinaigrette, balsamic (fat-free) | 2 tablespoons |
| Vinegar, balsamic | 2 tablespoons |

# EXTREME CYCLE ACCEPTABLE FOODS
# AND 100-CALORIE PORTIONS

## FATS

| | |
|---|---|
| Almond butter (with salt) | 1 tablespoon |
| Almond milk (unsweetened) | 2 cups |
| Almonds (raw, whole) | 2 tablespoons |
| Avocados | ½ medium |
| Butter | 1 tablespoon |
| Cheese | 1 ounce |
| Cream, heavy whipping | 2 tablespoons |
| Feta cheese/Ricotta cheese (regular) | ⅓ cup |
| Mayonnaise (regular) | 1 tablespoon |
| Oil, fish | 1 tablespoon |
| Oil, flaxseed | 1 tablespoon |
| Oil, olive | 1 tablespoon |
| Olives (large) | 10 olives |
| Peanut butter (powdered) | 4.5 tablespoons |
| Peanut butter (salted) | 1 tablespoon |
| Pecans (raw, chopped) | 2 tablespoons |
| Sunflower seeds | 2 tablespoons |
| Soy nuts (roasted, lightly salted) | 2 tablespoons |
| Walnuts (raw, chopped) | 2 tablespoons |

## HERBS & SPICES

| | |
|---|---|
| Basil | Unlimited! |
| Cayenne pepper | Unlimited! |
| Chili powder | Unlimited! |
| Cinnamon | Unlimited! |
| Cloves | Unlimited! |
| Cocoa powder | Unlimited! |
| Curry powder | Unlimited! |
| Garlic/Garlic powder | Unlimited! |
| Ginger | Unlimited! |
| Horseradish | Unlimited! |
| Salt-free spice blends | Unlimited! |
| Nutmeg | Unlimited! |
| Onion powder | Unlimited! |
| Oregano | Unlimited! |
| Paprika | Unlimited! |
| Parsley | Unlimited! |
| Pepper, black | Unlimited! |
| Peppers | Unlimited! |
| Rosemary | Unlimited! |
| Sea salt (high-sodium) | Unlimited! |
| Stevia | Unlimited! |
| Thyme | Unlimited! |
| Turmeric | Unlimited! |

## PROTEIN

| | |
|---|---|
| Egg substitutes | 1 cup |
| Egg whites | 5 whites |
| Egg yolks | 2 yolks |
| Whey/Egg/Pea/ Soy protein powder | 1 scoop |

### Beef

| | |
|---|---|
| Steak, cube | 2½ ounces |
| Steak, flank | 2 ounces |
| Steak, round | 2 ounces |

### Dairy

| | |
|---|---|
| Cottage cheese | 1 cup |
| Yogurt, fat-free plain Greek | 1 cup |

### Lean Meats

| | |
|---|---|
| Buffalo (ground) | 1½ ounces |
| Chicken breast (lean ground) | 2 ounces |
| Turkey (lean ground) | 3 ounces |
| Ostrich/Duck breast | 2 ounces |
| Venison/Elk | 2 ounces |

### Poultry

| | |
|---|---|
| Chicken breast | 4 ounces |
| Chicken broth (low-sodium) | 4 cups |
| Chicken thighs | 3 ounces |
| Turkey breast (not deli) | 3 ounces |
| Turkey (low-sodium deli) | 3½ ounces |

### Seafood

| | |
|---|---|
| Salmon (canned) | 3½ ounces |
| Salmon (fillet) | 2 ounces |
| Shellfish: Scallops/Crab/ Lobster/Shrimp | 4 ounces |
| Tuna (canned) | 3 ounces |
| Whitefish: Snapper/ Halibut/Cod/Tilapia | 2 ounces |

# EXTREME CYCLE ACCEPTABLE FOODS
# AND 100-CALORIE PORTIONS

## VEGETABLES

| | |
|---|---|
| Asparagus | Unlimited! |
| Broccoli | Unlimited! |
| Cabbage | Unlimited! |
| Carrots | Unlimited! |
| Cauliflower | Unlimited! |
| Celery | Unlimited! |
| Collard greens | Unlimited! |
| Cucumbers | Unlimited! |
| Eggplant | Unlimited! |
| Green beans | Unlimited! |
| Lettuces | Unlimited! |
| Mixed greens | Unlimited! |
| Mushrooms | Unlimited! |
| Onions | Unlimited! |
| Peppers | Unlimited! |
| Sprouts | Unlimited! |
| Squash | Unlimited! |
| Tomatoes | Unlimited! |
| Zucchini | Unlimited! |

# ACKNOWLEDGMENTS

A very special thank-you to the incredible team of stellar individuals who worked long and tireless hours to make this book possible: Billie Fitzpatrick, Simon Green, Ryan Levine, Jennifer Weaver, Molly Schoneveld, Hachette Books, Lisa LaFon, Erika Peterson, David Rushing, Allison Tyler Jones, Susan Kelley, and Jessie Dahling.

To our family and friends: Thank you for loving and supporting us unconditionally. Thank you for understanding our chaotic family life and work schedules. Even though we don't get to see much of one another these crazy days, we look forward to spending quality time together soon.

To ABC and our *Extreme Weight Loss* production crew: Thank you for your support, hard work, and friendship over the years. It has been a wild ride, but together we have been able to capture and share what the true journey of transformation looks like.

To our courageous *Extreme Weight Loss* participants: Thank you for letting us embark on the journey with you. Thank you for sharing your struggles and triumphs. Thank you for teaching us the real journey of transformation through your experiences. Because of you, we are able to share this guide with the world. Together, we will continue to change millions of lives.

# INDEX

# Want more inspiration and transformation?

Choose Chris Powell's other bestselling titles today!

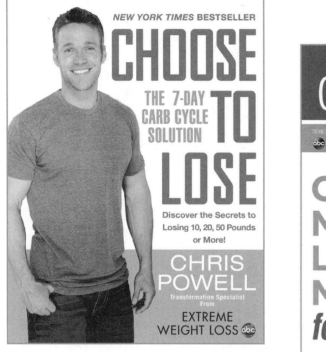

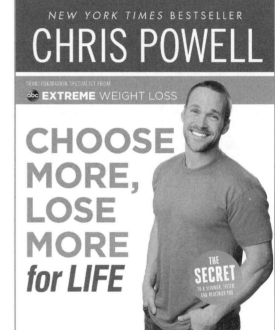

Also Available as eBooks and from
Hachette Audio

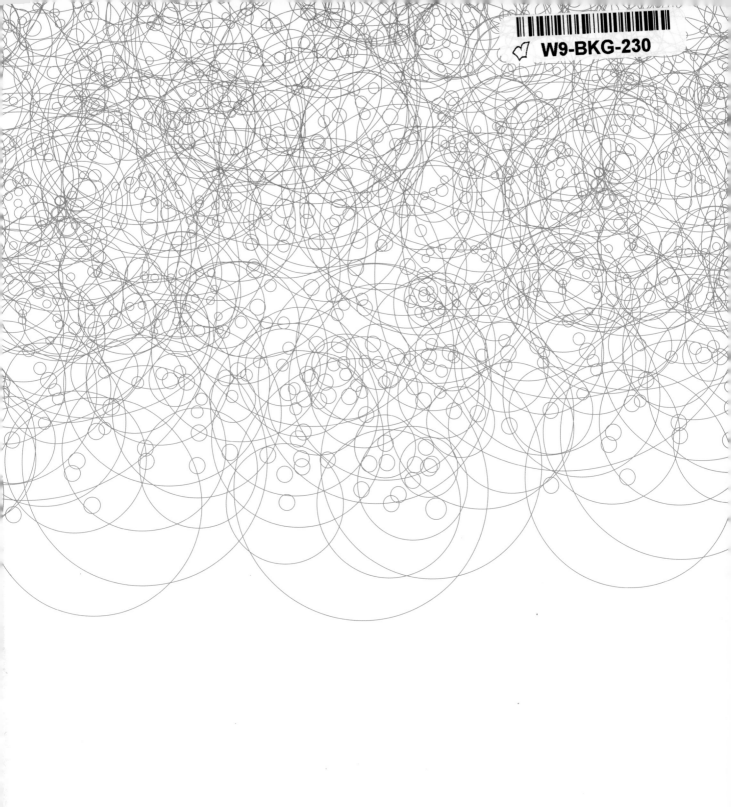

# GRAPHIC DESIGN

# THE NEW BASICS

ELLEN LUPTON AND JENNIFER COLE PHILLIPS

**Princeton Architectural Press, New York** and

**Maryland Institute College of Art, Baltimore**

Published by
Princeton Architectural Press
37 East Seventh Street
New York, New York 10003

For a free catalog of books, call
1.800.722.6657.
Visit our website at www.papress.com.

Library of Congress Cataloging-in-Publication Data
Lupton, Ellen.
  Graphic design : the new basics / Ellen Lupton and
Jennifer Cole Phillips.
    247 p. : ill. (chiefly col.) ; 23 cm.
  Includes bibliographical references and index.
  ISBN 978-1-56898-770-5 (hardcover : alk. paper)
  ISBN 978-1-56898-702-6 (paperback : alk. paper)
  1. Graphic arts.  I. Phillips, Jennifer C., 1960– II. Title.
  NC997.L87 2008
  741.6—dc22
                                    2007033805

eISBN 978-1-56898-947-1

**For Maryland Institute College of Art**

**Book Design**
Ellen Lupton and Jennifer Cole Phillips

**Contributing Faculty**
Ken Barber
Kimberly Bost
Jeremy Botts
Corinne Botz
Bernard Canniffe
Nancy Froehlich
Ellen Lupton
Al Maskeroni
Ryan McCabe
Abbott Miller
Jennifer Cole Phillips
James Ravel
Zvezdana Rogic
Nolen Strals
Mike Weikert
Bruce Willen
Yeohyun Ahn

**Visiting Artists**
Marian Bantjes
Nicholas Blechman
Alicia Cheng
Peter Cho
Malcolm Grear
David Plunkert
C. E. B. Reas
Paul Sahre
Jan van Toorn
Rick Valicenti

**For Princeton Architectural Press**

**Editor**
Clare Jacobson

**Special thanks to**
Nettie Aljian, Sara Bader, Dorothy Ball,
Nicola Bednarek, Janet Behning, Becca Casbon,
Penny (Yuen Pik) Chu, Russell Fernandez,
Pete Fitzpatrick, Wendy Fuller, Jan Haux,
Aileen Kwun, Nancy Eklund Later, Linda
Lee, Laurie Manfra, Katharine Myers, Lauren
Nelson Packard, Jennifer Thompson, Arnoud
Verhaeghe, Paul Wagner, Joseph Weston, and
Deb Wood — *Kevin C. Lippert, publisher*

# Contents

# Foreword

*Ellen Lupton and Jennifer Cole Phillips*

How do designers get ideas? Some places they look are design annuals and monographs, searching for clever combinations of forms, fonts, and colors to inspire their projects. For students and professionals who want to dig deeper into how form works, this book shows how to build richness and complexity around simple relationships. We created this book because we didn't see anything like it available for today's students and young designers: a concise, visually inspiring guide to two-dimensional design.

As educators with decades of combined experience in graduate and undergraduate teaching, we have witnessed the design world change and change again in response to new technologies. When we were students ourselves in the 1980s, classic books such as Armin Hofmann's *Graphic Design Manual* (published in 1965) had begun to lose their relevance within the restless and shifting design scene. Postmodernism was on the rise, and abstract design exercises seemed out of step with the current interest in appropriation and historicism.

During the 1990s, design educators became caught in the pressure to teach (and learn) software, and many of us struggled to balance technical skills with visual and critical thinking. Form sometimes got lost along the way, as design methodologies moved away from universal visual concepts toward a more anthropological understanding of design as a constantly changing flow of cultural sensibilities.

This book addresses the gap between software and visual thinking. By focusing on form, we have re-embraced the Bauhaus tradition and the pioneering work of the great formal design educators, from Armin Hofmann to some of our own teachers, including Malcolm Grear. We believe that a common ground of visual principles connects designers across history and around the globe.

We initiated this project in 2005, after stepping back and noticing that our students were not at ease building concepts abstractly. Although they were adept at working and reworking pop-culture vocabularies, they were less comfortable manipulating scale, rhythm, color, hierarchy, grids, and diagrammatic relationships.

In this book, you won't see exercises or demonstrations involving parody or cultural critique— not that there is anything wrong with those lines of inquiry. Designers and educators will always build personal meaning and social content into their work. With this book we chose to focus, however, on design's formal structures.

This is a book for students and emerging designers, and it is illustrated primarily with student work, produced within graduate and undergraduate design studios. Our school, Maryland Institute College of Art (MICA), became our laboratory. Numerous faculty and scores of students participated in our brave experiment over a two-year period. The work that emerged is varied and diverse, reflecting an organic range of skill levels and sensibilities. Unless otherwise noted, all the student examples were generated in the context of MICA's courses; a few projects originate from schools we visited or where our own graduate students are teaching.

Our student contributors come from China, India, Japan, Korea, Puerto Rico, Trinidad, Seattle, Minneapolis, Baltimore, rural Pennsylvania, and many other places. The book was manufactured in China and published with Princeton Architectural Press in New York City.

This book was thus created in a global context. The work presented within its pages is energized by the diverse backgrounds of its producers, whose creativity is shaped by their cultural identities as well as by their unique life experiences. A common thread that draws all these people together in one place is design.

The majority of student work featured here comes from the course we teach together at MICA, the Graphic Design MFA Studio. Our MFA program's first publishing venture was the book *D.I.Y.: Design It Yourself* (2006), directed at general readers who want to use design in their own lives. Currently underway is a guide to independent publishing, along with other titles devoted to expanding access to and the understanding of design processes.

The current volume, *Graphic Design: The New Basics*, marks the launch of MICA's Center for Design Thinking, an umbrella for organizing the college's diverse efforts in the area of practical design research. In addition to publishing books about design, the Center for Design Thinking will organize conferences and educational events to help build the design discourse while creating invaluable opportunities for MICA's students and faculty.

To complement the student work featured in this project, we have selected key examples from contemporary professional practice. These works demonstrate experimental, visually rich design approaches conducted at the highest possible level.

Many of the designers featured, including Marian Bantjes, Alicia Cheng, Peter Cho, Malcolm Grear, David Plunkert, C. E. B. Reas, Paul Sahre, Rick Valicenti, and Jan van Toorn, have worked with our students as visiting artists at MICA. Some conducted special workshops whose results are included in this volume.

*Graphic Design: The New Basics* lays out the elements of a visual language whose forms are employed by individuals, institutions, and locales that are increasingly connected in a global society. We hope the book will inspire more thought and creativity.

## Acknowledgments

My work creating this book constituted my degree project in the Doctorate in Communication Design program at the University of Baltimore. I thank my advisors, Stuart Moulthrop, Sean Carton, and Amy Pointer. I also thank my colleagues at MICA, including Fred Lazarus, President; Ray Allen, Provost; Leslie King Hammond, Dean of Graduate Studies; and my longtime friend and collaborator, Jennifer Cole Phillips. Special thanks go to the dozens of students whose work enlivens these pages.

Editor Clare Jacobson and the team at Princeton Architectural Press helped make the book real.

My whole family is an inspiration, especially my parents Bill, Shirley, Mary Jane, and Ken; my children Jay and Ruby; my sisters Julia and Michelle; and my husband Abbott.

*Ellen Lupton*

My contribution to this book is dedicated to Malcolm Grear, my lifelong mentor and friend.

The culture at MICA is a joy in which to work, thanks in large part to the vision and support of Fred Lazarus, President; Ray Allen, Provost; and Leslie King Hammond, Dean of Graduate Studies; and our savvy and talented faculty colleagues. Many thanks to our student contributors, especially the Graphic Design MFA group; this book exudes their energy. I hold heartfelt gratitude for my friend and close collaborator, Ellen Lupton, for her generosity and grace.

Clare Jacobson and Wendy Fuller at Princeton Architectural Press were invaluable with their expertise.

My family, especially my parents Ann and Jack and my sisters Lanie and Jodie, are a constant source of encouragement and support.

*Jennifer Cole Phillips*

# Back to the Bauhaus

*Ellen Lupton*

The idea of searching out a shared framework in which to invent and organize visual content dates back to the origins of modern graphic design. In the 1920s, institutions such as the Bauhaus in Germany explored design as a universal, perceptually based "language of vision," a concept that continues to shape design education today around the world.

This book reflects on that vital tradition in light of profound shifts in technology and global social life. Whereas the Bauhaus promoted rational solutions through planning and standardization, designers and artists today are drawn to idiosyncrasy, customization, and sublime accidents as well as to standards and norms. The modernist preference for reduced, simplified forms now coexists with a desire to build systems that yield unexpected results. Today, the impure, the contaminated, and the hybrid hold as much allure as forms that are sleek and perfected. Visual thinkers often seek to spin out intricate results from simple rules or concepts rather than reduce an image or idea to its simplest parts.

**The Bauhaus Legacy** In the 1920s, faculty at the Bauhaus and other schools analyzed form in terms of basic geometric elements. They believed this language would be understandable to everyone, grounded in the universal instrument of the eye.

Bauhaus faculty pursued this idea from different points of view. Wassily Kandinsky called for the creation of a "dictionary of elements" and a universal visual "grammar" in his Bauhaus textbook *Point and Line to Plane*. His colleague László Moholy-Nagy sought to uncover a rational vocabulary ratified by a shared society and a common humanity. Courses taught by Josef Albers emphasized systematic thinking over personal intuition, objectivity over emotion.

Albers and Moholy-Nagy forged the use of new media and new materials. They saw that art and design were being transformed by technology—photography, film, and mass production. And yet their ideas remained profoundly humanistic, always asserting the role of the individual over the absolute authority of any system or method. Design, they argued, is never reducible to its function or to a technical description.

Since the 1940s, numerous educators have refined and expanded on the Bauhaus approach, from Moholy-Nagy and Gyorgy Kepes at the New Bauhaus in Chicago; to Johannes Itten, Max Bill, and Gui Bonsiepe at the Ulm School in Germany; to Emil Ruder and Armin Hofmann in Switzerland; to the "new typographies" of Wolfgang Weingart, Dan Friedman, and Katherine McCoy in Switzerland and the United States. Each of these revolutionary educators articulated structural approaches to design from distinct and original perspectives.

Some of them also engaged in the postmodern rejection of universal communication. According to postmodernism, which emerged in the 1960s, it is futile to look for inherent meaning in an image or object because people will bring their own cultural biases and personal experiences to the process of interpretation. As postmodernism itself became a dominant ideology in the 1980s and '90s, in both the academy and in the marketplace, the design process got mired in the act of referencing cultural styles or tailoring messages to narrowly defined communities.

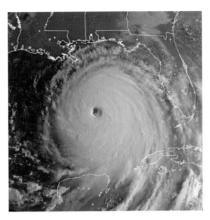

**Transparency and Layers** The Google Earth interface allows users to manipulate the transparency of overlays placed over satellite photographs of Earth. Here, Hurricane Katrina hovers over the Gulf Coast of the U.S. Storm: University of Wisconsin, Madison Cooperative Institute for Meteorogical Satellite Studies, 2005. Composite: Jack Gondela.

**The New Basics** Designers at the Bauhaus believed not only in a universal way of *describing* visual form, but also in its universal *significance*. Reacting against that belief, postmodernism discredited formal experiment as a primary component of thinking and making in the visual arts. Formal study was considered to be tainted by its link to universalistic ideologies. This book recognizes a difference between description and interpretation, between a potentially universal language of making and the universality of meaning.

Today, software designers have realized the Bauhaus goal of describing (but not interpreting) the language of vision in a universal way. Software organizes visual material into menus of properties, parameters, filters, and so on, creating tools that are universal in their social ubiquity, cross-disciplinarity, and descriptive power. Photoshop, for example, is a systematic study of the features of an image (its contrast, size, color model, and so on). InDesign and QuarkXpress are structural explorations of typography: they are software machines for controlling leading, alignment, spacing, and column structures as well as image placement and page layout.

In the aftermath of the Bauhaus, textbooks of basic design have returned again and again to elements such as point, line, plane, texture, and color, organized by principles of scale, contrast, movement, rhythm, and balance. This book revisits those concepts as well as looking at some of the new universals emerging today.

What are these emerging universals? What is new in basic design? Consider, for example, transparency—a concept explored in this book. Transparency is a condition in which two or more surfaces or substances are visible through each other. We constantly experience transparency in the physical environment: from water, glass, and smoke to venetian blinds, slatted fences, and perforated screens. Graphic designers across the modern period have worked with transparency, but never more so than today, when transparency can be instantly manipulated with commonly used tools.

What does transparency *mean*? Transparency can be used to construct thematic relationships. For example, compressing two pictures into a single space can suggest a conflict or synthesis of ideas (East/West, male/female, old/new). Designers also employ transparency as a compositional (rather than thematic) device, using it to soften edges, establish emphasis, separate competing elements, and so on.

Transparency is crucial to the vocabulary of film and motion-based media. In place of a straight cut, an animator or editor diminishes the opacity of an image over time (fade to black) or mixes two semitransparent images (cross dissolve). Such transitions affect a film's rhythm and style. They also modulate, in subtle ways, the message or content of the work. Although viewers rarely stop to interpret these transitions, a video editor or animator understands them as part of the basic language of moving images.

Layering is another universal concept with rising importance. Physical printing processes use layers (ink on paper), and so do software interfaces (from layered Photoshop files to sound or motion timelines).

Transparency and layering have always been at play in the graphic arts. In today's context, what makes them new again is their omnipresent accessibility through software. Powerful digital tools are commonly available to professional artists and designers but also to children, amateurs, and tinkerers of every stripe. Their language has become universal.

Software tools provide models of visual media, but they don't tell us what to make or what to say. It is the designer's task to produce works that are relevant to living situations (audience, context, program, brief, site) and to deliver meaningful messages and rich, embodied experiences. Each producer animates design's core structures from his or her own place in the world.

# Beyond the Basics

*Jennifer Cole Phillips*

Even the most robust visual language is useless without the ability to engage it in a living context. While this book centers around formal structure and experiment, some opening thoughts on process and problem solving are appropriate here, as we hope readers will reach not only for more accomplished form, but for form that resonates with fresh meaning.

Before the Macintosh, solving graphic design problems meant outsourcing at nearly every stage of the way: manuscripts were sent to a typesetter; photographs—selected from contact sheets—were printed at a lab and corrected by a retoucher; and finished artwork was the job of a paste-up artist, who sliced and cemented type and images onto boards. This protocol slowed down the work process and required designers to plan each step methodically.

By contrast, powerful, off-the-shelf software now allows designers and users of all ilks to endlessly edit their work in the comfort of a personal or professional workspace.

Yet, as these digital technologies afford greater freedom and convenience, they also require ongoing education and upkeep. This recurring learning curve, added to already overloaded schedules, often cuts short the creative window for concept development and formal experimentation.

In the college context, students arrive ever more digitally facile. Acculturated by iPods, Playstations, and PowerBooks, design students command the technical savvy that used to take years to build. Being plugged in, however, has not always profited creative thinking.

Too often, the temptation to turn directly to the computer precludes deeper levels of research and ideation—the distillation zone that unfolds beyond the average appetite for testing the waters and exploring alternatives. People, places, thoughts, and things become familiar through repeated exposure. It stands to reason, then, that initial ideas and, typically, the top tiers of a Google search turn up only cursory results that are often tired and trite.

Getting to more interesting territory requires the perseverance to sift, sort, and assimilate subjects and solutions until a fresh spark emerges and takes hold.

**Visual Thinking** Ubiquitous access to image editing and design software, together with zealous media inculcation on all things design, has created a tidal wave of design makers outside our profession. Indeed, in our previous book, *D.I.Y.: Design It Yourself*, we extolled the virtues of learning and making, arguing that people acquire pleasure, knowledge, and power by engaging with design at all levels.

With this volume we shift the climate of the conversation. Instead of skimming the surface, we dig deeper. Rather than issuing instructions, we frame problems and suggest possibilities. Inside, you will find many examples, by students and professionals, that balance and blend idiosyncrasy with formal discipline.

Rather than focus on practical problems such as how to design a book, brochure, logo, or website, this book encourages readers to experiment with the visual language of design. By "experiment," we mean the process of examining a form, material, or process in a methodical yet open-ended way. To experiment is to isolate elements of an operation, limiting some variables in order to better study others. An experiment asks a question or tests a hypothesis whose answer is not known in advance.

Choose your corner, pick away at it carefully, intensely and to the best of your ability and that way **you might change the world.** Charles Eames

The book is organized around some of the formal elements and phenomena of design. In practice, those components mix and overlap, as they do in the examples shown throughout the book. By focusing attention on particular aspects of visual form, we encourage readers to recognize the forces at play behind strong graphic solutions. Likewise, while a dictionary studies specific words in isolation, those words come alive in the active context of writing and speaking.

Filtered through formal and conceptual experimentation, design thinking fuses a shared discipline with organic interpretation.

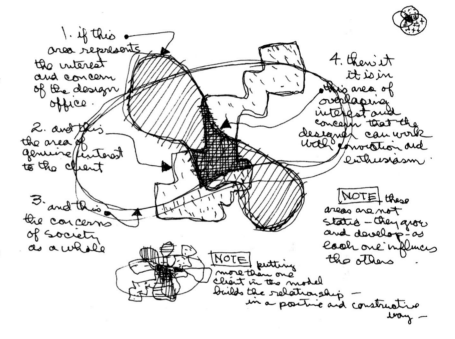

**Diagramming Process** Charles Eames drew this diagram to explain the design process as achieving a point where the needs and interests of the client, the designer, and society as a whole overlap. Charles Eames, 1969, for the exhibition "What is Design" at the Musée des Arts décoratifs, Paris, France. © 2007 Eames Office LLC.

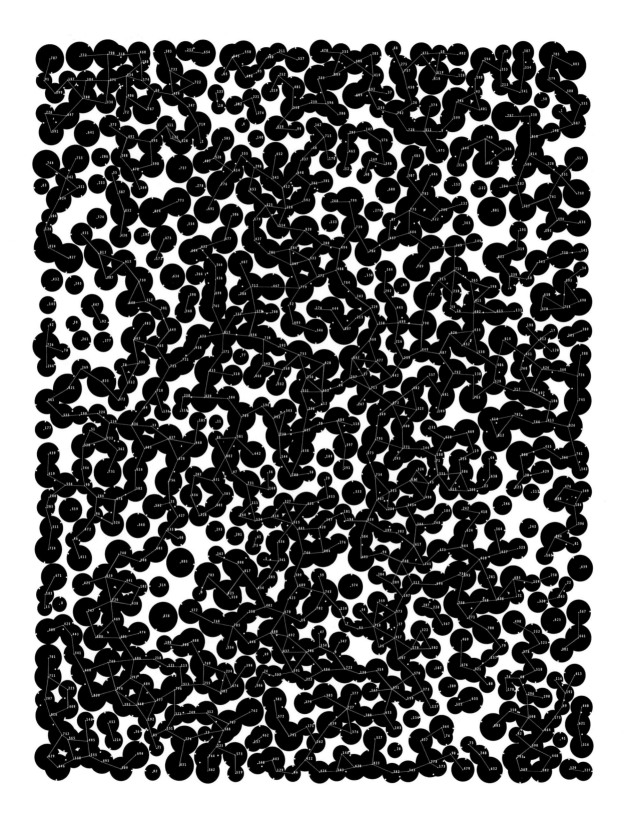

# Point, Line, Plane

A line is the track made by the moving point... It is created by movement—specifically through the destruction of the intense, self-contained repose of the point. Wassily Kandinsky

Point, line, and plane are the building blocks of design. From these elements, designers create images, icons, textures, patterns, diagrams, animations, and typographic systems. Indeed, every complex design shown in this book results at some level from the interaction of points, lines, and planes.

Diagrams build relationships among elements using points, lines, and planes to map and connect data. Textures and patterns are constructed from large groups of points and lines that repeat, rotate, and otherwise interact to form distinctive and engaging surfaces. Typography consists of individual letters (points) that form into lines and fields of text.

For hundreds of years, printing processes have employed dots and lines to depict light, shadow, and volume. Different printing technologies support distinct kinds of mark making. To produce a woodcut, for example, the artist carves out material from a flat surface. In contrast to this subtractive process, lithography allows the artist to make positive, additive marks across a surface. In these processes, dots and lines accumulate to build larger planes and convey the illusion of volume.

Photography, invented in the early 1800s, captures reflected light automatically. The subtle tonal variations of photography eliminated the intermediary mesh of point and line.

Yet reproducing the tones of a photographic image requires translating it into pure graphic marks, because nearly every mechanical printing method—from lithography to laser printing—works with solid inks. The halftone process, invented in the 1880s and still used today, converts a photograph into a pattern of larger and smaller dots, simulating tonal variation with pure spots of black or flat color. The same principle is used in digital reproduction.

Today, designers use software to capture the gestures of the hand as data that can be endlessly manipulated and refined. Software describes images in terms of point, line, plane, shape, and volume as well as color, transparency, and other features. There are numerous ways to experiment with these basic elements of two-dimensional design: observing the environment around you, making marks with physical and digital tools, using software to create and manipulate images, or writing code to generate form with rules and variables.

```
Id       0        1        2        3
X        224.543  715.448  227.491  313.495
Y        247.001  879.651  839.485  291.144
Size     20.000   20.024   20.048   20.072
Angle    1.429    1.000    4.141    0.144
Others   2        1        2        1

29       30       31       32       33
396.477  386.946  655.302  347.761  158.650
396.899  468.870  242.406  625.749  466.553
20.691   20.715   20.739   20.763   20.787
4.687    5.715    5.395    3.691    6.245
1        3        2        2        1

59       60       61       62       63
388.065  450.679  302.301  18.621   9.702
269.422  795.973  319.802  598.880  782.143
21.406   21.430   21.454   21.478   21.502
2.471    2.117    1.626    0.988    3.603
1        1        2        1        2

89       90       91       92       93
247.620  67.441   13.802   90.058   440.551
450.361  388.695  920.408  602.967  200.302
22.122   22.145   22.169   22.193   22.217
2.354    0.952    2.805    0.112    2.384
4        3        2        1        2
```

**Point to Line** Processing is a programming language created by C. E. B. Reas and Benjamin Fry. In this digital drawing by Reas, the lines express a relationship among the points, derived from numerical data. C. E. B. Reas. *Process 4 (Form/Data 1)*, 2005 (detail).

•
x = 4.5521 in
y = 0.997 in

## Point

A point marks a position in space. In pure geometric terms, a point is a pair of x, y coordinates. It has no mass at all. Graphically, however, a point takes form as a dot, a visible mark. A point can be an insignificant fleck of matter or a concentrated locus of power. It can penetrate like a bullet, pierce like a nail, or pucker like a kiss. Through its scale, position, and relationship to its surroundings, a point can express its own identity or melt into the crowd.

A series of points forms a line. A mass of points becomes texture, shape, or plane. Tiny points of varying size create shades of gray.

The tip of an arrow points the way, just as the crossing of an X marks a spot.

In typography, the point is a period—the definitive end of a line. Each character in a field of text is a singular element, and thus a kind of point, a finite element in a series.

# end of a line.

In typography, each character in a field of text is a point, a finite element represented by a single key stroke. The letter occupies a position in a larger line or plane of text. At the end of the line is a period. The point is a sign of closure, of finality. It marks the end.

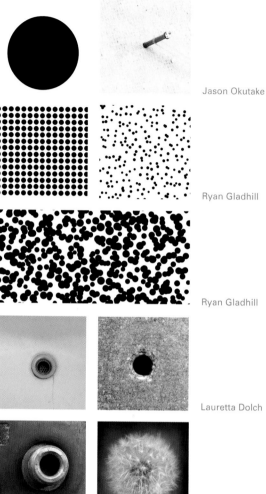

Jason Okutake

Ryan Gladhill

Ryan Gladhill

Lauretta Dolch

Lauretta Dolch
Summer Underwood

Robert Ferrell

Digital Imaging. Al Maskeroni, faculty.

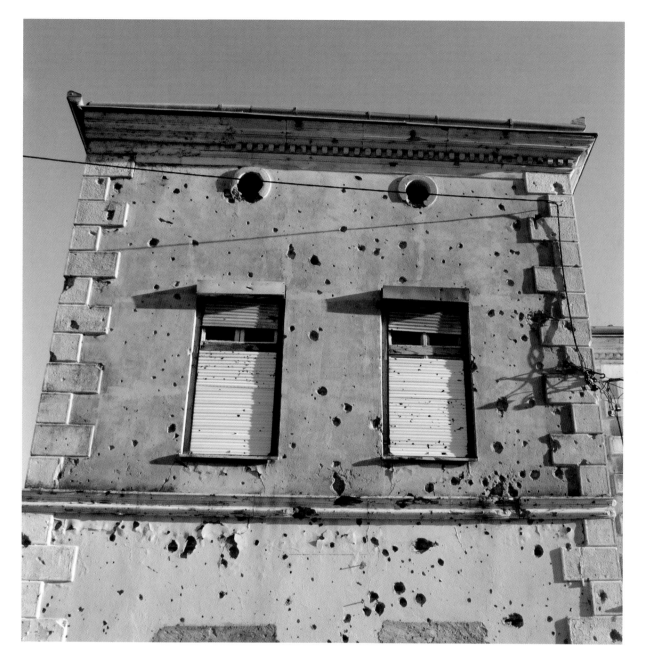

**Destructive Points** Never underestimate the power of a point. This damaged facade was photographed in the war-torn city of Mostar, on the Balkan Peninsula in Bosnia and Herzegovina. Nancy Froehlich.

length = .9792 in

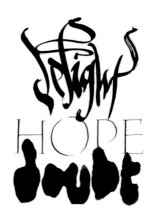

Jeremy Botts

Lines express emotions.

Josh Sims
Bryan McDonough

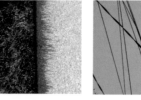

Alex Ebright
Justin Lloyd

Digital Imaging.
Nancy Froehlich,
faculty.

Lines describe structure and edges.

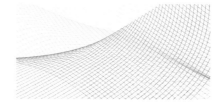

Allen Harrison

Lines turn and multiply to describe planes.

## Line

A line is an infinite series of points. Understood geometrically, a line has length, but no breadth. A line is the connection between two points, or it is the path of a moving point.

A line can be a positive mark or a negative gap. Lines appear at the edges of objects and where two planes meet.

Graphically, lines exist in many weights; the thickness and texture as well as the path of the mark determine its visual presence. Lines are drawn with a pen, pencil, brush, mouse, or digital code. They can be straight or curved, continuous or broken. When a line reaches a certain thickness, it becomes a plane. Lines multiply to describe volumes, planes, and textures.

A graph is a rising and falling line that describes change over time, as in a waveform charting a heart beat or an audio signal.

In typographic layouts, lines are implied as well as literally drawn. Characters group into lines of text, while columns are positioned in blocks that are flush left, flush right, and justified. Imaginary lines appear along the edges of each column, expressing the order of the page.

Type sits on a baseline.

Typographic alignment refers to the organization of text into columns with a hard or soft edge. A justified column is even along both the left and right sides.

The crisp edge of a column is implied by the even starting or ending points of successive lines of type. The eye connects the points to make a line. Such typographic lines are implied, not drawn.

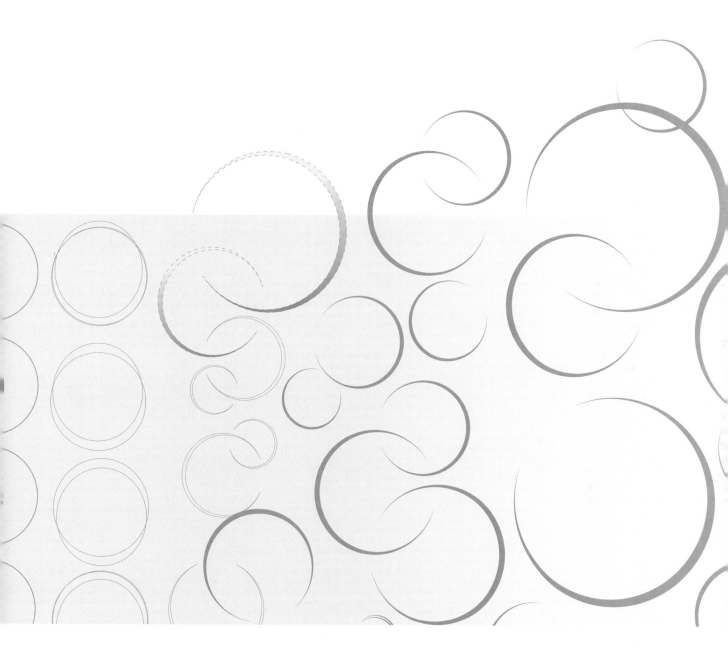

**Line/Shape Study** Vector-based software uses a closed line to define a shape. Here, new lines are formed by the intersection of shapes, creating a swelling form reminiscent of the path of a steel-point pen. Ryan Gladhill, MFA Studio.

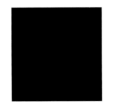

width = 0.9792 in
height = 0.9792 in

## Plane

A plane is a flat surface extending in height and width. A plane is the path of a moving line; it is a line with breadth. A line closes to become a shape, a bounded plane. Shapes are planes with edges. In vector-based software, every shape consists of line and fill. A plane can be parallel to the picture surface, or it can skew and recede into space. Ceilings, walls, floors, and windows are physical planes. A plane can be solid or perforated, opaque or transparent, textured or smooth.

A field of text is a plane built from points and lines of type. A typographic plane can be dense or open, hard or soft. Designers experiment with line spacing, font size, and alignment to create different typographic shapes.

In typography, letters gather into lines, and lines build up into planes. The quality of the plane—its density or opacity, its heaviness or lightness on the page—is determined by the size of the letters, the spacing between lines, words, and characters, and the visual character of a given typeface.

Hard, closed shape

In typography, letters gather into lines, and lines build up into planes. The quality of the plane—its density, its opacity, its weight on the page—is determined by the size of the letters, the spacing between lines, words, and characters, and the visual character of a given typeface.

Soft, open shape

**Plane Letters** A plane can be described with lines or with fields of color. These letterforms use ribbons of color to describe spatial planes. Kelly Horigan, Experimental Typography. Ken Barber, faculty.

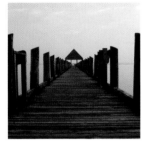

**Parallel Lines
Converge**
Summer
Underwood

## Space and Volume
A graphic object that encloses three-dimensional space has volume. It has height, width, and depth. A sheet of paper or a computer screen has no real depth, of course, so volume is represented through graphic conventions.

Linear perspective simulates optical distortions, making near objects appear large as far objects become small, receding into nothing as they reach the horizon. The angle at which elements recede reflects the position of the viewer. Are the objects above or below the viewer's eye level? Camera lenses replicate the effects of linear perspective, recording the position of the camera's eye.

Axonometric projections depict volume without making elements recede into space. The scale of elements thus remains consistent as objects move back into space. The result is more abstract and impersonal than linear perspective.

Architects often use axonometric projections in order to keep a consistent scale across the page. Digital game designers often use this technique as well, creating maps of simulated worlds rather than depicting experience from the ground.

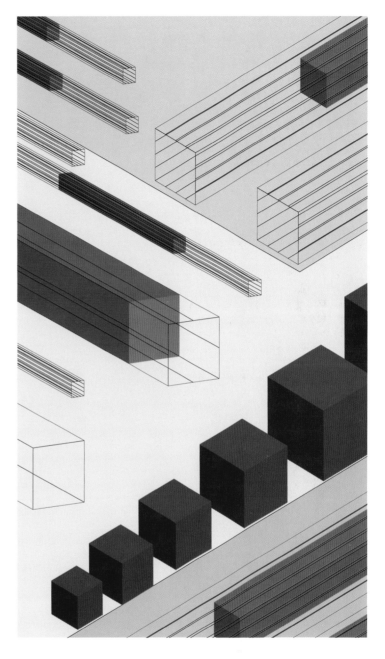

**Projection Study** This idealized landscape uses axonometric projection, in which scale is consistent from the front to back of the image. As seen on a map or computer game, this space implies a disembodied, godlike viewer rather than a physical eye positioned in relation to a horizon. Visakh Menon, MFA Studio.

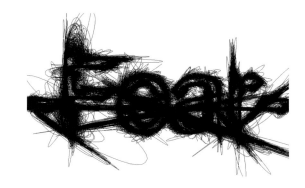

Yeohyun Ahn

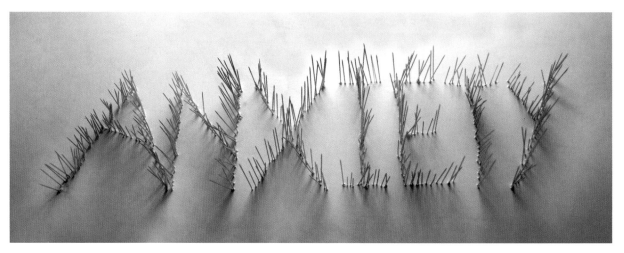

Visakh Menon

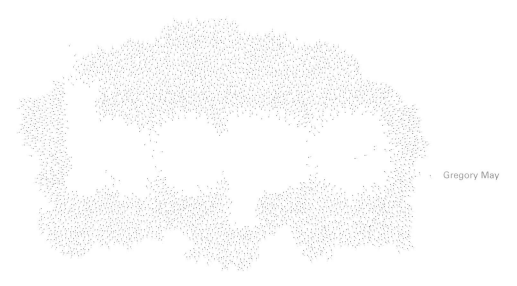

Gregory May

Yeohyun Ahn

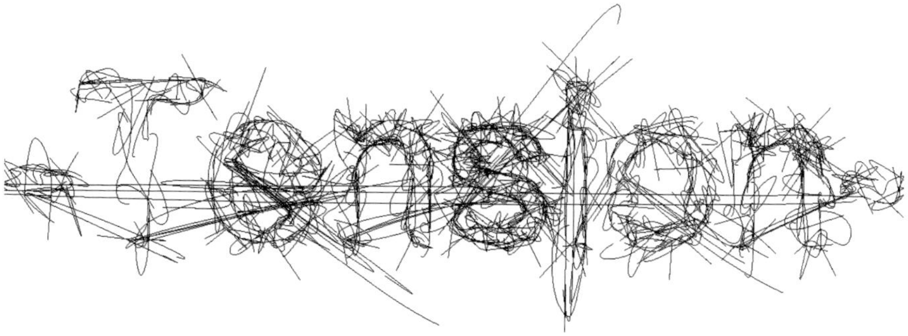

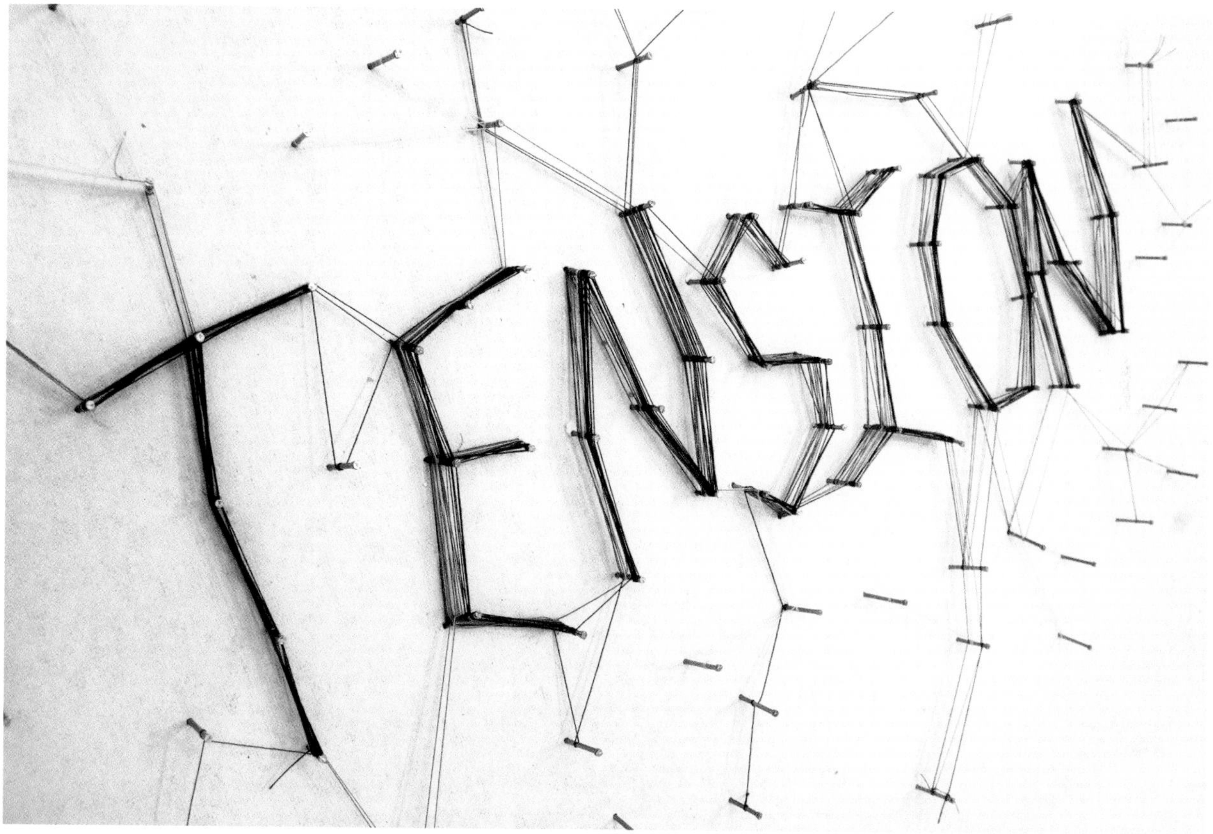

Jason Okutake

**Point and Line: Physical and Digital** In the lettering experiments shown here, each word is written with lines, points, or both, produced with physical elements, digital illustrations, or code-generated vectors. MFA Studio. Marian Bantjes, visiting faculty.

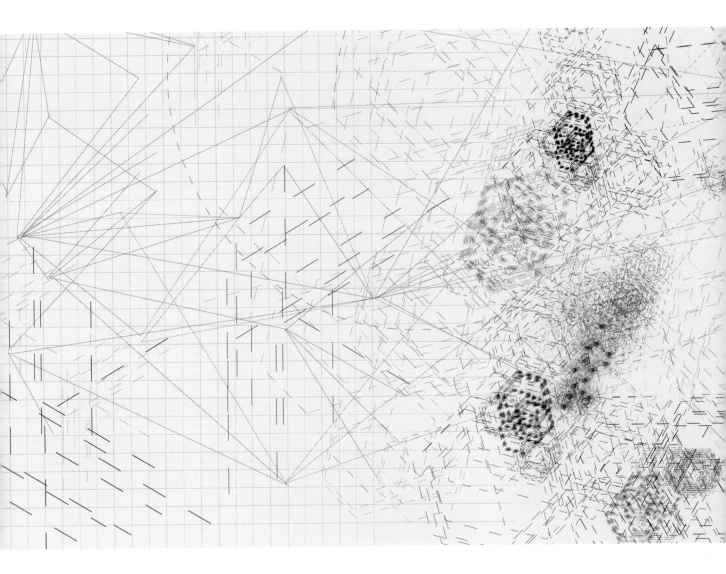

**Line Study: Order and Disorder** Inspired
by maps of population density, this digital
drawing uses lines to describe shapes and
volumes as well as to form dense splotches
of texture. The drawing originates from
the center with a series of hexagons. As the
hexagons migrate to the left, they become
more open. As they migrate to the right,
they erode, becoming soft and organic. Ryan
Gladhill, MFA Studio.

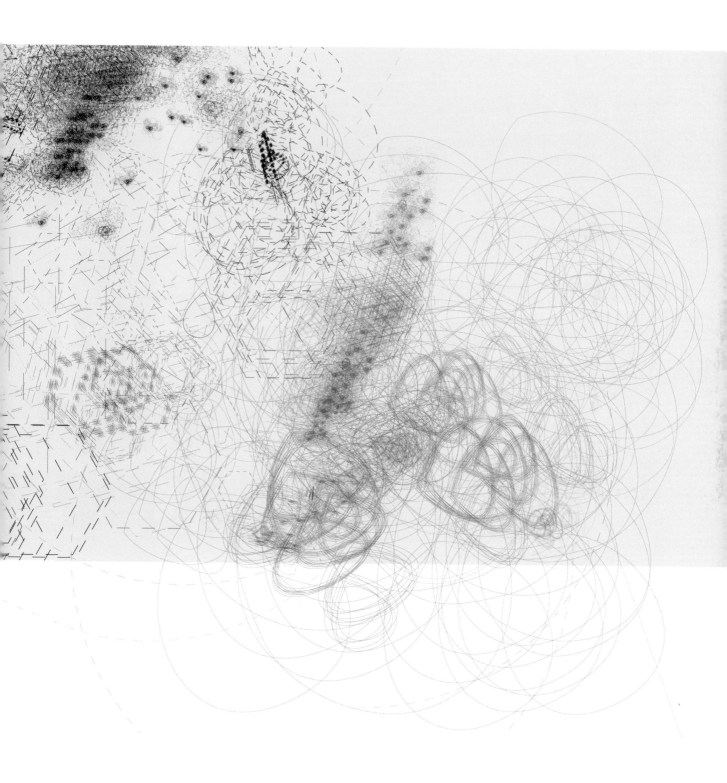

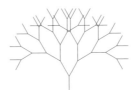

BinaryTree(400,600,400,550,30,1);

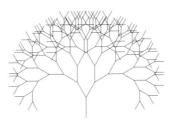

BinaryTree(400,600,400,550,30,3);

## Drawing with Code

The drawings shown here were created with Processing, an open-source software application. The designs are built from a binary tree, a basic data structure in which each node spawns at most two offspring. Binary trees are used to organize information hierarchies, and they often take a graphical form. The density of the final drawing depends on the angle between the "children" and the number of generations.

The larger design is created by repeating, rotating, inverting, connecting, and overlapping the tree forms. In code-based drawing, the designer varies the results by changing the inputs to the algorithm.

BinaryTree(400,600,400,550,30,5);

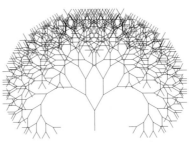

BinaryTree(400,600,400,550,30,7);

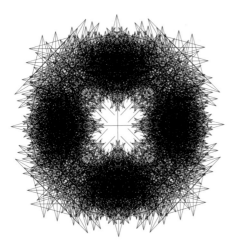

BinaryTree(400,600,400,550,30,9);

**Binary Tree** The drawing becomes denser with each generation. The last number in the code indicates the number of iterations. Yeohyun Ahn, MFA Studio.

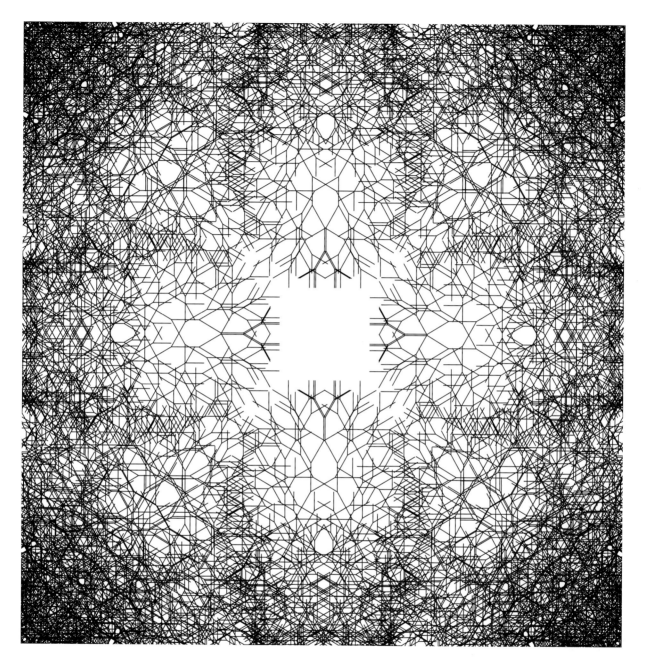

**Binary Tree Pattern** Produced with code, this textured drawing employs techniques that have been used across history to produce rhythmic patterns: copying, repeating, rotating, inverting, and connecting. Yeohyun Ahn, MFA Studio.

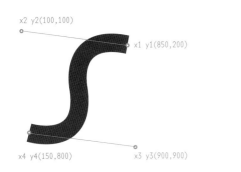

x2 y2(100,100)

x1 y1(850,200)

x4 y4(150,800)

x3 y3(900,900)

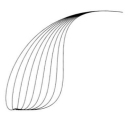

bezier(850,200,100,100,900,900,150,800);

for(int i=0; i<900; i=i+100)
{bezier(850,200,100,100,i,900,150,800);}

### Bézier Curves

A Bézier curve is a line defined by
a set of anchor and control points.
Designers are accustomed to
drawing curves using vector-based
software and then modifying
the curve by adding, subtracting,
and repositioning the anchor and
control points.

The drawings shown here were
created with the open-source software application Processing. The
curves were drawn directly in code:

```
bezier(x1,y1,x2,y2,x3,y3,x4,y4);
```

The first two parameters (x1, y1)
specify the first anchor point, and
the last two parameters (x4, y4)
specify the other anchor point.
The middle parameters locate the
control points that define the curve.

Curves drawn with standard
illustration software are fundamentally the same as curves drawn
in code, but we understand and
control them with different means.
The designer varies the results by
changing the inputs to the algorithm.

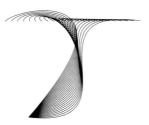

for(int i=0;i<900; i=i+40)
{bezier(i,200,100,100,900,i,150,800);}

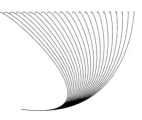

for(int i=0;i<900;i=i+40)
{bezier(i,200,i,100,900,900,150,800);}

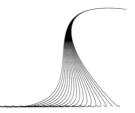

for(int i=0; i<900; i=i+50)
{bezier(900,200,100,100,900,900,i,800);}

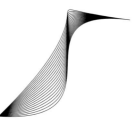

for(int i=0; i<900; i=i+100)
{bezier(900,200,100,100,900,i,50,800);}

**Repeated Bézier Curve** The designer has
written a function that repeats the curve in
space according to a given increment (i).
The same basic code was used to generate
all the drawings shown above, with varied
inputs for the anchor and control points. A
variable (i) defines the curve. Yeohyun Ahn,
MFA Studio.

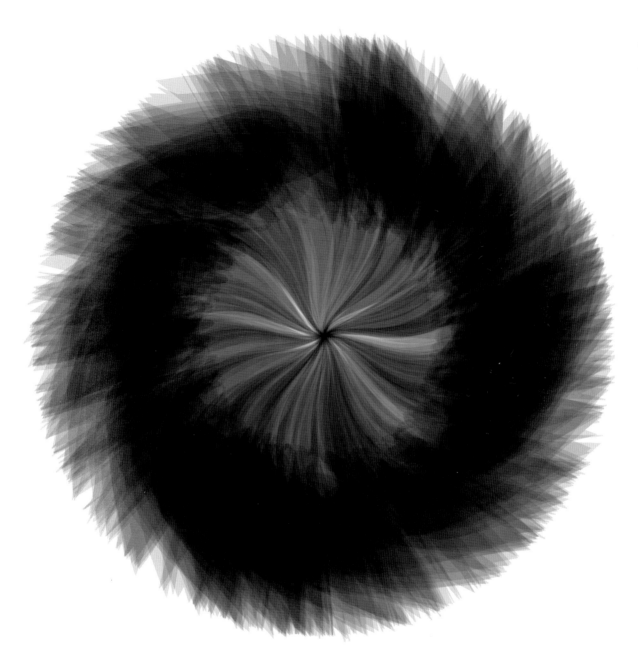

```
beginShape(POLYGON);
vertex(30,20);
bezierVertex(80,0,80,75,30,75);
bezierVertex(50,80,60,25,30,20);
endShape()
```

**Black Flower** A Bézier vertex is a shape created by closing a Bézier curve. This design was created by rotating numerous Bézier vertices around a common center, with varying degrees of transparency.
Yeohyun Ahn, MFA Studio.

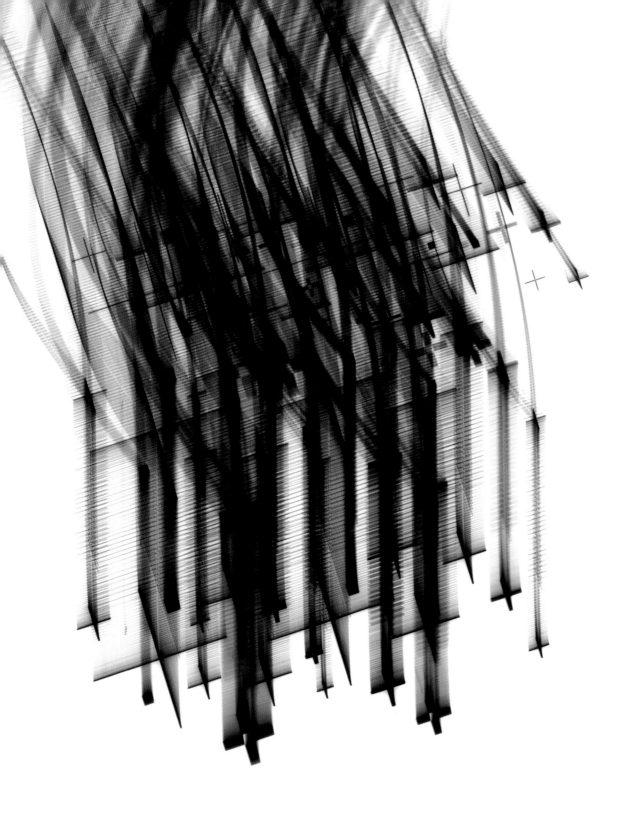

# Rhythm and Balance

I pay close attention to the variety of shapes and sizes, and place the objects so that **the lines and edges create a rhythm** that guides the viewer's eye around the image and into the focal point. Sergei Forostovskii

Balance is a fundamental human condition: we require physical balance to stand upright and walk; we seek balance among the many facets of our personal and professional lives; the world struggles for balance of power. Indeed, balance is a prized commodity in our culture, and it is no surprise that our implicit, intuitive relationship with it has equipped us to sense balance—or imbalance—in the things we see, hear, smell, taste, and touch.

In design, balance acts as a catalyst for form—it anchors and activates elements in space. Do you ever notice your eye getting stuck in a particular place when looking at an unresolved design? This discord usually occurs because the proportion and placement of elements in relation to each other and to the negative space is off—too big, too tight, too flat, misaligned, and so on.

Relationships among elements on the page remind us of physical relationships. Visual balance occurs when the weight of one or more things is distributed evenly or proportionately in space. Like arranging furniture in a room, we move components around until the balance of form and space feels just right. Large objects are a counterpoint to smaller ones; dark objects to lighter ones.

A symmetrical design, which has the same elements on at least two sides along a common axis, is inherently stable. Yet balance need not be static. A tightrope walker achieves balance while traversing a precarious line in space, continually shifting her weight while staying in constant motion. Designers employ contrasting size, texture, value, color, and shape to offset or emphasize the weight of an object and achieve the acrobat's dynamic sense of balance.

Rhythm is a strong, regular, repeated pattern: the beating of drums, the patter of rain, the falling of footsteps. Speech, music, and dance all employ rhythm to express form over time. Graphic designers use rhythm in the construction of static images as well as in books, magazines, and motion graphics that have duration and sequence. Although pattern design usually employs unbroken repetition, most forms of graphic design seek rhythms that are punctuated with change and variation. Book design, for example, seeks out a variety of scales and tonal values across its pages, while also preserving an underlying structural unity.

Balance and rhythm work together to create works of design that pulse with life, achieving both stability and surprise.

**Rhythm and Repetition** This code-driven photogram employs a simple stencil plus sign through which light is projected as the photo paper shifts minutely and mechanically across the span of hours. The visual result has the densely layered richness of a charcoal drawing. Tad Takano. Photographed for reproduction by Dan Meyers.

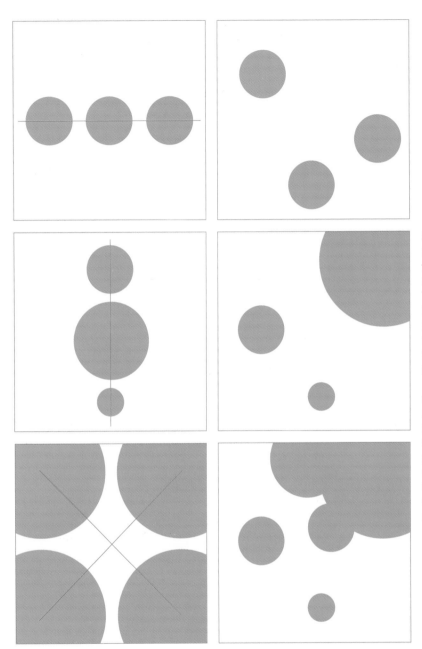

## Symmetry and Asymmetry

Symmetry can be left to right, top to bottom, or both. Many natural organisms have a symmetrical form. The even weighting of arms and legs helps insure a creature's safe mobility; a tree develops an even distribution of weight around its core to stand erect; and the arms of a starfish radiate from the center.

Symmetry is not the only way to achieve balance, however. Asymmetrical designs are generally more active than symmetrical ones, and designers achieve balance by placing contrasting elements in counterpoint to each other, yielding compositions that allow the eye to wander while achieving an overall stability.

**Symmetry** The studies above demonstrate basic symmetrical balance. Elements are oriented along a common axis; the image mirrors from side to side along that axis. The configurations shown here are symmetrical from left to right and/or from top to bottom.

**Asymmetry** These studies use asymmetry to achieve compositional balance. Elements are placed organically, relying on the interaction of form and negative space and the proximity of elements to each other and to the edges of the field, yielding both tension and balance.

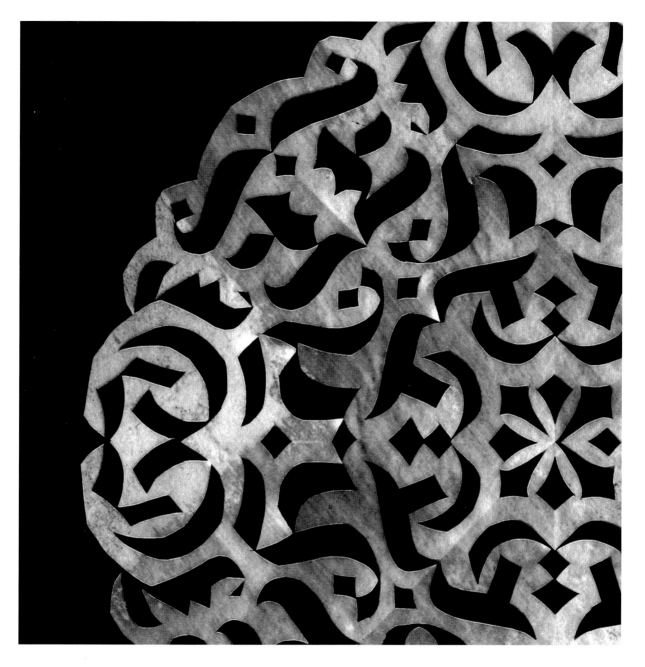

**Symmetry and Asymmetry** The designer
has cropped a symmetrical form in order to
create an asymmetrical composition.
A rhythm of repeated elements undulates
across the surface. The larger ornamental
form has been shifted dramatically off center,
yielding dynamic balance. Jeremy Botts,
MFA Studio.

Highway Overpasses, Houston, Texas

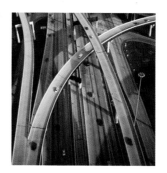

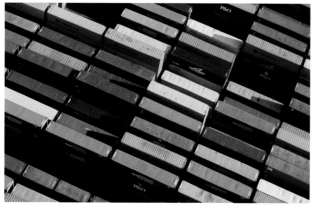

## Repetition and Change

From the flowing contours of a farmer's fields to a sea of cars tucked into the lined compartments of a parking lot, repetition is an endless feature of the human environment. Like melodic consonance and fervent discord in music, repetition and change awaken life's visual juxtapositions. Beauty arises from the mix.

Shipping Containers, Norfolk, Virginia

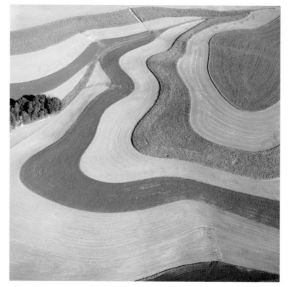

Contour Farming, Meyersville, Maryland

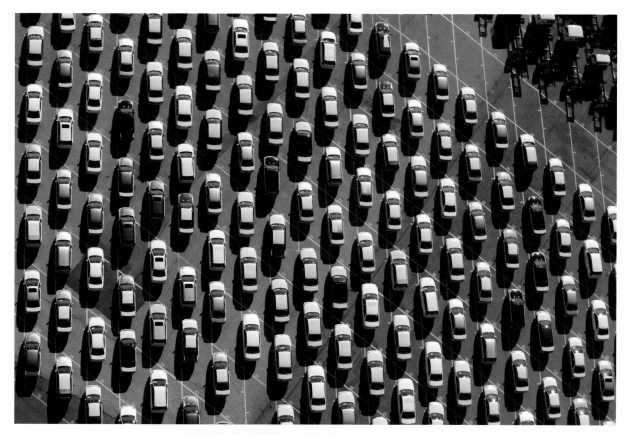

Port of Baltimore, Maryland

Arlington National Cemetery,
Washington, D.C.

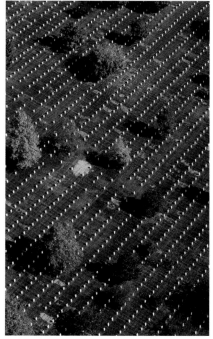

**Observed Rhythm** Aerial photographs are
fascinating and surprising because we
are not accustomed to seeing landscapes
from above. The many patterns, textures,
and colors embedded in both man-made
and natural forms—revealed and concealed
through light and shadow—yield intriguing
rhythms. Cameron Davidson.

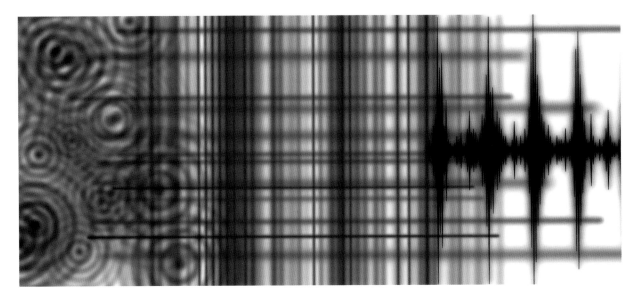

Jason Okutake, MFA Studio

## Rhythm and Time

We are familiar with rhythm from the world of sound. In music, an underlying pattern changes in time. Layers of pattern occur simultaneously in music, supporting each other and providing aural contrast. In audio mixing, sounds are amplified or diminished to create a rhythm that shifts and evolves over the course of a piece.

Graphic designers employ similar structures visually. The repetition of elements such as circles, lines, and grids creates rhythm, while varying their size or intensity generates surprise. In animation, designers must orchestrate both audio and visual rhythms simultaneously.

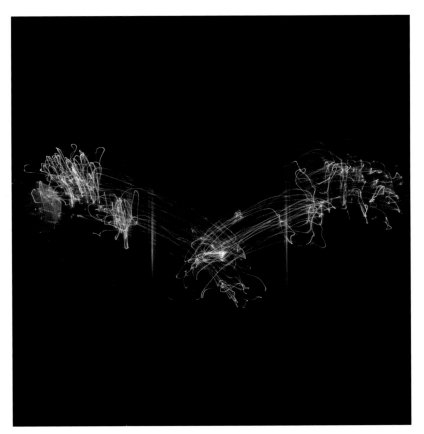

**Frozen Rhythms** Long-exposure photography records physical movements in time on a two-dimensional surface. Sketching with light yields a rhythmic line of changing intensity. Jason Okutake, MFA Studio.

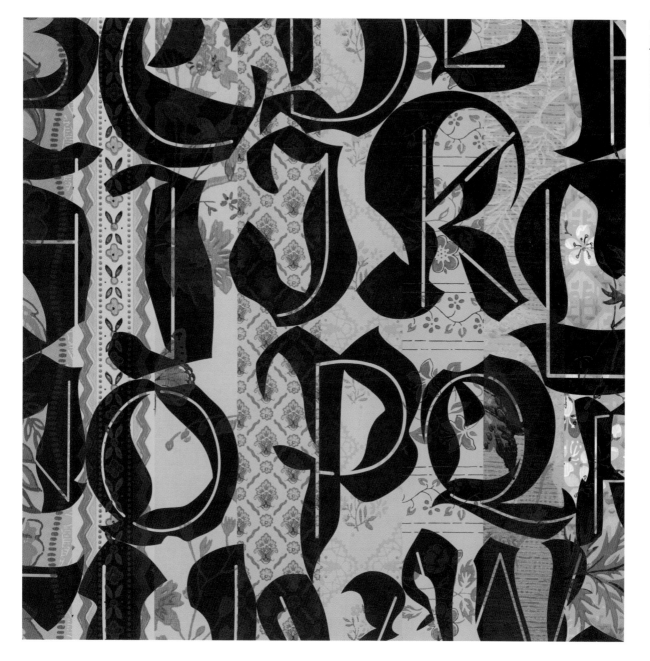

**Pattern Dissonance** Letterforms with abruptly
shifting features are built around a thin
skeleton. The strange anatomy of the letters
plays against the comfortable, gentle rhythms
of the old-fashioned wallpaper behind them.
Jeremy Botts, MFA Studio.

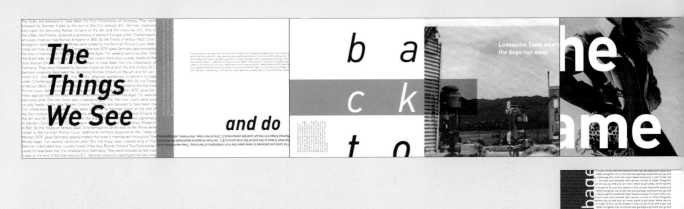

Lonesome Town where
the dogs run away

**Rhythm and Pacing**

Designers often work with content distributed across many pages. As in a single-page composition, a sequential design must possess an overall coherence. Imagery, typography, rules, color fields, and so on are placed with mindful intention to create focal points and to carry the viewer's eye through the piece. An underlying grid helps bring order to a progression of pages. Keeping an element of surprise and variation is key to sustaining interest.

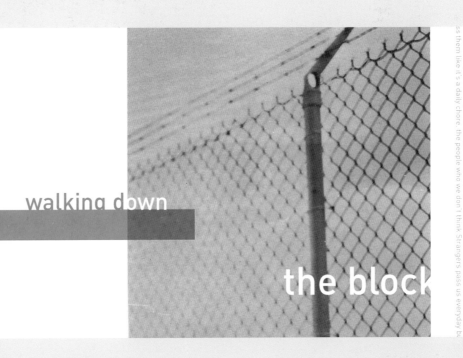

followed by German pes at the end of the nd century B.C. Ger-invasions destroyed he declining Roman mpire in the 4th and n centuries A.D. One e tribes, the Franks, tained supremacy in estern Europe under arlemagne, who was rowned Holy Roman mperor in 800. By the eaty of Verdun (843), emagne's lands east e Rhine were ceded o the German Prince Additional territory quired by the Treaty f Mersen (870) gave many approximately e area it maintained roughout the Middle s. For several centu-after Otto the Great rowned king in ions troyed the declining an Empire in the 4th nd 5th centuries A.D. One of the tribes, the

walking down

the block

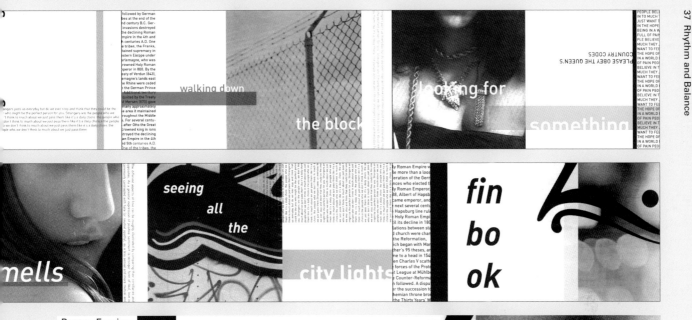

**Found Rhythms** In this project, designers cut a 2.5-inch square cleanly through a magazine, yielding dozens of unexpected compositions. Each designer used ten of these small squares as imagery in an accordion book. The squares were scanned at 200% and placed into a page layout file (formatted in 5-inch-square pages) and paired with a text gathered from Wikipedia.

Each designer created a visual "story" by considering the pacing and scale of the images and text within each spread and across the entire sequence. Working with found or accidental content frees designers to think abstractly. Molly Hausmann, Typography I. Jeremy Botts, faculty.

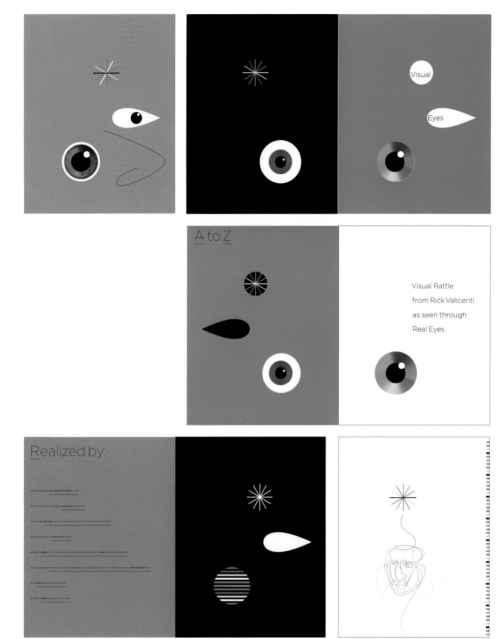

**Graceful Entry** These pages serve as the cover, lead in, and close of a lavishly designed and illustrated alphabet book. The simple, well-balanced elements are introduced, then animated with color and context, and finally returned to abstraction, creating a playful and compelling progression that belies the complexity of the book's interior. Rick Valicenti, Thirst.

Beautiful

Michael ) in this book
m 1976 to 1982
rietta, Ohio;
llinois; or
lle, Virginia.

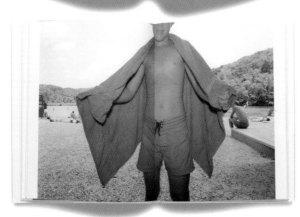

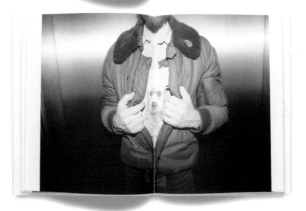

The pictures
were taken fror
in either Ma Northrup
Chicago, I
Charlottesvi

l Ecstasy

**Spinal Orientation** This collection of photographs by Michael Northrup includes many images with a prominent central feature. Designer Paul Sahre responded to this condition by splitting the title and other opening text matter between the front and back of the book, thus creating surprise for and increased interaction with the reader. Paul Sahre, Office of Paul Sahre. Book photographed by Dan Meyers.

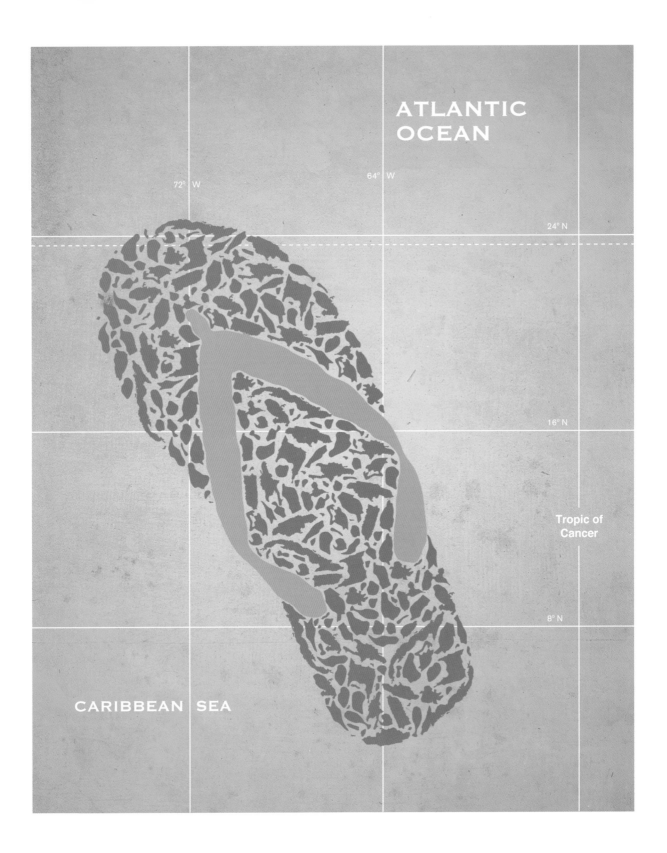

ATLANTIC
OCEAN

72° W

64° W

24° N

16° N

Tropic of
Cancer

8° N

CARIBBEAN SEA

# Scale

Miss Darcy was tall, and on **a larger scale** than Elizabeth; and, though little more than sixteen, her figure was formed, and her appearance womanly and graceful. Jane Austen

A printed piece can be as small as a postage stamp or as large as a billboard. A logo must be legible both at a tiny size and from a great distance, while a film might be viewed in a huge stadium or on a handheld device. Some projects are designed to be reproduced at multiple scales, while others are conceived for a single site or medium. No matter what size your work will ultimately be, it must have its own sense of scale.

What do designers mean by scale? Scale can be considered both objectively and subjectively. In objective terms, scale refers to the literal dimensions of a physical object or to the literal correlation between a representation and the real thing it depicts. Printed maps have an exact scale: an increment of measure on the page represents an increment in the physical world. Scale models re-create relationships found in full-scale objects. Thus a model car closely approximates the features of a working vehicle, while a toy car plays with size relationships, inflating some elements while diminishing others.

Subjectively, scale refers to one's impression of an object's size. A book or a room, for example, might have a grand or intimate scale, reflecting how it relates to our own bodies and to our knowledge of other books and other rooms. We say that an image or representation "lacks scale" when it has no cues that connect it to lived experience, giving it a physical identity. A design whose elements all have a similar size often feels dull and static, lacking contrast in scale.

Scale can depend on context. An ordinary piece of paper can contain lettering or images that seem to burst off its edges, conveying a surprising sense of scale. Likewise, a small isolated element can punctuate a large surface, drawing importance from the vast space surrounding it.

Designers are often unpleasantly surprised when they first print out a piece that they have been designing on screen; elements that looked vibrant and dynamic on screen may appear dull and flaccid on the page. For example, 12pt type generally appears legible and appropriately scaled when viewed on a computer monitor, but the same type can feel crude and unwieldy as printed text. Developing sensitivity to scale is an ongoing process for every designer.

**Big Picture from Small Parts** This design represents Caribbean culture as the colloquy of numerous small islands. The meaning of the image comes directly from the contrast in scale. Robert Lewis, MFA Studio.

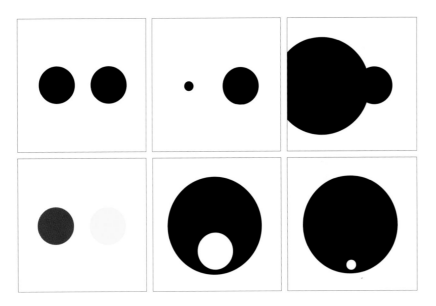

## Scale is Relative

A graphic element can appear larger or smaller depending on the size, placement, and color of the elements around it. When elements are all the same size, the design feels flat. Contrast in size can create a sense of tension as well as a feeling of depth and movement. Small shapes tend to recede; large ones move forward.

**Cropping to Imply Scale**
The larger circular form seems especially big because it bleeds off the edges of the page.

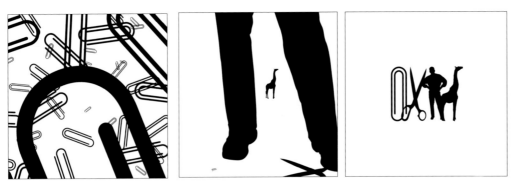

**Familiar Objects, Familiar Scale** We expect some objects to be a particular scale in relation to each other. Playing with that scale can create spatial illusions and conceptual relationships. Gregory May, MFA Studio.

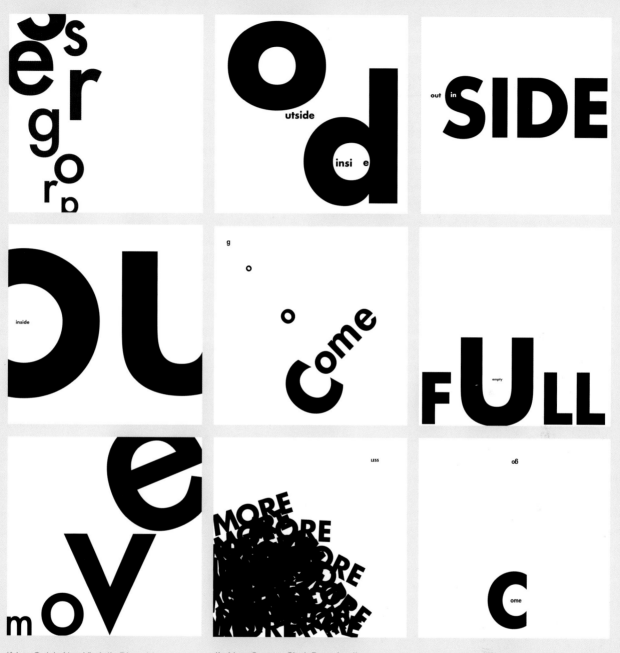

Krista Quick, Nan Yi, Julie Diewald

Jie Lian, Sueyun Choi, Ryan Artell

Jenn Julian, Nan Yi, Sueyun Choi

**Scale, Depth, and Motion** In the typographic compositions shown here, designers worked with one word or a pair of words and used changes in scale as well as placement on the page to convey the meaning of the word or word pair. Contrasts in scale can imply motion or depth as well as express differences in importance.

Typography I and Graphic Design I. Ellen Lupton and Zvezdana Rogic, faculty.

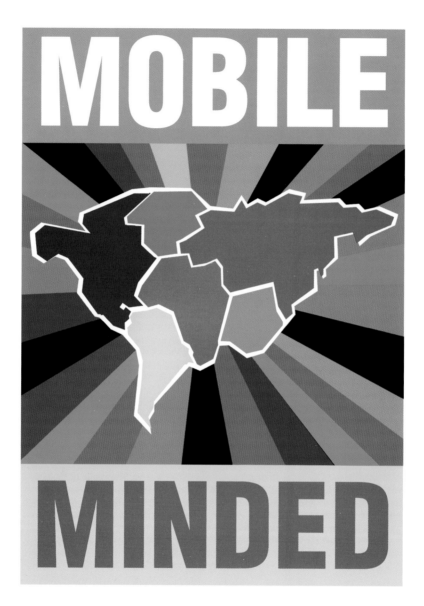

**Big Type, Small Pages** In this book designed
by Mieke Gerritzen, the small trim size of
the page contrasts with the large-scale type.
The surprising size of the text gives the
book its loud and zealous voice. The cover
is reproduced here at actual size (1:1 scale).
Mieke Gerritzen and Geert Lovink, *Mobile
Minded*, 2002.

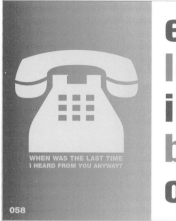

WHEN WAS THE LAST TIME
I HEARD FROM YOU ANYWAY?

058

e mobil
le mobi
ile mob
bile mo
obi lem

MILBI TOY

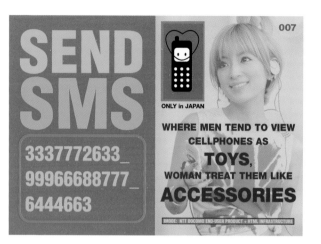

SEND
SMS

3337772633_
99966688777_
6444663

MODE: NTT DOCOMO END-USER PRODUCT + HTML INFRASTRUCTURE

007

ONLY in JAPAN

WHERE MEN TEND TO VIEW
CELLPHONES AS
**TOYS,**
WOMAN TREAT THEM LIKE
**ACCESSORIES**

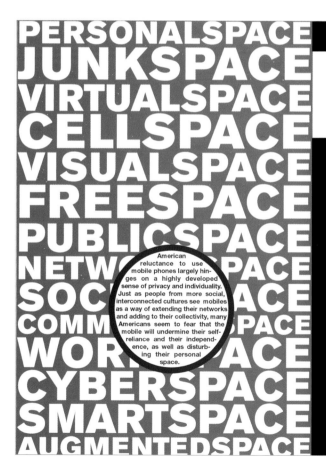

PERSONALSPACE
JUNKSPACE
VIRTUALSPACE
CELLSPACE
VISUALSPACE
FREESPACE
PUBLICSPACE
NETWORKSPACE
SOCIALSPACE
COMMSPACE
WORKSPACE
CYBERSPACE
SMARTSPACE
AUGMENTEDSPACE

American reluctance to use mobile phones largely hinges on a highly developed sense of privacy and individuality. Just as people from more social, interconnected cultures see mobiles as a way of extending their networks and adding to their collectivity, many Americans seem to fear that the mobile will undermine their self-reliance and their independence, as well as disturbing their personal space.

## THE 1990'S WERE ABOUT THE VIRTUAL:

VIRTUAL REALITY
VIRTUAL WORLDS
CYBERSPACE
AND DOT COMS

The image of an escape into a virtual world which would leave the physical space useless dominated the decade. The new decade brings with it a new emphasis on a physical space augmented with electronic, network and computer technologies: GPG; the omnipresence of video surveillance; "cellspace" applications; objects and buildings sending information to your cellphone or PDA when you are in their vicinity; and gradual dissemination of larger and flatter computer/video displays in public spaces.

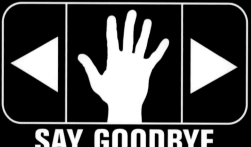

**SAY GOODBYE,
VIRTUAL SPACE.
PREPARE TO LIVE IN
AUGMENTED SPACE.**

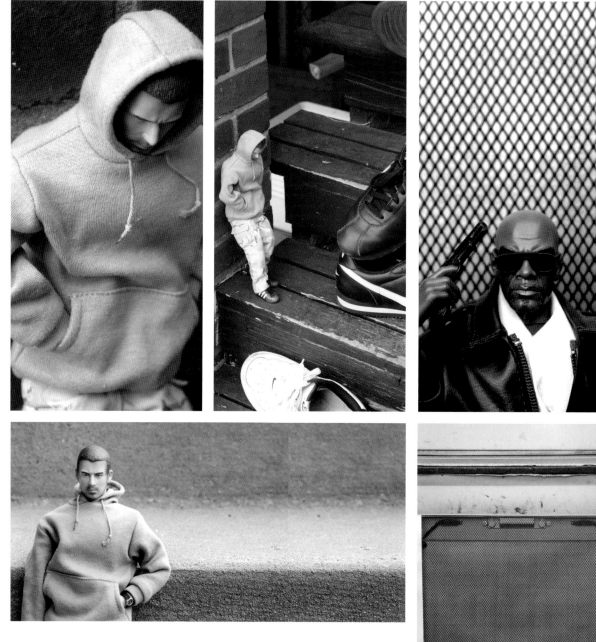

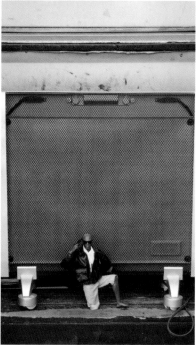

**Ambiguous Scale** These portraits of toy action figures play with the viewer's expectations about scale. Spatial cues reveal the actual scale of the figures; cropping out recognizable objects keeps the illusion alive. Yong Seuk Lee, MFA Studio. Abbott Miller, faculty.

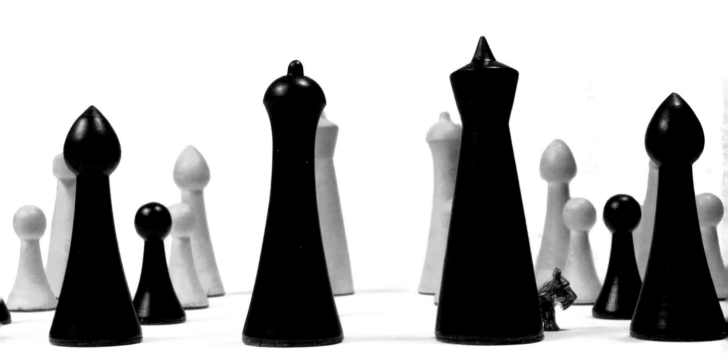

**Point of View** Photographing small objects up close and from a low vantage point creates an illusion of monumentality. Kim Bentley, MFA Studio. Abbott Miller, faculty.

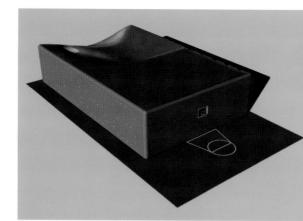

**Absence of Scale** This electrical utility building designed by NL Architects in Utrecht, Netherlands, has no windows or doors to indicate its scale relative to human beings or to familiar building types. The basketball hoop is the only clue to the size of this enigmatic structure. NL Architects, Netherlands, in cooperation with Bureau Nieuwbouw Centrales UNA N.V., 1997–98.

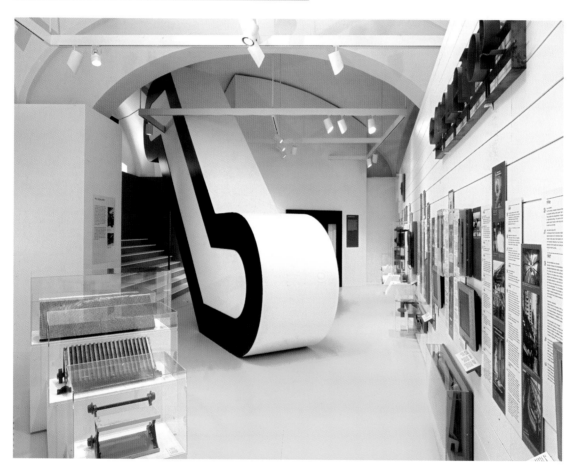

**Inflated Scale** In this design for an exhibition about the history of elevators and escalators, a graphic icon is blown up to an enormous scale, becoming the backdrop for a screening area in the gallery. Abbott Miller and Jeremy Hoffman, Pentagram.

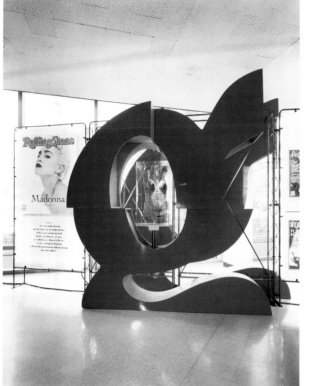

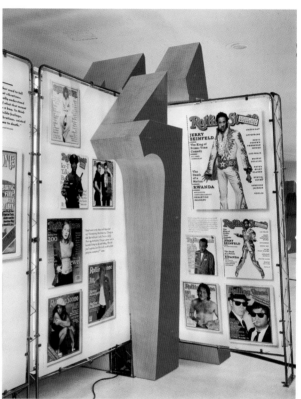

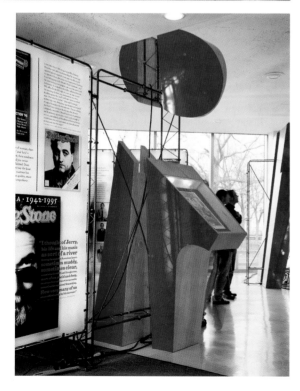

**Environmental Typography** For an exhibition celebrating the history of *Rolling Stone*, the designers made showcases out of large-scale letterforms taken from the magazine's distinctive logotype. Abbott Miller and James Hicks, Pentagram.

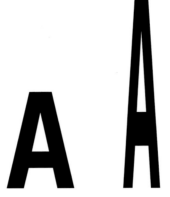

### Scale is a Verb

To scale a graphic element is to change its dimensions. Software makes it easy to scale photographs, vector graphics, and letterforms. Changing the scale of an element can transform its impact on the page or screen. Be careful, however: it's easy to distort an element by scaling it disproportionately.

Vector graphics are scalable, meaning that they can be enlarged or reduced without degrading the quality of the image. Bitmap images cannot be enlarged without resulting in a soft or jaggy image.

In two-dimensional animation, enlarging a graphic object over time can create the appearance of a zoom, as if the object were moving closer to the screen.

**Scaling Letterforms** If the horizontal and vertical dimensions of a letter are scaled unevenly, the resulting form looks distorted. With vertical scaling, the horizontal elements become too thick, while vertical elements get too skinny.

With horizontal scaling, vertical elements become disproportionately heavy, while horizontal elements get thin.

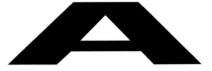

**Full-Range Type Family** Many typefaces include variations designed with different proportions. The Helvetica Neue type family includes light, medium, bold, and black letters in normal, condensed, and extended widths. The strokes of each letter appear uniform. That effect is destroyed if the letters are unevenly scaled.

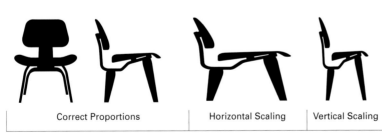

| Correct Proportions | Horizontal Scaling | Vertical Scaling |

**Scaling Images and Objects** Uneven scaling distorts images as well as typefaces. Imagine if you could scale a physical object, stretching or squashing it to make it fit into a particular space. The results are not pretty. Eric Karnes.

**Extreme Heights** In the poster at right for a lecture at a college, designer Paul Sahre put his typography under severe pressure, yielding virtually illegible results. (He knew he had a captive audience.) Paul Sahre.

PAUL SAHRE: EXERCISES IN FUTILITY, PART IV

APRIL 7, 2000 4PM BUNTING 110 M.I.C.A.

FREE

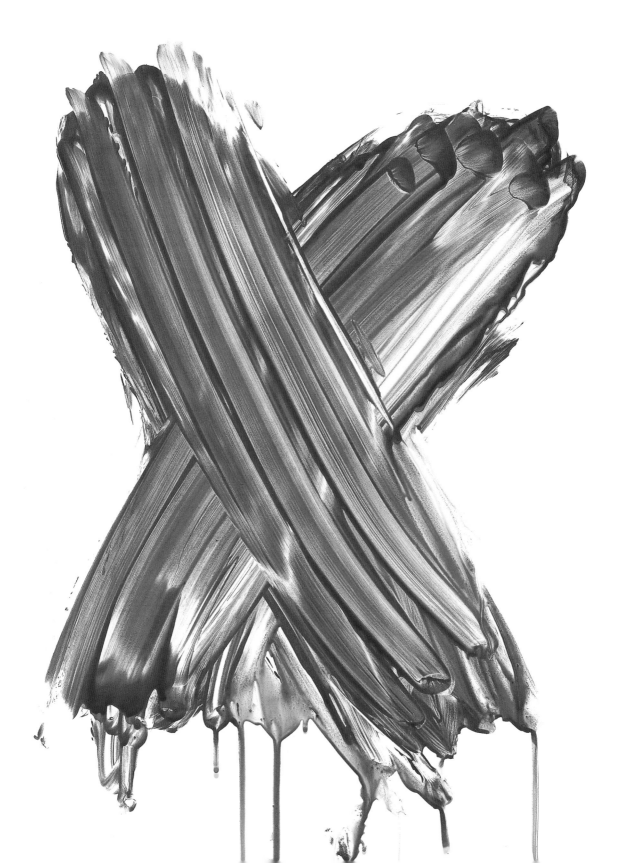

# Texture

If you touch something (it is likely) someone will feel it.
If you feel something (it is likely) **someone will be touched.**

Rick Valicenti

Texture is the tactile grain of surfaces and substances. Textures in our environment help us understand the nature of things: rose bushes have sharp thorns to protect the delicate flowers they surround; smooth, paved roads signal safe passage; thick fog casts a veil on our view.

The textures of design elements similarly correspond to their visual function. An elegant, smoothly patterned surface might adorn the built interior or printed brochure of a day spa; a snaggle of barbed wire could stand as a metaphor for violence or incarceration.

In design, texture is both physical and virtual. Textures include the literal surface employed in the making of a printed piece or physical object as well as the optical appearance of that surface. Paper can be rough or smooth, fabric can be nubby or fine, and packaging material can be glossy or matte. Physical textures affect how a piece feels to the hand, but they also affect how it looks. A smooth or glossy surface, for example, reflects light differently than a soft or pebbly one.

Many of the textures that designers manipulate are not physically experienced by the viewer at all, but exist as optical effect and representation. Texture adds detail to an image, providing an overall surface quality as well as rewarding the eye when viewed up close.

Whether setting type or depicting a tree, the designer uses texture to establish a mood, reinforce a point of view, or convey a sense of physical presence. A body of text set in Garamond italic will have a delicately irregular appearance, while a text set in Univers roman will appear optically smooth with even tonality. Likewise, a smoothly drawn vector illustration will have a different feel from an image taken with a camera or created with code.

As in life, the beauty of texture in design often lies in its poignant juxtaposition or contrast: prickly/soft, sticky/dry, fuzzy/smooth, and so on. By placing one texture in relation to its opposite, or a smart counterpart, the designer can amplify the unique formal properties of each one.

This chapter presents a wide spectrum of textures generated by hand, camera, computer, and code. They are abstract and concrete, and they have been captured, configured, sliced, built, and brushed. They were chosen to remind us that texture has a genuine, visceral, wholly seductive capacity to reel us in and hold us.

**High-Tech Finger Paint** The letterforms in Rick Valicenti's Touchy Feely alphabet were painted on vertical glass and recorded photographically with a long exposure from a digital, large-format Hasselblad camera. Rick Valicenti, Thirst.

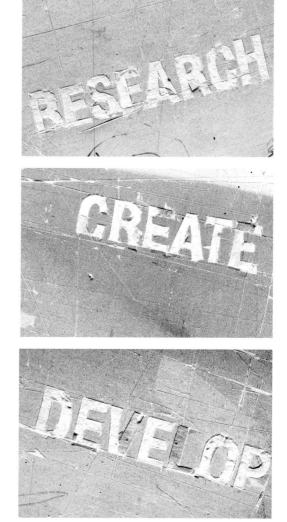

### Concrete Texture

The physical quality resulting from repeated slicing, burning, marking, and extracting creates concrete textural surfaces with robust appeal. The studies to the right grew out of a studio exercise where the computer was prohibited in the initial stages of concept and formal development. Turbulence (below), an alphabet by Rick Valicenti, similarly evokes a raw physicality. The alphabet began with vigorous hand-drawn, looping scribbles that were then translated into code.

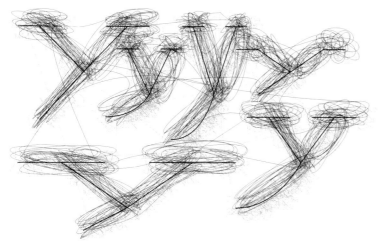

**Surface Manipulation** The textural physicality of these type studies artfully reflects the active processes featured in the words. The crisscrossing lines of an artist's cutting board resemble an urban street grid. Jonnie Hallman, Graphic Design I. Bernard Canniffe, faculty.

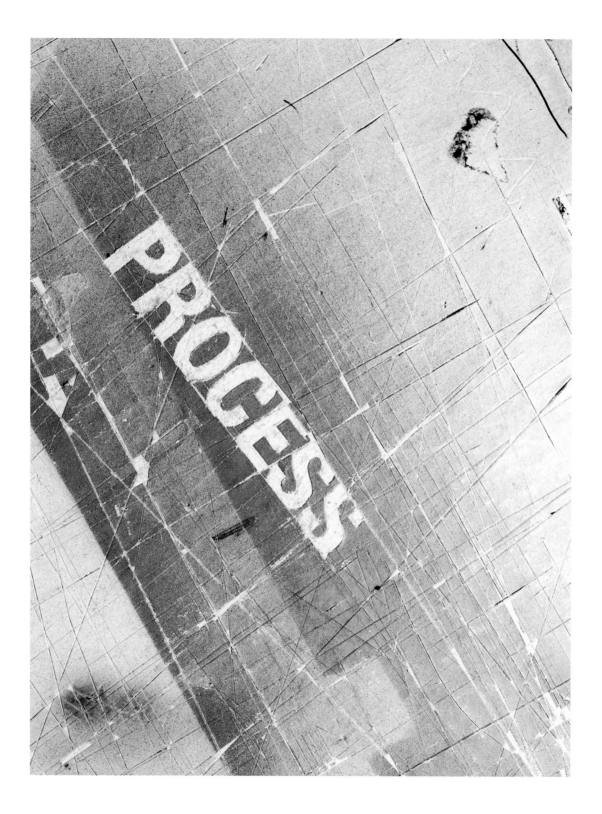

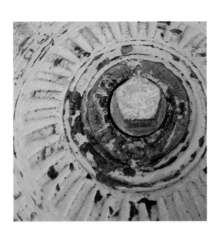

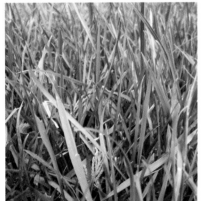

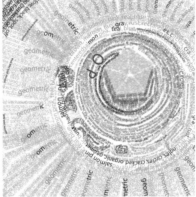

### Physical and Virtual Texture
This exercise builds connections between physical and virtual texture (the feel and look of surfaces). Designers used digital cameras to capture compelling textures from the environment. Next, they wrote descriptive paragraphs about each of the textures, focusing on their images' formal characteristics.

Using these descriptive texts as content, the designers re-created the textures typographically in Adobe Illustrator, employing repetition, scale, layers, and color. Typeface selection was open, but scale distortion was not permitted.
Graphic Design I. Mike Weikert, faculty.

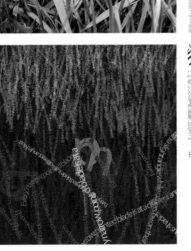

Hayley Griffin

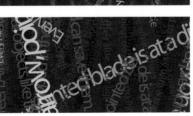

Grey Haas

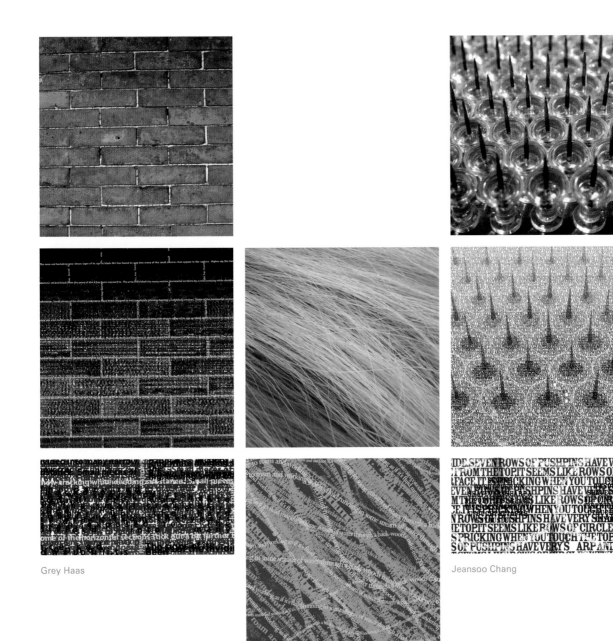

Grey Haas

Jeansoo Chang

Tim Mason

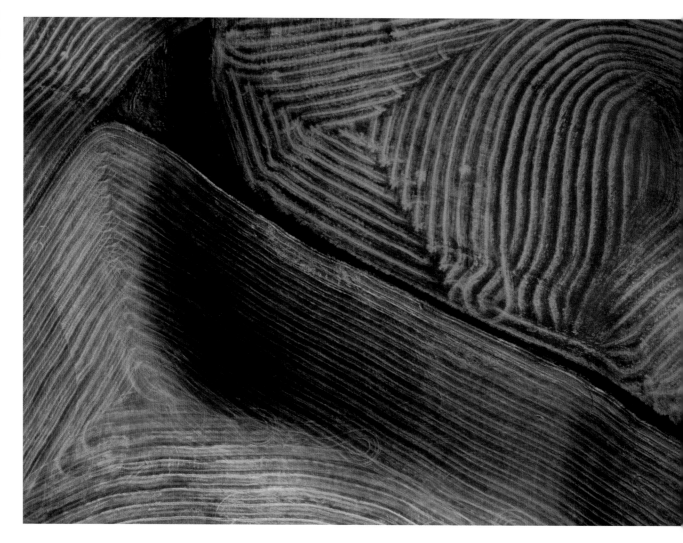

**Topographic Landscape** Aerial photograph of harvested wheat fields shows indexical traces of the process through many incised, looping and overlapping lines. Cameron Davidson.

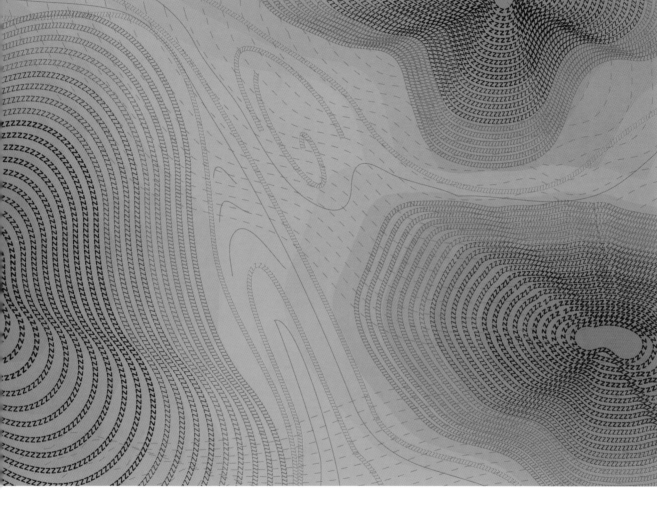

**Typographic Landscape** Curving lines of
text serve to build up a typographic surface,
creating the illusion of a topographic
landscape. Visakh Menon, MFA Studio.

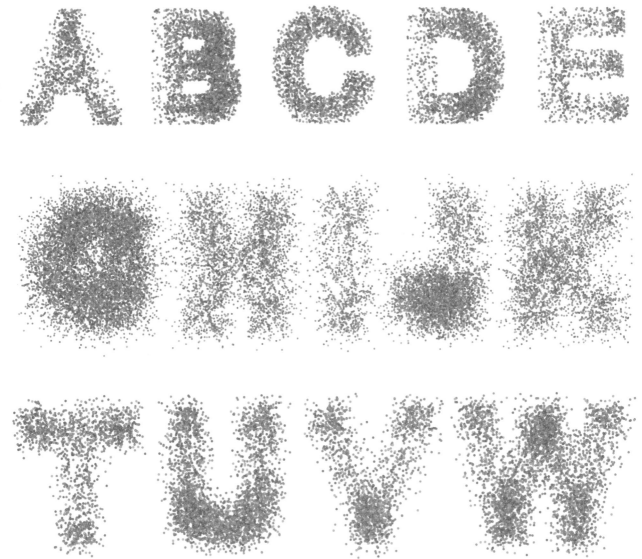

**Code-Driven Texture** The Swiss typographer
Emil Ruder once claimed that vital and
individual typographic rhythms are alien
to machines. The code-driven letterforms
shown here prove otherwise. Generated
in the computer language Processing, these
forms are effervescent, organic, and, indeed,
vital. Yeohyun Ahn, MFA Studio.

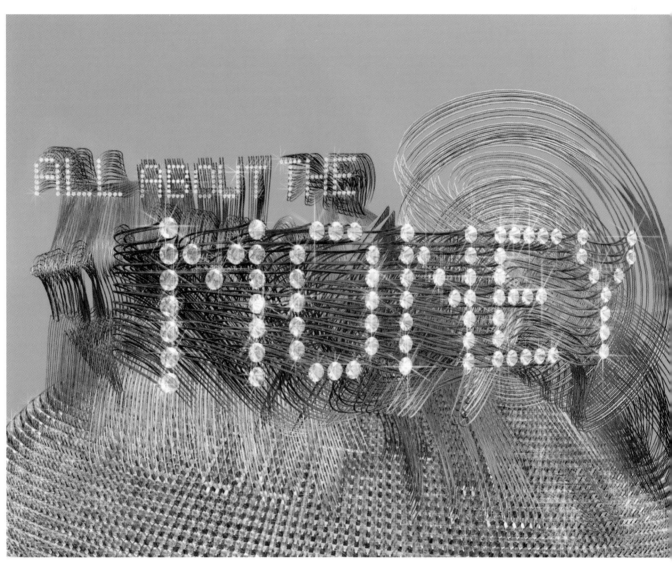

**All About the Money** The textured letters in this editorial illustration are rendered in 3D imaging software. The rhinestone-studded text is set against a Tiffany-blue sky, providing what designer Rick Valicenti calls "a suburban white male's version of the pixel pusher/gangsta aesthetic." Designer: Rick Valicenti, Thirst. Programmer: Matt Daly, Luxworks.

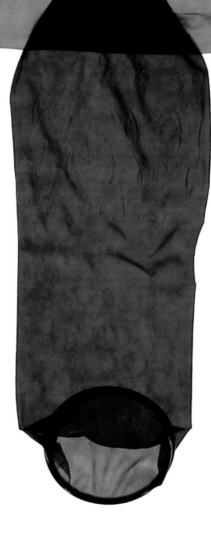

**Textural Harmony and Contrast**
Surface details can have harmonic or
contrasting characteristics, yielding
distinct visual effects. Some textures
have a high degree of contrast
and are built from relatively large
elements; others are low contrast and
have a fine, delicate grain. A rubbery,
baggy condom contrasts with
the soft, bruised skin of a banana.
Letterforms can be made with
sweeping, gooey brush forms
or with crisp strips of paper, each
technique imbuing the page with
a particular physical quality.

Satoru Nihei

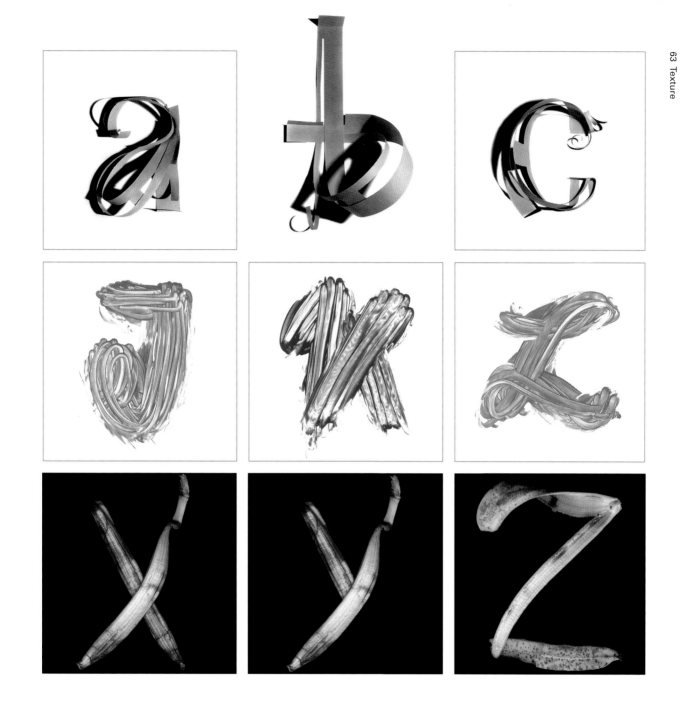

**Alphabetic Texture** These alphabets are from a diverse collection created for Rick Valicenti's Playground experiment, where letters are constructed from physical objects and processes. Designers top to bottom: Michelle Bowers, Rick Valicenti, Jenn Stucker.

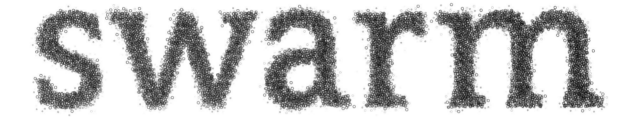

Abbott Miller and Kristen Spilman, Pentagram

**Textured Logotypes** The logotypes shown here, designed by Pentagram, use textured surfaces to convey ideas of movement and change. In a logo for an exhibition about the idea of "swarming" in contemporary art, thousands of tiny elements flock together to create a larger structure. In Pentagram's visual identity for MICA, patterning provides a rich patina that resonates with the school's urban neighborhood. The main typographic mark gracefully balances tradition and innovation. Solid historical letterforms are punctuated by a modern linear framework, referencing the two architecturally significant buildings that anchor the campus—one building is classical and cubic, while the other is dramatically angled. The texture makes the logo light and engaging when it is used at a large scale.

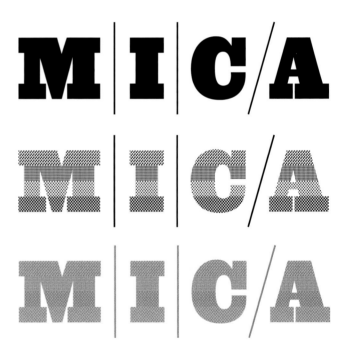

Abbott Miller and Kristen Spilman, Pentagram

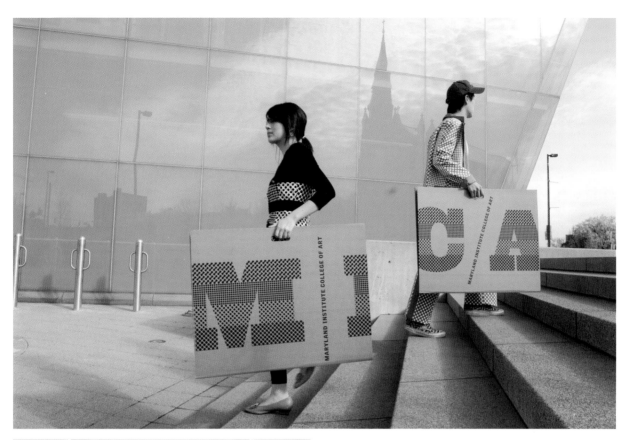

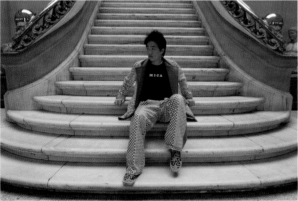

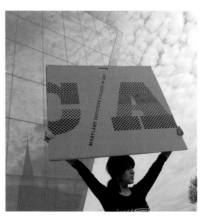

**Textural Applications** The MICA mark and pattern breathe life into a cardboard portfolio. The same pattern appears on works of street couture. Abbott Miller and Kristen Spilman, Pentagram. Photography: Nancy Froehlich.

**Five Squares Ten Inches** All typefaces have an innate optical texture that results from the accumulation of attributes such as serifs, slope, stroke width, and proportion. Those attributes interact on the page with the size, tracking, leading, and paragraph style selected by the designer, yielding an overall texture.

In this exercise, designers composed five justified squares of type inside a ten-inch frame. Variation of type style, texture, and value were achieved by combining contrasting characteristics such as old style italic serifs, uniformly weighted sans serifs, geometric slab serifs, and so on. Light to dark value (typographic color) was controlled through the combination of stroke width, letterspacing, and paragraph leading.

Finally, students manipulated the scale and placement of the squares to achieve compositional balance, tension, and depth. Squares were permitted to bleed off the edges, reinforcing the illusion of amplification and recession. Typography I. Jennifer Cole Phillips, faculty.

Julie Diewald

Anna Eshelman

ny, that hath to instrument
e never surfeited sea hath
land where man doth not
unfit to live. I have made
our men hang and drown
ny fellows are ministers of
ords are temper'd, may as
bemock'd—at stabs kill the
dowle that's in my plume
erable. If you could hurt
ur strengths and will not
ny business to you, that you
Prospero, exposed unto the
s innocent child: for which
rgetting, have incensed the
against your peace. Thee
and do pronounce by me
death can be at once, shall
vs, whose wraths to guard
esolate isle, else falls upon
row and a clear life ensuing.

never may believe these antique
fables, nor these fairy toys. Lovers
and madmen have such seething
brains, such shaping fantasies, that
apprehend more than cool reason ever
comprehends. One sees more devils
than vast hell can hold, that is, the
madman. The lover, all as frantic, sees
Helen's beauty in a brow of Egypt: the
poet's eye, in fine frenzy rolling, doth
glance from heaven to earth, from
earth to heaven; and as imagination
bodies forth the forms of things
unknown, the poet's pen turns them
to shapes and gives to airy nothing
a local habitation and a name. Such
tricks hath strong imagination, that if
it would but apprehend some joy, it
comprehends some bringer of that joy

**Anna Eshelman**

vy mouth tastes like menthol, newly minted coins, and
blood. the flavor of clean. flossed and metallic, french
kissing a robot. You told me something wednesday night
hat made me chirp and glow. Do you know you do
hat? Your love is one to revel in. You mean so many subtle
hings. Like the way wassail burns the back of your throat
vet draws you back for more. Like waking up and keeping
your eyes closed and your heartrate low. Like the color of
he sky when it snows. Like that second when the blades
on a ceiling fan finally come to a smooth halt. you embody
everything i have ever known, loved, and stored
n mind If I were a transformer, I'd fold into a cat. Maybe.

**My mouth tastes like menthol, newly minted
coins, and blood. the flavor of clean. flossed
and metallic, french kissing a robot. You told
me something wednesday night that made me
chirp and glow. Do you know you do that?
Your love is one to revel in. You mean so
many subtle things. Like the way wassail
burns the back of your throat, but draws you
back for more. like waking up and keeping
your eyes closed and your heartrate low. like
the color of the sky when it snows. like that
second when the blades on a ceiling fan finally
burns the back of your throat, but draws you
back for more. like waking up and keeping
your eyes closed and your heartrate low. like
burns the back of your throat, but draws
closed and your heartrate low. like come**

My mouth tastes like menthol, newly minted
coins, and blood. the flavor of clean. flossed and metallic, french
kissing a robot. You told me something wednesday night that made me chirp
and glow. Do you know you do that? Your love is one to revel in. You mean so many
subtle things. Like the way wassail burns the
back of your throat, but draws you back for
more. like waking up and keeping your eyes
closed and your heartrate low. like the color
of the sky when it snows. like that second when
the blades on a ceiling fan finally come to a
smooth halt. you embody everything i have
ever known, loved, and stored in mind. If I
were a transformer, I'd fold into a cat. Maybe

MY MOUTH TASTES LIKE MENTHOL, NEWL
MINTED COINS, AND BLOOD. THE FLAVO
OF CLEAN. FLOSSED AND METALLIC, FRENC
KISSING A ROBOT. YOU TOLD ME SOMETHIN
WEDNESDAY NIGHT THAT MADE ME CHIR
AND GLOW. DO YOU KNOW YOU DO THAT?
YOUR LOVE IS ONE TO REVEL IN. YOU MEAN
SO MANY SUBTLE THINGS. LIKE THE WA
WASSAIL BURNS THE BACK OF YOUR THROAT
BUT DRAWS YOU BACK FOR MORE. LIKE WAKIN
UP AND KEEPING YOUR EYES CLOSED AN
YOUR HEARTRATE LOW. LIKE THE COLOR O
THE SKY WHEN IT SNOWS. LIKE THAT SECON
WHEN THE BLADES ON A CEILING FA
FINALLY COME TO A SMOOTH HALT. YO
EMBODY EVERYTHING I HAVE EVER KNOWN
LOVED, AND STORED IN MIND. IF I WERE A
TRANSFORMER, I'D FOLD INTO A CAT. MAYB

**Ellen Kling**

**At the Pentagon, Defense Secretary Donald H
Rumsfeld said that while it was unclear what
role the U.S. military might take in enforcing
new U.N. sanctions, he did not expect the United
States or any other nation to do so unilaterally
At the Pentagon, Defense Secretary Donald H
Rumsfeld said that while it was unclear what
role the U.S. military might take in enforcing
new U.N. sanctions, he did not expect the United
States or any other nation to do so unilaterally
At the Pentagon, Defense Secretary Donald H
Rumsfeld said that while it was unclear what
role the U.S. military might take in enforcing
new U.N. sanctions, he did not expect the United
States or any other nation to do so unilaterally
At the Pentagon, Defense Secretary Donald H
Rumsfeld said that while it was unclear what
role the U.S. military might take in enforcing
new U.N. sanctions, he did not expect the United**

*At the Pentagon, Defense Secretary Donald H Rumsfeld
said that while it was unclear what role the U.S. military
might take in enforcing new U.N. sanctions, he did
not expect the United States or any other nation to do so
At the Pentagon, Defense Secretary Donald H Rumsfeld
said that while it was unclear what role the U.S. military
might take in enforcing new U.N. sanctions, he did
not expect the United States or any other nation to do so
At the Pentagon, Defense Secretary Donald H Rumsfeld
said that while it was unclear what role the U.S. military
might take in enforcing new U.N. sanctions, he did
not expect the United States or any other nation to do so
At the Pentagon, Defense Secretary Donald H Rumsfeld
said that while it was unclear what role the U.S. military
might take in enforcing new U.N. sanctions, he did*

**HyunSoo Lim**

On Wednesday, owners and workers downtown
boom shattering glass Everyone first feared add
another These fears were quickly dispelled mad
when sources noise traveled into sight fighters a
Witnesses couldn't believe their eyes Building its
sized vegetables were bouncing down the foxes
street smashing things that got into their wand
Small found throughout city had begun vegetable
their Suddenly some unseen force dervish fusion
levitated tarnish and into the streets water cared
humongous siblings Fire trucks and cops sandy
shoot down hose down, and rope down every wand
traffic hazards Nothing worked. vegetables after
only leaked lifesize seeds tons of juice onto most
buildings, pedestrians streets. The parade of lost
vegetables apparently was first spotted upper
Manhattan and traveled all the way to the Statue
Liberty, where they then moved out to sea. Mast
three hours the parade had managed structurally
damage thirty five buildings, scare the population
of the New York City, and leave them without add
vegetables for potentially a week is scary thought

ss, and tell the face thou viewest Now
face should form another Whose fresh
thou not renewest Thou dost beguile
bless some mother For where is she so
near'd womb Disdains the tillage of
Or who is he so fond will be the tomb
, to stop posterity Thou art thy mother's
e in thee Calls back the lovely April
o thou through windows of thine age
te of wrinkles this thy golden time But
member'd not to be Die single, and
ies with thee Look in thy glass, tell the

day Thou art more lovely and m
temperate Rough winds do shav
the darling buds of May And m
summer's lease hath all too shor
a date Sometime too hot the e
of heaven shines And often is
gold complexion dimm'd And ev
fair from fair sometime declines
chance or nature's changing cou
untrimm'd But thy eternal summ
shall not fade Nor lose possess
of that fair thou owest Nor shal
Death brag thou wander'st in th
shade When in eternal lines to t
thou growest So long as men ca
breathe or eyes can see So long
lives this and this gives life to th

**Julie Diewald**

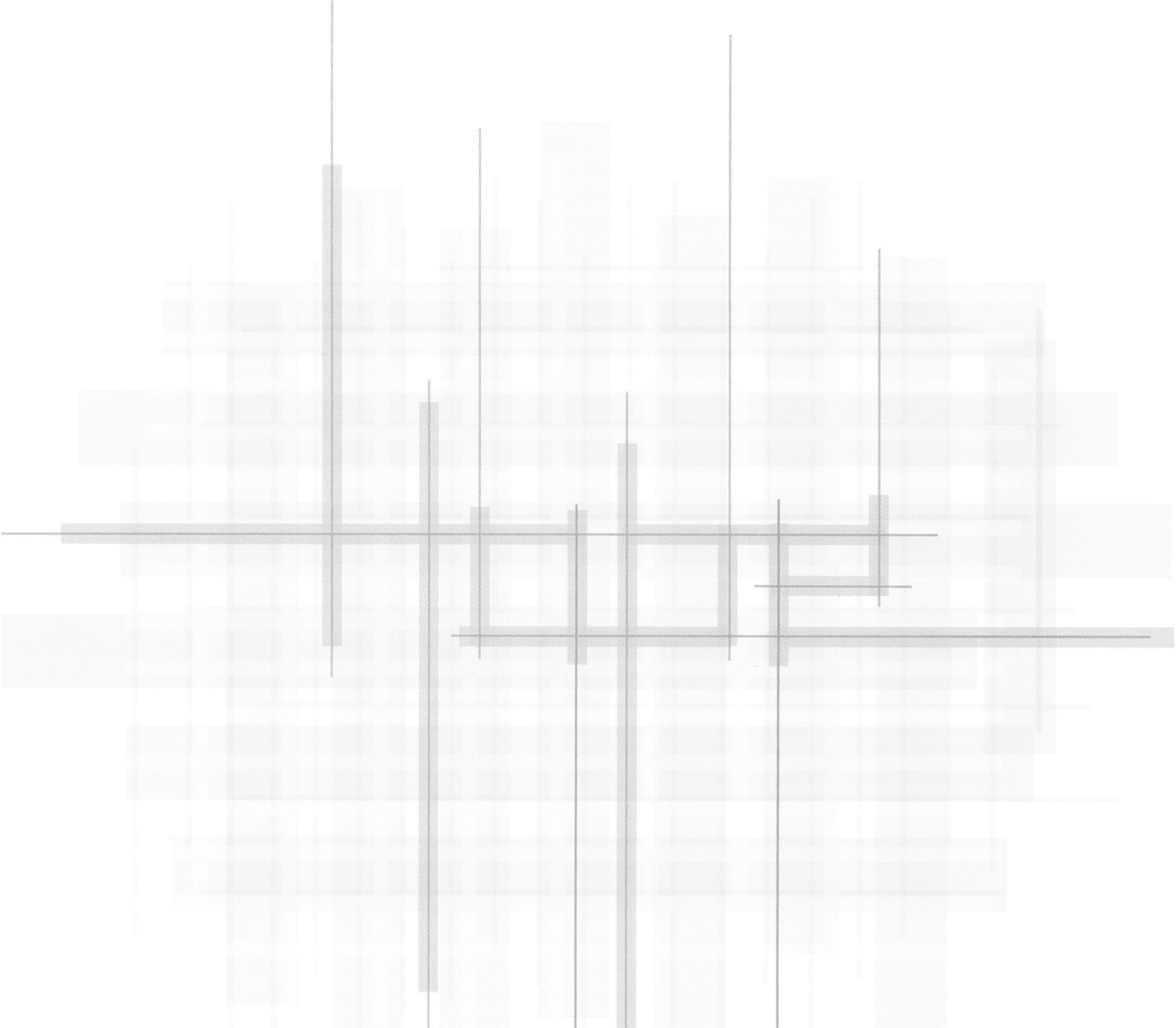

**Using Texture to Create Emphasis**
A field of individual marks becomes
a texture when the overall surface
pattern becomes more important
than any single mark. A texture
generally serves as ground, not as
figure, serving a supporting role to
a primary image or form. This role
is not passive, however. Used well
(as shown here), the background
texture supports the main image and
furthers the visual concept. Used
poorly, texture distracts and confuses
the eye, adding unwelcome noise to
a composition.

**Conveying a Mood** A texture can be
generated in response to a central image
(hope) or in opposition to it (anxiety).
Kelley McIntyre and Kim Bentley, MFA
Studio. Marian Bantjes, visiting faculty.

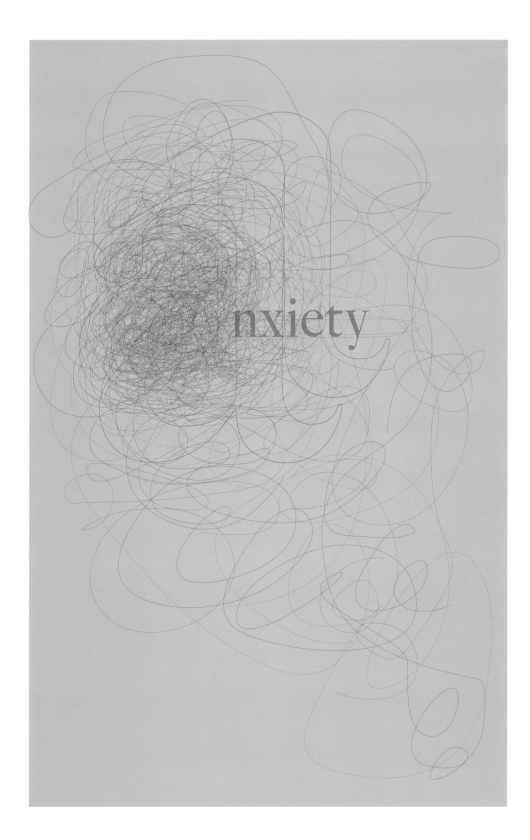

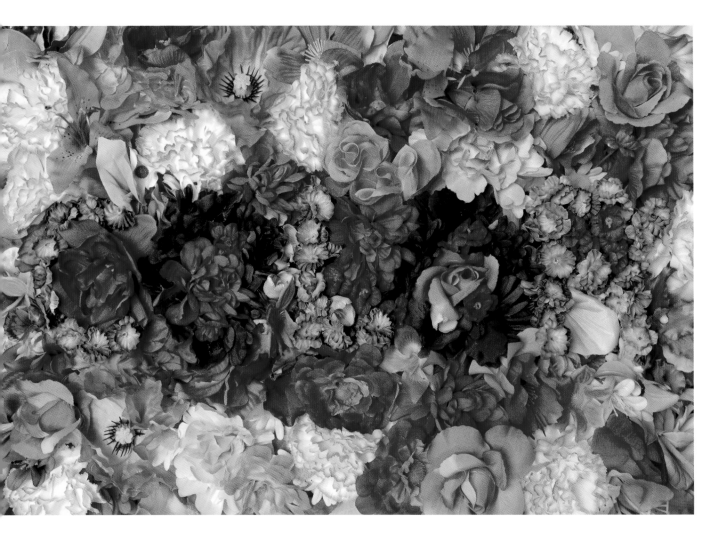

# Color

All colors are the friends of their neighbors and the **lovers of their opposites**. Marc Chagall

Color can convey a mood, describe reality, or codify information. Words like "gloomy," "drab," and "glittering" each bring to mind a general climate of colors, a palette of relationships. Designers use color to make some things stand out (warning signs) and to make other things disappear (camouflage). Color serves to differentiate and connect, to highlight and to hide.

Graphic design was once seen as a fundamentally black-and-white enterprise. This is no longer the case. Color has become integral to the design process. Color printing, once a luxury, has become routine. An infinite range of hues and intensities bring modern media to life, energizing the page, the screen, and the built environment with sensuality and significance. Graphics and color have converged.

According to the classical tradition, the essence of design lies in linear structures and tonal relationships (drawing and shading), not in fleeting optical effects (hue, intensity, luminosity). Design used to be understood as an abstract armature that underlies appearances. Color, in contrast, was seen as subjective and unstable.

And, indeed, it is. Color exists, literally, in the eye of the beholder. We cannot perceive color until light bounces off an object or is emitted from a source and enters the eye.

Our perception of color depends not solely on the pigmentation of physical surfaces, but also on the brightness and character of ambient light. We also perceive a given color in relation to the other colors around it. For example, a light tone looks lighter against a dark ground than against a pale one.

Likewise, color changes meaning from culture to culture. Colors carry different connotations in different societies. White signals virginity and purity in the West, but it is the color of death in Eastern cultures. Red, worn by brides in Japan, is considered racy and erotic in Europe and the United States. Colors go in and out of fashion, and an entire industry has emerged to guide and predict its course.

To say, however, that color is a shifting phenomenon—both physically and culturally—is not to say that it can't be described or understood. A precise vocabulary has been established over time that makes it possible for designers, software systems, printers, and manufacturers to communicate to one another with some degree of clarity. This chapter outlines the basic terms of color theory and shows ways to build purposeful relationships among colors.

**Opposites Attract** Strong color contrasts add visual energy to this dense physical montage made from flowers. Blue and purple stand out against pink, orange, and red. Nancy Froehlich and Zvezdana Rogic.

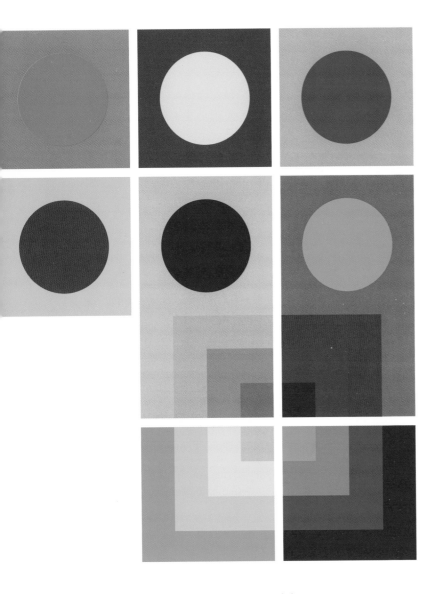

## Basic Color Theory

In 1665 Sir Isaac Newton discovered that a prism separates light into the spectrum of colors: red, orange, yellow, green, blue, indigo, and violet. He organized the colors around a wheel very much like the one artists use today to describe the relationships among colors.[1]

Why is the color wheel a useful design tool? Colors that sit near each other on the spectrum or close together on the color wheel are analogous. Using them together provides minimal color contrast and an innate harmony, because each color has some element in common with others in the sequence. Analogous colors also have a related color temperature. Two colors sitting opposite each other on the wheel are complements. Each color contains no element of the other, and they have opposing temperatures (warm versus cool). Deciding to use analogous or contrasting colors affects the visual energy and mood of any composition.

**Complementary and Analogous Colors**
This diagram shows combinations of primary, secondary, and tertiary colors.
Robert Lewis, MFA Studio.

1. On basic color theory and practice, see Tom Fraser and Adam Banks, *Designer's Color Manual* (San Francisco: Chronicle Books, 2004).

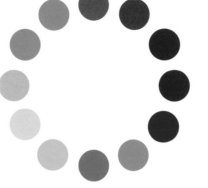

**The Color Wheel**
This basic map shows relationships among colors. Children learn to mix colors according to this model, and artists use it for working with pigments (oil paint, watercolor, gouache, and so on).

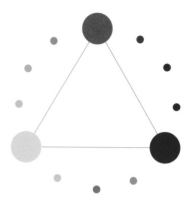

**Primary Colors**
Red, yellow, and blue are pure; they can't be mixed from other colors. All of the other colors on the wheel are created by mixing primary colors.

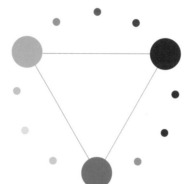

**Secondary Colors**
Orange, purple, and green each consist of two primaries mixed together.

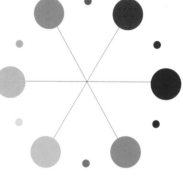

**Tertiary Colors**
Colors such as red orange and yellow green are mixed from one primary and one secondary color.

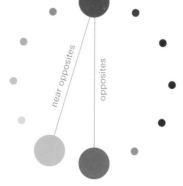

**Complements**
Red/green, blue/orange, and yellow/purple sit opposite each other on the color wheel. For more subtle combinations, choose "near opposites," such as red plus a tertiary green, or a tertiary blue and a tertiary orange.

near opposites

opposites

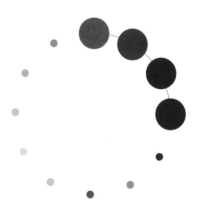

**Analogous Colors**
Color schemes built from hues that sit near to each other on the color wheel (analogous colors) have minimal chromatic differences.

**Hue** is the place of the color within the spectrum. A red hue can look brown at a low saturation, or pink at a pale value.

**Intensity** is the brightness or dullness of a color. A color is made duller by adding black or white, as well as by neutralizing it toward gray (lowering its saturation).

**Value** is the light or dark character of the color, also called its luminance, brightness, lightness, or tone. Value is independent of the hue or intensity of the color. When you convert a color image to black and white, you eliminate its hue but preserve its tonal relationships.

**Shade** is a variation of a hue produced by the addition of black.

**Tint** is a variation of a hue produced by the addition of white.

**Saturation** (also called chroma) is the relative purity of the color as it neutralizes to gray.

## Aspects of Color

Every color can be described in relation to a range of attributes. Understanding these characteristics can help you make color choices and build color combinations. Using colors with contrasting values tends to bring forms into sharp focus, while combining colors that are close in value softens the distinction between elements.

These colors are close in value and intensity, and just slightly different in hue.

These colors are close in hue and value but different in intensity.

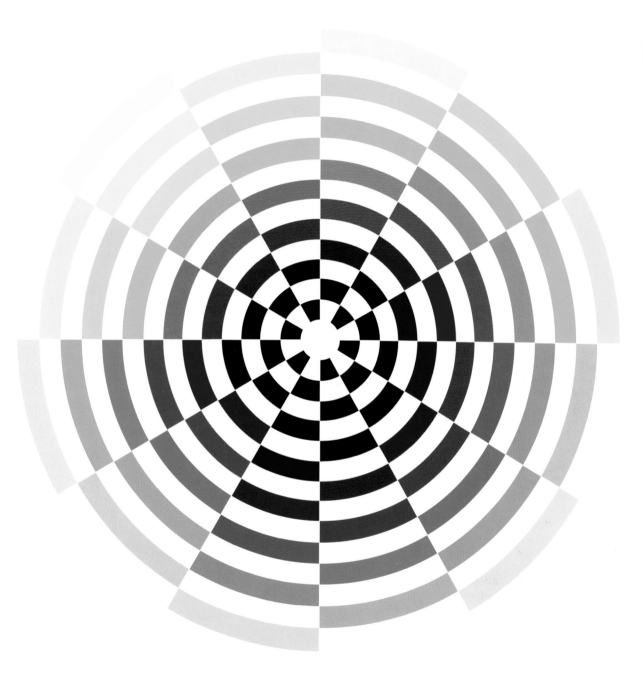

**Graduated Color Wheel** Each hue on the color wheel is shown here in a progressive series of values (shades and tints). Note that the point of greatest saturation is not the same for each hue. Yellow is of greatest intensity toward the lighter end of the value scale, while blue is more intense in the darker zone.

Use the graduated color wheel to look for combinations of colors that are similar in value or saturation, or use it to build contrasting relationships. Robert Lewis, MFA Studio.

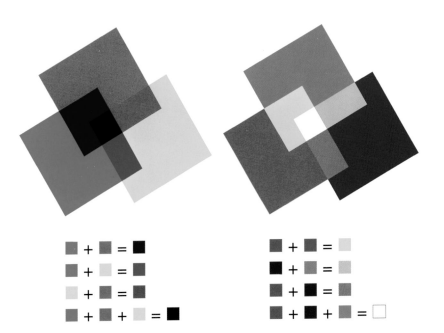

## Color Models

Surfaces absorb certain light waves and reflect back others onto the color receptors (cones) in our eyes. The light reflected back is the light we see. The true primaries of visible light are red, green, and blue. The light system is called "additive" because the three primaries together create all the hues in the spectrum.

In theory, combining red and green paint should produce yellow. In practice, however, these pigments combine into a blackish brown. This is because pigments absorb more light than they reflect, making any mix of pigments darker than its source colors. As more colors are mixed, less light is reflected. Thus pigment-based color systems are called "subtractive."

Offset and desktop printing methods use CMYK, a subtractive system. Nonstandard colors are used because the light reflected off cyan and magenta pigments mixes more purely into new hues than the light reflected off of blue and red pigments.

**CYMK** is used in the printing process. While painters use the basic color wheel as a guide for mixing paint, printing ink uses a different set of colors: cyan, magenta, yellow, and black, which are ideal for reproducing the range of colors found in color photographs. C, M, Y, and K are known as the "process colors," and full-color printing is called "four-color process." Ink-jet and color laser printers use CMYK, as does the commercial offset printing equipment used to print books such as this one.

In principle, C, M, and Y should produce black, but the resulting mix is not rich enough to reproduce color images with a full tonal range. Thus black is needed to complete the four-color process.

**RGB** is the additive system used for designing on screen. Different percentages of red, green, and blue light combine to generate the colors of the spectrum. White occurs when all three colors are at full strength. Black occurs when zero light (and thus zero color) is emitted.

Any given color can be described with both CMYK and RGB values, as well as with other color models. Each model (called a "color space") uses numbers to convey color information uniformly around the globe and across media. Different monitors, printing conditions, and paper stocks all affect the appearance of the final color, as does the light in the environment where the color is viewed. Colors look different under fluorescent, incandescent, and natural light. Colors rarely translate perfectly from one space to another.

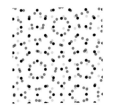

**Transparent Ink** Printer's inks are transparent, so color mixing occurs as colors show through each other. Color mixing is also performed optically when the image is broken down into tiny dots of varying size. The resulting colors are mixed by the eye.

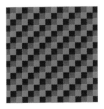

**Transparent Light** The medium of light is also transparent. The colors of an emitted image are generated when different colors of light mix directly, as well as when tiny adjacent pixels combine optically.

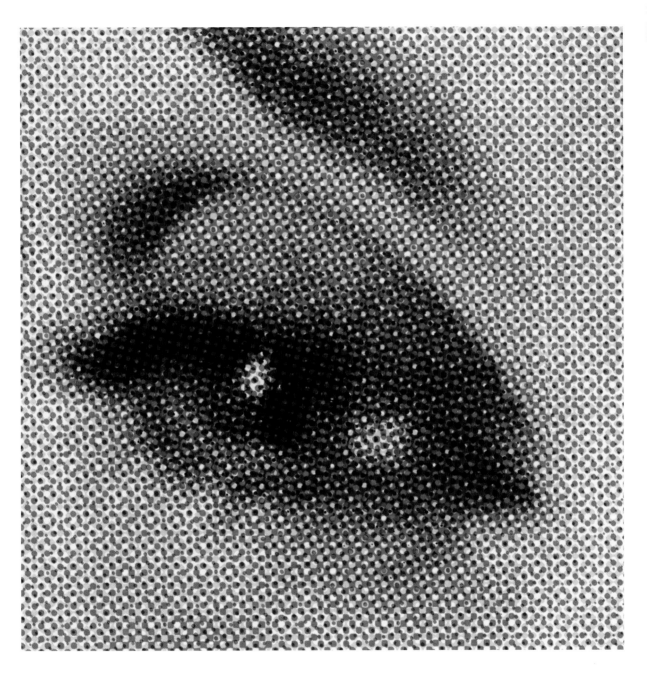

**Optical Color Mixing** This detail from a printed paper billboard shows the principle of four-color process printing (CMYK). Viewed from a distance, the flecks of color mix together optically. Seen up close, the pattern of dots is strongly evident.

Whatever color model your software is using, if you are viewing it on screen, it is RGB. If you are viewing it in print, it is CMYK.

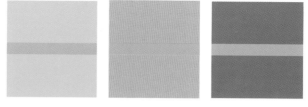

**One Color, Different Effects** The neutral tone passing through these three squares of color is the same in each instance. It takes on a slightly different hue or value depending on its context.

**Bezold Effect** Johann Friedrich Wilhelm von Bezold was a German physicist working in the nineteenth century. Fascinated with light and color, he also was an amateur rug maker. He noticed that by changing a color that interwove with other colors in a rug, he could create entirely different results. Adding a darker color to the carpet would create an overall darker effect, while adding a lighter one yielded a lighter carpet. This effect is known as optical mixing.

**Vibration and Value** When two colors are very close in value, a glowing effect occurs; on the left, the green appears luminous and unstable. With a strong value difference, as seen on the right, the green appears darker.

## Interaction of Color

Josef Albers, a painter and designer who worked at the Bauhaus before emigrating the United States, studied color in a rigorous manner that influenced generations of art educators.[2] Giving his students preprinted sheets of colored paper with which to work, he led them to analyze and experience how the perception of color changes in relation to how any given color is juxtaposed with others.

Colors are mixed in the eye as well as directly on the painter's palette or the printing press. This fact affects how designers create patterns and textures, and it is exploited in digital and mechanical printing methods, which use small flecks of pure hue to build up countless color variations.

Designers juxtapose colors to create specific climates and qualities, using one color to diminish or intensify another. Understanding how colors interact helps designers control the power of color and systematically test variations of an idea.

2. See Josef Albers, *Interaction of Color* (1963; repr., New Haven: Yale University Press, 2006).

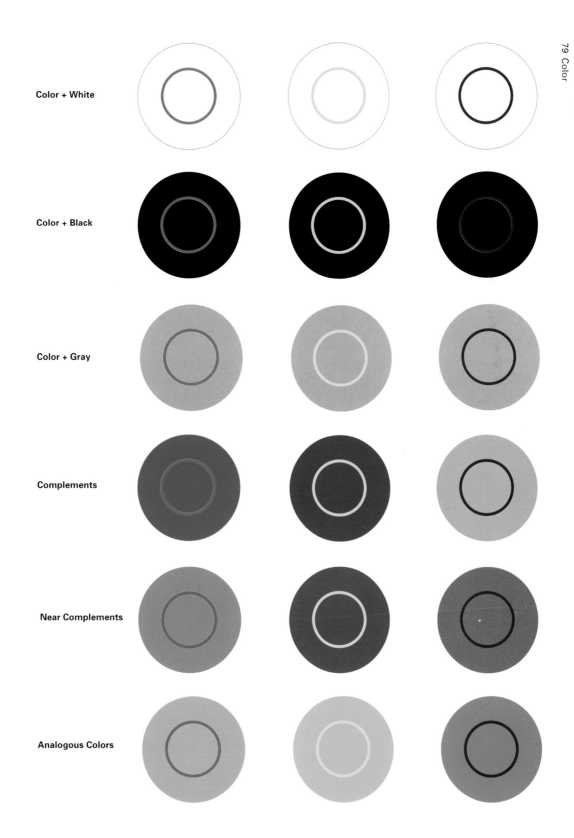

Color + White

Color + Black

Color + Gray

Complements

Near Complements

Analogous Colors

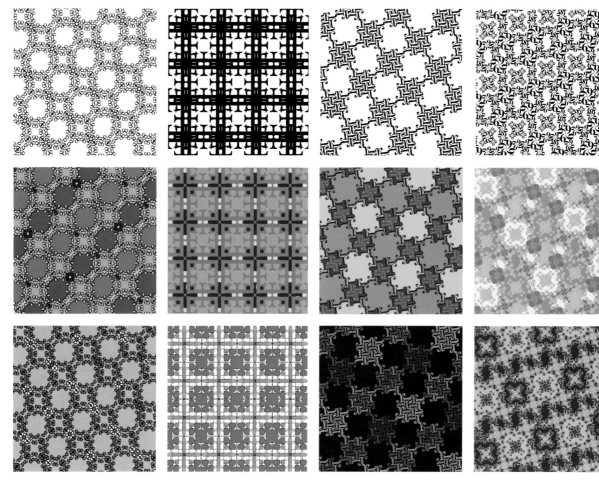

Joanna Marshall

Katie Evans

Ellen Kling

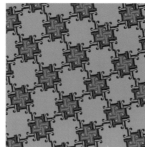

Elizabeth Tipson

Neutral earth tones
combine to make a
quiet overall pattern,
while a palette with
strong contrasts of
value and hue yields
a more linear effect.

By changing the
colors of background
and foreground
elements, completely
new forms appear
and disappear.

Colors close in value
but different in hue
create a vibrant yet
soft effect. The effect
becomes even softer
when analogous
colors are used.

**Selective Emphasis** These studies use
typographic pattern to explore how color
alters not just the mood of a pattern, but
the way its shapes and figures are perceived.
Color affects both the parts and the whole.
Each study begins with a black and white
pattern built from a single font and letterform.

Experiments with hue, value, and saturation,
as well as with analogous, complementary,
and near complementary color juxtapositions,
affect the way the patterns feel and behave.
Through selective emphasis, some elements
pull forward and others recede. Typography I.
Jennifer Cole Phillips, faculty.

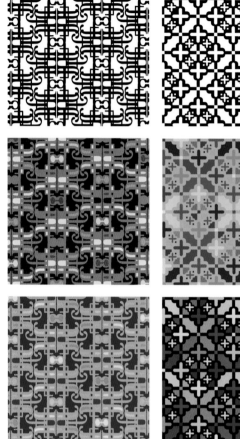

Anna Eshelman

The similarly muted hues of olive and brown sit back, allowing a pale yellow pattern to come forward. Next, gradations of yellow, orange, and red weave through a green background of equivalent value, causing the dark blue shapes to command attention.

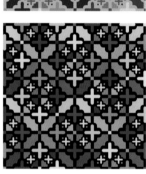

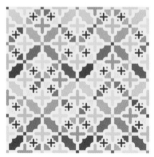

Anna Eshelman

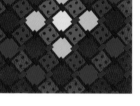

Julie Diewald

In the first color study above, the complementary orange and blue squares vibrate against each other, while the analogous yellow and green play a more passive role. In the second study, the dark blue and burgundy tones frame and push forward the brighter blues in the center.

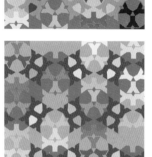

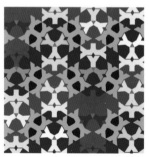

Anna Eshelman

The muted neutral hues allow the forms to gently commingle, while contrasting hues and values break the elements apart.

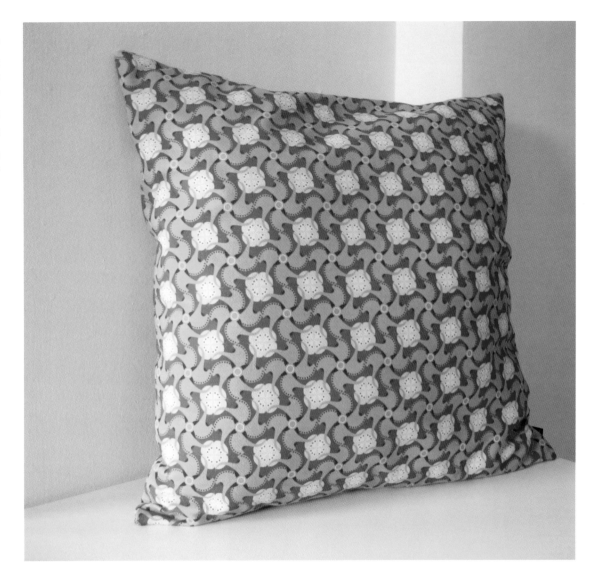

**Passion, Palettes, and Products** What began as a love for Portuguese tile patterns on a trip to Lisbon evolved into an intensive investigation into pattern, form, and color, manifesting itself in an MFA thesis project and now an online business.

Textile designers often create numerous color ways for a single pattern, allowing the same printing plates or weaving templates to generate diverse patterns. Different color palettes make different elements of the pattern come forward or recede. Jessica Pilar, MFA Studio.

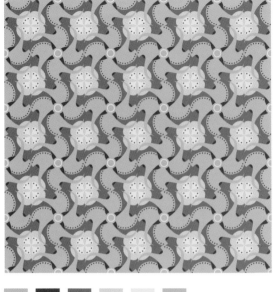
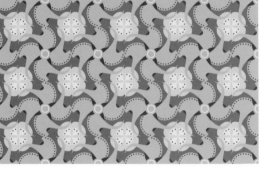
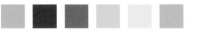

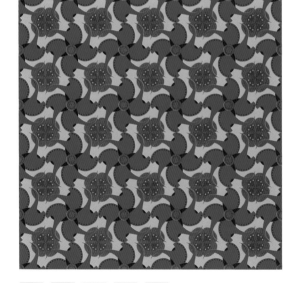

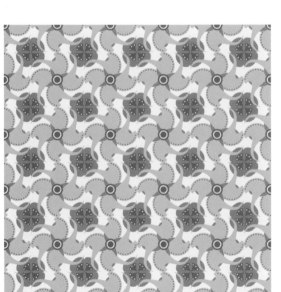

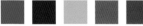

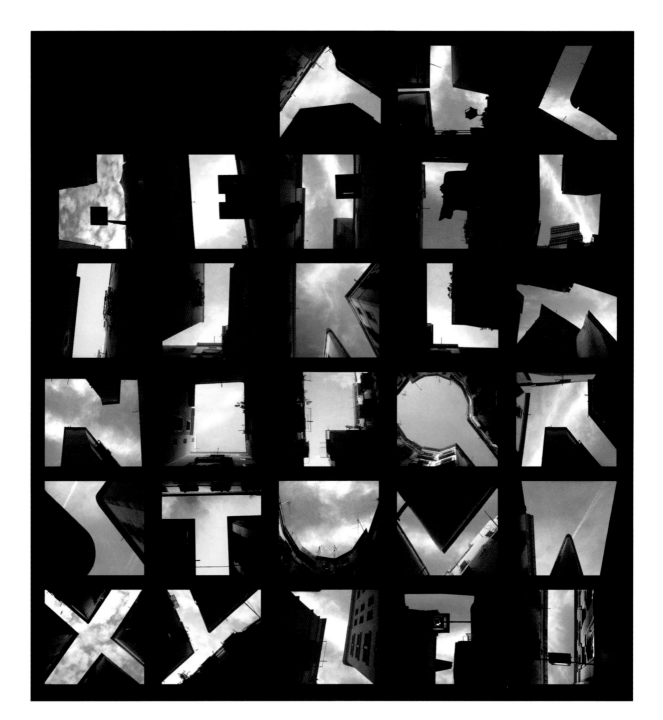

# Figure/Ground

The form of an object is not more important than the form of the space surrounding it. **All things exist in interaction with other things.** In music, are the separations between notes less important than the notes themselves? Malcolm Grear

Figure/ground relationships shape visual perception. A figure (form) is always seen in relation to what surrounds it (ground, or background)—letters to a page, a building to its site, a sculpture to the space within it and around it, the subject of a photograph to its setting, and so on. A black shape on a black field is not visible; without separation and contrast, form disappears.

People are accustomed to seeing the background as passive and unimportant in relation to a dominant subject. Yet visual artists quickly become attuned to the spaces around and between elements, discovering their power to shape experience and become active forms in their own right.

Graphic designers often seek a balance between figure and ground, using this relationship to bring energy and order to form and space. They build contrasts between form and counterform in order to construct icons, illustrations, logos, compositions, and patterns that stimulate the eye. Creating figure/ground tension or ambiguity adds visual energy to an image or mark. Even subtle ambiguity can invigorate the end result and shift its direction and impact.

Figure/ground, also known as positive and negative space, is at work in all facets of graphic design. In the design of logotypes and symbols, the distillation of complex meaning into simplified but significant form often thrives on the taut reciprocity of figure and ground. In posters, layouts, and screen designs, what is left out frames and balances what is built in. Similarly, in time-based media, including multipage books, the insertion and distribution of space across time affects perception and pacing.

The ability to create and evaluate effective figure/ground tension is an essential skill for graphic designers. Train your eye to carve out white space as you compose with forms. Learn to massage the positive and negative areas as you adjust the scale of images and typography. Look at the shapes each element makes and see if the edges frame a void that is equally appealing. Notice how as the value of a text block becomes darker, its shape becomes more defined when composed with other elements.

Recognizing the potency of the ground, designers strive to reveal its constructive necessity. Working with figure/ground relationships gives designers the power to create—and destroy—form.

**Figure Sky** These photographs use urban buildings to frame letterforms. The empty sky becomes the dominant figure, and the buildings become the background that makes them visible. Lisa Rienermann, University of Essen, Germany.

Stable

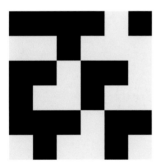

Reversible

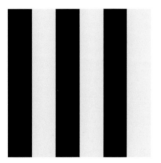

Ambiguous

**Stable, Reversible, Ambiguous**
A stable figure/ground relationship exists when a form or figure stands clearly apart from its background. Most photography functions according to this principle, where someone or something is featured within a setting.

Reversible figure/ground occurs when positive and negative elements attract our attention equally and alternately, coming forward, then receding, as our eye perceives one first as dominant and next as subordinate. Reversible figure ground motifs can be seen in the ceramics, weaving, and crafts of cultures around the globe.

Images and compositions featuring ambiguous figure/ground challenge the viewer to find a focal point. Figure is enmeshed with ground, carrying the viewer's eye in and around the surface with no discernable assignment of dominance. The Cubist paintings of Picasso mobilize this ambiguity.

**Interwoven Space**
Designers, illustrators, and photographers often play with figure/ground relationships to add interest and intrigue to their work. Unlike conventional depictions where subjects are centered and framed against a background, active figure/ground conditions churn and interweave form and space, creating tension and ambiguity.

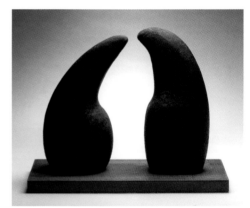

**Form and Counterform** Sculpture—like buildings in a landscape—displaces space, creating an active interplay between the form and void around it. Here, the distilled shapes and taut tension pay homage to Henry Moore, with whom this artist studied in the **1930s.** Reuben Kramer, 1937. Photographed by Dan Meyers.

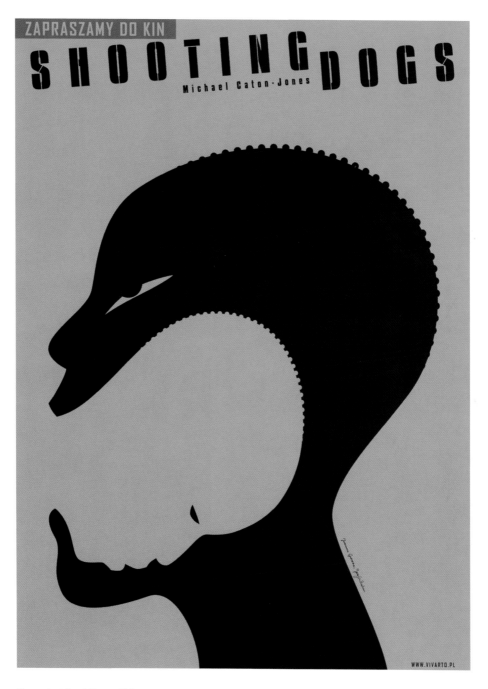

**Figure Inside of Figure** This poster reveals its subject at second glance. One head takes form as the void inside the other. The tension between figure and ground acquires an ominous energy. Joanna Górska and Jerzy Skakun, Homework.

**Letterform Abstraction** In this introduction to letterform anatomy, students examined the forms and counterforms of the alphabet in many font variations, eventually isolating just enough of each letter to hint at its identity. Each student sought to strike a balance between positive and negative space. Typography I. Jennifer Cole Phillips, faculty.

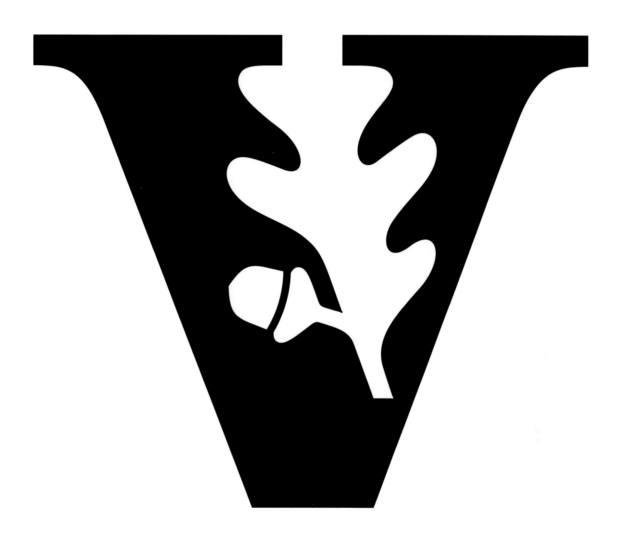

**Optical Interplay** This mark for Vanderbilt University employs a strong contrast between rigid form and organic counterform. The elegant oak leaf alternately sinks back, allowing the letterform to read, and comes forward, connoting growth, strength, and beauty. Malcolm Grear, Malcolm Grear Designers.

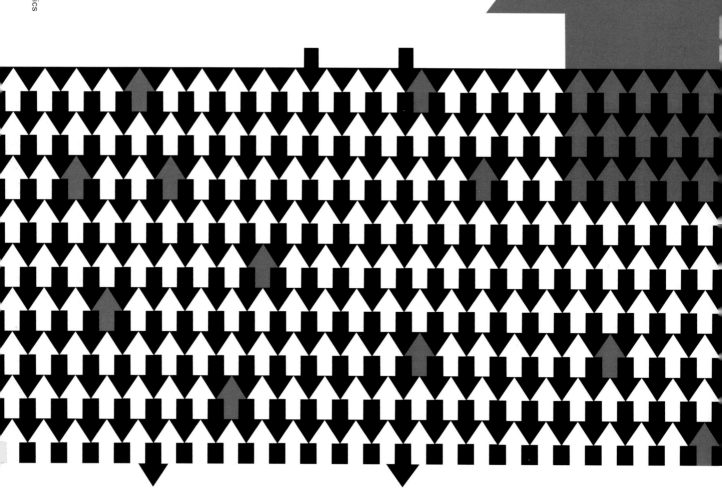

**Figure/Ground Battalion** These marching positive and negative arrows commingle and break away from the pack. The dynamic use of scale, direction, rhythm, and color ushers the viewer's eye in and around the composition. Superforms take shape out of the crowd. Yong Seuk Lee, MFA Studio.

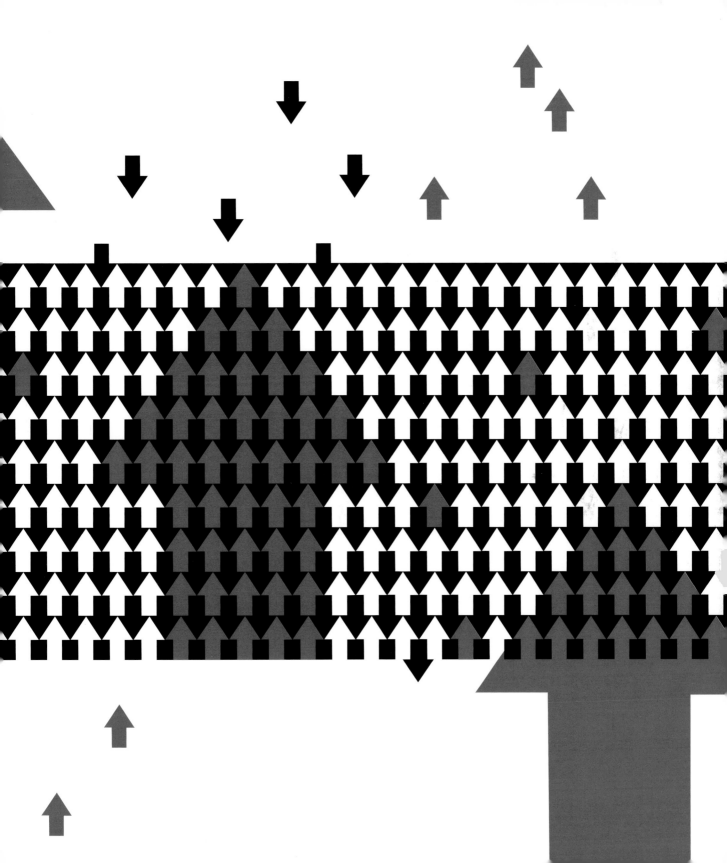

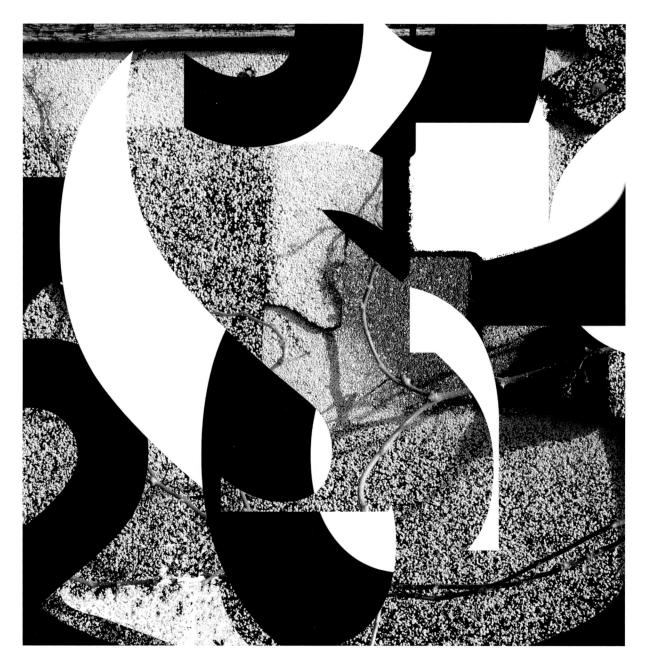

**Photo Letter Mesh** In this abstract study of type and texture, black and white letterforms are skillfully interwoven with granular, high-contrast imagery, creating an ambiguous figure/ground condition. Jeremy Botts, MFA Studio.

**Contrast and Composition.** In this project, students explored principles of visual contrast, homing in on letterform details to illuminate unique anatomical and stylistic features. Each study focuses on one pair of contrasting letterforms, which the designer could crop, combine, repeat, rotate, enlarge, and reduce. The final designs celebrate formal differences as well as distribute positive and negative space into fluid, balanced compositions. Typography I. Jennifer Cole Phillips, faculty.

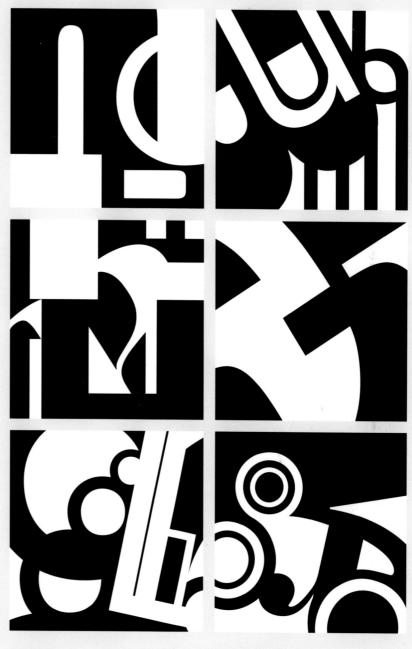

Zey Akay
Anna Eshelman
HyunSoo Lim

Lindsay Petrick
Elizabeth Tipson
Lindsay Petrick

The Guggenheim Museum

**Artful Reduction** A minimal stack of carefully shaped forms, in concert with exacting intervals of spaces, instantly evokes this sculptural landmark. Malcolm Grear, Malcolm Grear Designers.

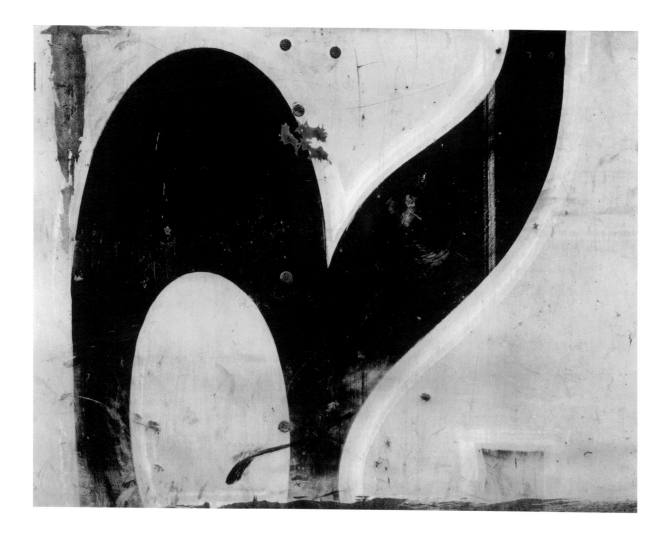

**Capturing Tension** Aaron Siskind (1903–1991),
known for his profound contribution to abstract
expressionist photography, was a master of
figure/ground relationships. *Chicago 30, 1949,*
above, challenges the viewer to choose figure
or ground as the tension between black and
white is continually shifting. ©Aaron Siskind
Foundation. Image courtesy of Robert
Mann Gallery.

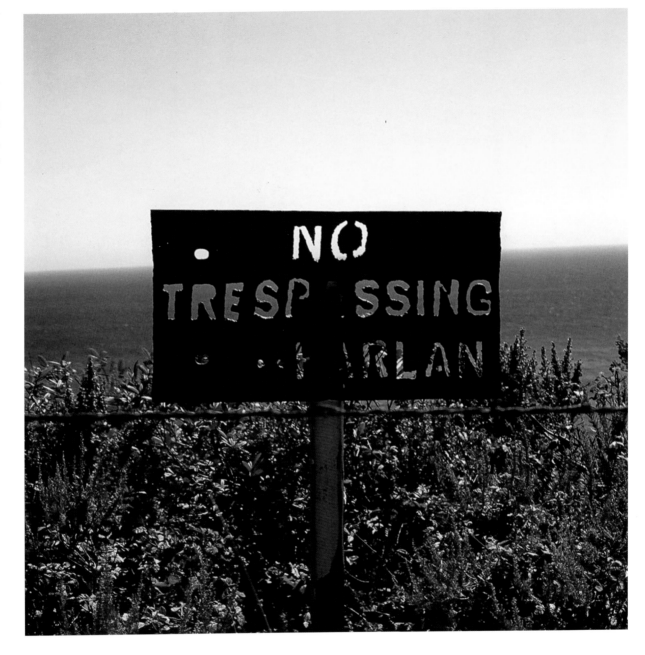

**No Entry** These crudely punched letters are readable against the sky and sea, whose contrasting value lights up the message. Jayme Odgers.

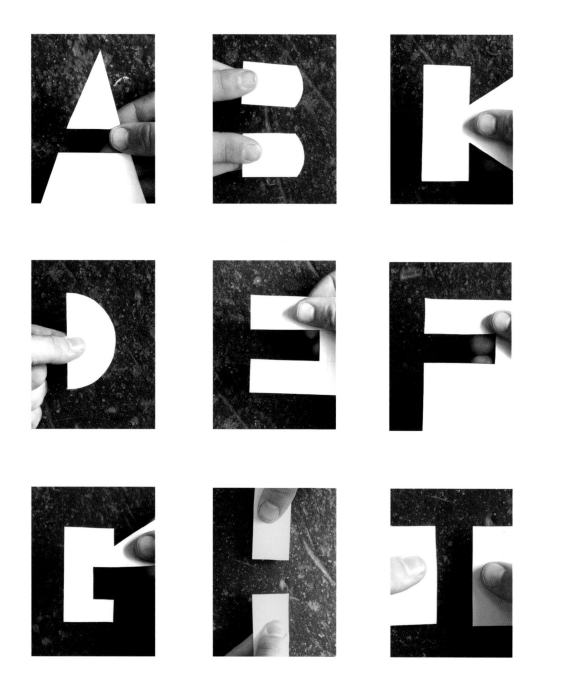

**Counter Hand** The simple device of cut white
paper held against a contrasting ground
defines the alphabet with quirky style and
spatial depth. FWIS Design.

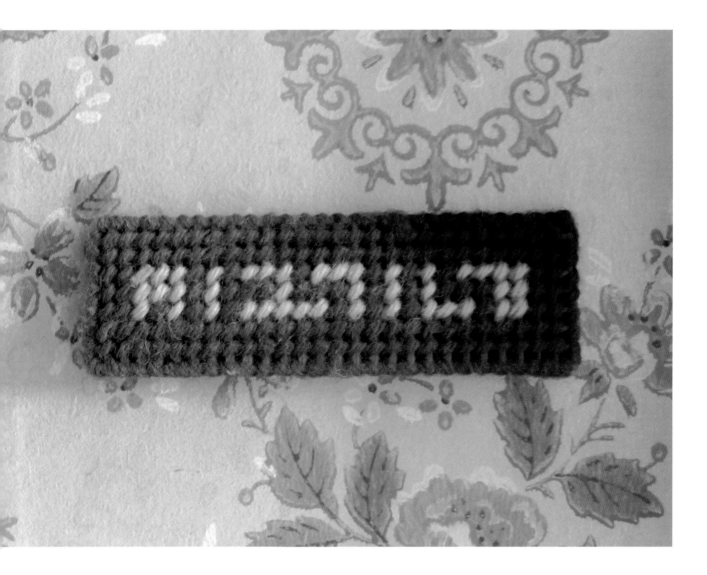

**Seeing Jesus** Simple stitches spell out a series of letters, which take form as the viewer's eye allows the background to move forward. The light stitches become counterforms for the dark letters. Needlepoint: Ralph Emerson Pierce (1912–1992). Photograph: Jeremy Botts, MFA Studio.

**Inspired by Jesus** The designer has interwoven the words "figure" and "ground" across each horizontal band. One word serves as the background or frame for the other, forcing the eye to shuttle between two conflicting readings. This complex study was inspired by the needlework at left. Jeremy Botts, MFA Studio.

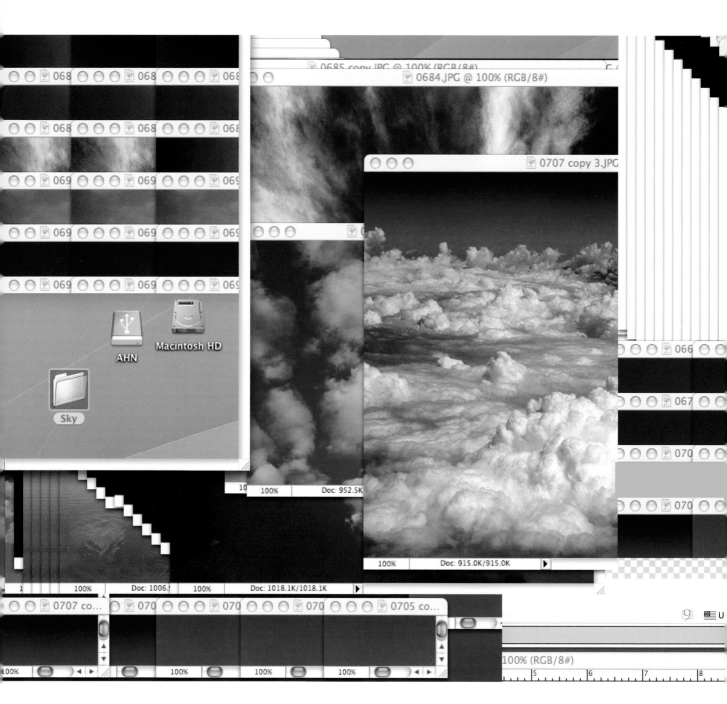

**Interface Overload** Graphic interfaces are
a constant presence throughout the design
process. Here, the interface itself—and
its excessive accumulation of windows—
becomes a design object. Yeohyun Ahn,
MFA Studio.

# Framing

[The frame] disappears, buries itself, melts away at the moment it deploys its greatest energy. **The frame is in no way a background... but neither is its thickness as margin a figure.** Or at least it is a figure which comes away of its own accord. Jacques Derrida

Frames are everywhere. A picture frame sets off a work of art from its surroundings, bringing attention to the work and lifting it apart from its setting. Shelves, pedestals, and vitrines provide stages for displaying objects. A saucer frames a tea cup, and a place mat outlines the pieces of a table setting.

Modern designers often seek to eliminate frames. A minimalist interior avoids moldings around doors or woodwork where walls meet the floor, exposing edge-to-edge relationships. The full-bleed photography of a sleek magazine layout eliminates the protective, formal zone of the white margin, allowing the image to explode off the page and into reality.

In politics, "framing" refers to explaining an issue in terms that will influence how people interpret it. The caption of a picture is a frame that guides its interpretation. A billboard is framed by a landscape, and a product is framed by its retail setting. Boundaries and fences mark the frames of private property.

Cropping, borders, margins, and captions are key resources of graphic design. Whether emphasized or erased, frames affect how we perceive information.

Frames create the conditions for understanding an image or object. The philosopher Jacques Derrida defined framing as a structure that is both present and absent.[1] The frame is subservient to the content it surrounds, disappearing as we focus on the image or object on view, and yet the frame shapes our understanding of that content. Frames are part of the fundamental architecture of graphic design. Indeed, framing is one of the most persistent, unavoidable, and infinitely variable acts performed by the graphic designer.

An interface is a kind of frame. The buttons on a television set, the index of a book, or the toolbars of a software application exist outside the central purpose of the product, yet they are essential to our understanding of it. A hammer with no handle or a cell phone with no controls is useless.

Consider the ubiquity of interfaces in the design process. The physical box of the computer screen provides a constant frame for the act of designing, while the digital desktop is edged with controls and littered with icons. Numerous windows compete for our attention, each framed by borders and buttons.

A well-designed interface is both visible and invisible, escaping attention when not needed while shifting into focus on demand. Once learned, interfaces disappear from view, becoming second nature.

Experimental design often exposes or dramatizes the interface: a page number or a field of white space might become a pronounced visual element, or a navigation panel might assume an unusual shape or position. By pushing the frame into the foreground, such acts provoke the discovery of new ideas.

This chapter shows how the meaning and impact of an image or text changes depending on how it is bordered or cropped. Frames typically serve to contain an image, marking it off from its background in order to make it more visible. Framing can also penetrate the image, rendering it open and permeable rather than stable and contained. A frame can divide an image from its background, but it can also serve as a transition from inside to outside, figure to ground.

1. Jacques Derrida, *The Truth in Painting*, trans. Geoff Bennington and Ian McLeod (Chicago: University of Chicago Press, 1987).

## Camera Frames

The mechanical eye of the camera cuts up the field of vision in a way that the natural eye does not. Every time you snap a picture with a camera, you make a frame. In contrast, the eye is in constant motion, focusing and refocusing on diverse stimuli in the environment.

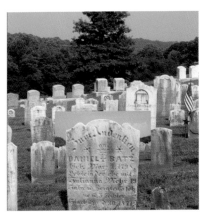

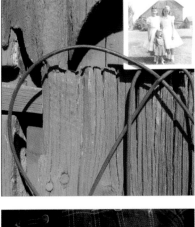

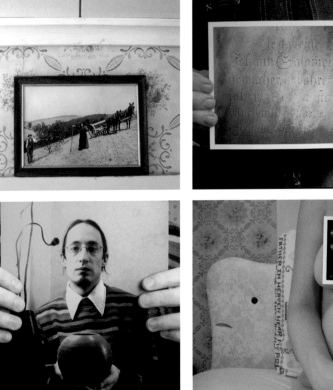

**Frames Inside of Frames** Frames exist throughout the environment. The photographs shown here use the tool of the camera to create not only the outer frame of the shot, but to discover inner frames as well. Sarah Joy Jordahl Verville, MFA Studio.

**Framing and Reframing** Here, the artist rephotographed pictures collected from the history and future of his own family in environments that are endowed with both historic and contemporary detail. Jeremy Botts, MFA Studio. Corinne Botz, faculty.

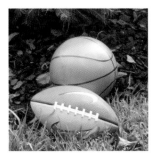

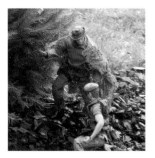

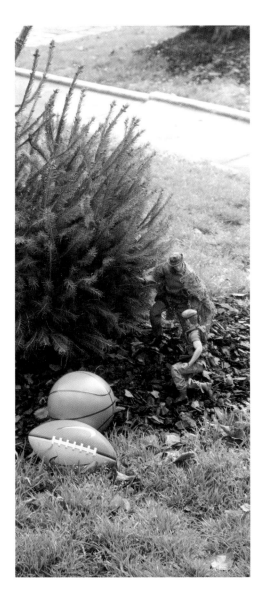

## Cropping

By cropping a photograph or illustration, the designer redraws its borders and alters its shape, changing the scale of its elements in relation to the overall picture. A vertical image can become a square, a circle, or a narrow ribbon, acquiring new proportions. By closing in on a detail, cropping can change the focus of a picture, giving it new meaning and emphasis.

By cropping a picture, the designer can discover new images inside it. Experiment with cropping by laying two L-shaped pieces of paper over an image, or look at the picture through a window cut from a piece of paper. Working digitally, move an image around inside the picture frame in a page-layout program, changing its scale, position, and orientation.

**New Frame, New Meaning** The way an image is cropped can change its meaning completely. Yong Seuk Lee, MFA Studio.

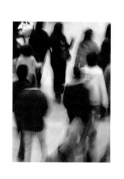

**Margin** A margin creates a protective zone around an image, presenting it as an object on a stage, a figure against a ground. Margins can be thick or thin, symmetrical or asymmetrical. A wider margin can add formality to the image it frames.

## Margins and Bleeds

Margins affect the way we perceive content by providing open spaces around texts and images. Wider margins can emphasize a picture or a field of text as an object, calling our attention to it. Narrower margins can make the content seem larger than life, bursting at its own seams.

Margins provide a protective frame around the contents of a publication. They also provide space for information such as page numbers and running heads. A deep margin can accommodate illustrations, captions, headings, and other information.

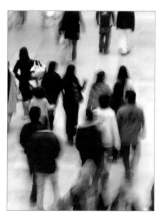

**Full Bleed** An image "bleeds" when it runs off the edges of a page. The ground disappears, and the image seems larger and more active.

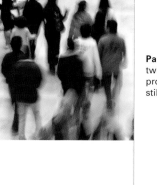

**Partial Bleed** An image can bleed off one, two, or three sides. Here, the bottom margin provides a partial border, yet the photograph still has a larger-than-life quality.

**Bleeds** The picture above is reproduced at the same scale in each instance, but its intimacy and impact change as it takes over more or less of the surrounding page.

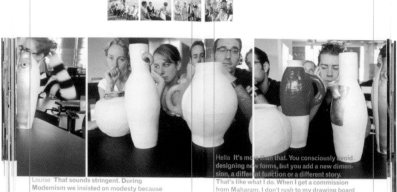

Louise **That sounds stringent. During Modernism we insisted on modesty because we believed it would help us penetrate further and further into the essence of things. The art of omission.**

Hella **It's more than that. You consciously avoid designing new forms, but you add a new dimension, a different function or a different story. That's like what I do. When I get a commission from Maharam, I don't rush to my drawing board to design a snazzy new pattern. I pore through the archives, use existing patterns, and add a new concept to them.**

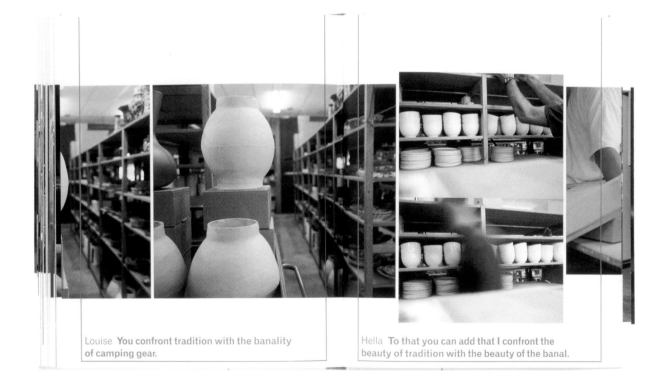

Louise **You confront tradition with the banality of camping gear.**

Hella **To that you can add that I confront the beauty of tradition with the beauty of the banal.**

**Using Margins and Bleeds** Designed by COMA, this book about the Dutch product designer Hella Jongerius uses margins, bleeds, rules, and other framing devices in distinctive ways. The photographs bleed off the left and right edges of each page, while the top and bottom margins are kept clear as an open territory that sometimes includes text and additional pictures. Tightly spaced together, the pictures create a strong horizontal movement, like a strip of film marching through the center of the book. Countering this horizontal motion are gold boxes printed on top of the pictures. Whereas boxes traditionally serve to neatly enclose an area, these boxes are open at the top, and their shape doesn't match the pictures underneath. The designers have thus used many of the standard components of book design in an unconventional way. Cornelia Blatter and Marcel Hermans, COMA. *Hella Jongerius*, 2003. Photographers: Joke Robaard with Maarten Theuwkens.

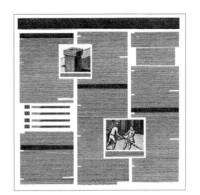

Shannon Snyder

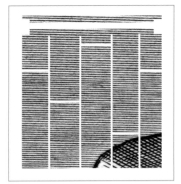

Jessica Alvarado

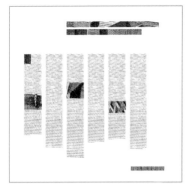

Melanie M. Rodgers

Lindsay Olson

**Using Images Typographically** How can an image be arranged, like type, into words, lines, columns, and grids? This exercise invited designers to think abstractly about both image and type. Each designer created a new visual "text" by mining lines, shapes, and textures from a larger picture. Typography is experienced in terms of blocks of graphic tone and texture that are framed by the margins and gutters of the page. Different densities of texture suggest hierarchies of contrasting typefaces. Headlines, captions, quotations, lists, illustrations, and other material take shape in relation to bodies of running text. Advanced Design Workshop, York College. Ellen Lupton, visiting faculty.

The exercises on this spread incorporate a high-resolution scan of an original eighteenth-century engraving from Denis Diderot's *Encyclopedia*. Shown here is the full image.

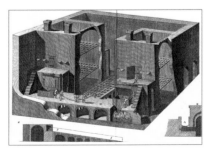

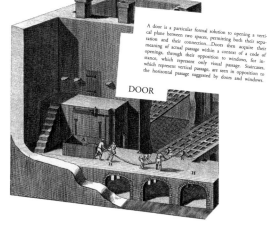

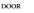

Luke Williams

Jessica Neil

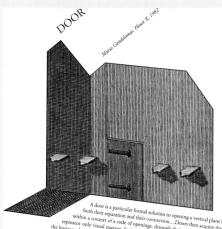

Jonnie Hallman

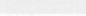

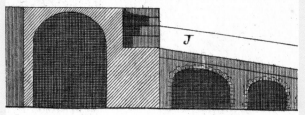

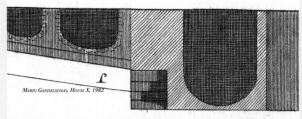

Lindsey Sherman

**Framing Text and Image** In this project, designers edited, framed, and cropped a picture in relation to a passage of text. The challenge was to make the text an equal player in the final composition, not a mere caption or footnote to the picture.

Designers approached the image abstractly as well as figuratively. Is the picture flat or three-dimensional? How does it look upside down? Designers edited the image by blocking out parts of it, changing the shape of the frame, or blowing up a detail.

They found lines, shapes, and planes within the picture that suggested ways to position and align the text. The goal was to integrate the text with the image without letting the text disappear. Typography I. Ellen Lupton, faculty.

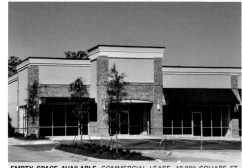

EMPTY SPACE AVAILABLE. COMMERCIAL LEASE, 10,000 SQUARE FT.

### Framing Image and Text

An image seen alone, without any words, is open to interpretation. Adding text to a picture changes its meaning. Written language becomes a frame for the image, shaping the viewer's understanding of it both through the content of the words and the style and placement of the typography. Likewise, pictures can change the meaning of a text.

Text and image combine in endless ways. Text can be subordinate or dominant to a picture; it can be large or small, inside or outside, opaque or transparent, legible or obscure. Text can respect or ignore the borders of an image.

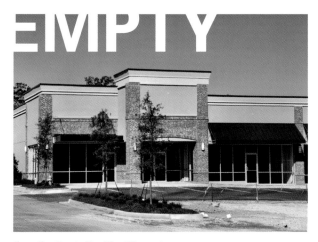

**From Caption to Headline** When a large-scale word replaces an ordinary caption, the message changes. What is empty? The sky, the store, or the larger social reality suggested by the landscape?

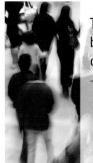
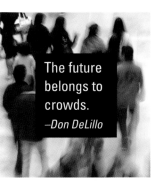
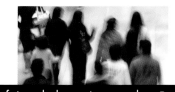
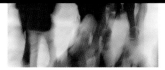

**Text Over Image** Putting type on top of a high-contrast image poses legibility conflicts. Boxes, bars, and transparent color fields are some of the ways designers deal with the problem of separating text from image.

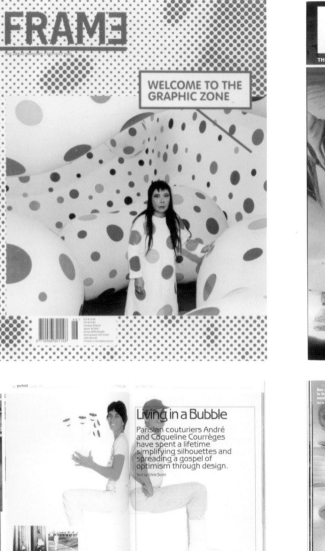

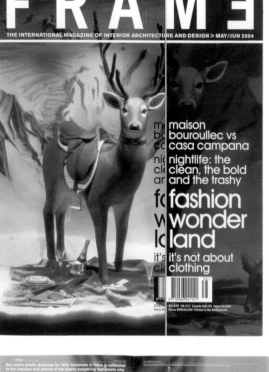

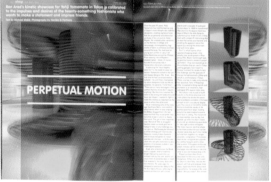

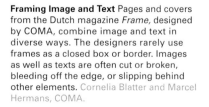

**Framing Image and Text** Pages and covers from the Dutch magazine *Frame,* designed by COMA, combine image and text in diverse ways. The designers rarely use frames as a closed box or border. Images as well as texts are often cut or broken, bleeding off the edge, or slipping behind other elements. Cornelia Blatter and Marcel Hermans, COMA.

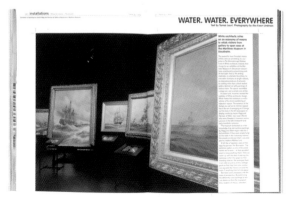

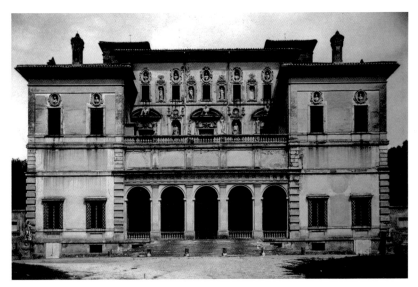

**Villa Borghese**, Rome, 1615. The ornament on this Renaissance palazzo frames the windows, doors, and niches as well as delineates the building's principal volumes and divisions. Architect: Giovanni Vasanzio. Vintage photograph.

**Marking Space** A frame can mark off a space with just a few points. Territory can be defined from the outside in (as in crop marks for trimming a print), or from the inside out (an x drawn from the center of a space to its four corners).

## Borders

A border is the frontier between inside and outside, marking the edge of a territory. A border naturally appears where an image ends and its background begins.

While many images hold their own edges (a dark picture on a white background), a graphic border can help define an image that lacks an obvious edge (a white background on a white page). A graphic border can emphasize an outer boundary, or it can frame off a section inside an image. Some borders are simple lines; others are detailed and complex. Around the world and across history, people have created elaborate frames, rules, cartouches, and moldings to frame pictures and architectural elements.

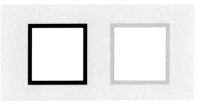

Whether simple or decorative, a border creates a transition between image and background. Against the pale wall of a room, for example, a black picture frame sharply separates a work of art from its surroundings. Alternatively, a frame whose color is close to that of the wall blends the work of art with the room around it. Graphic designers make similar decisions when framing visual elements, sometimes seeking to meld them with their context, and sometimes seeking to set them sharply apart. A frame can serve to either emphasize or downplay its contents.

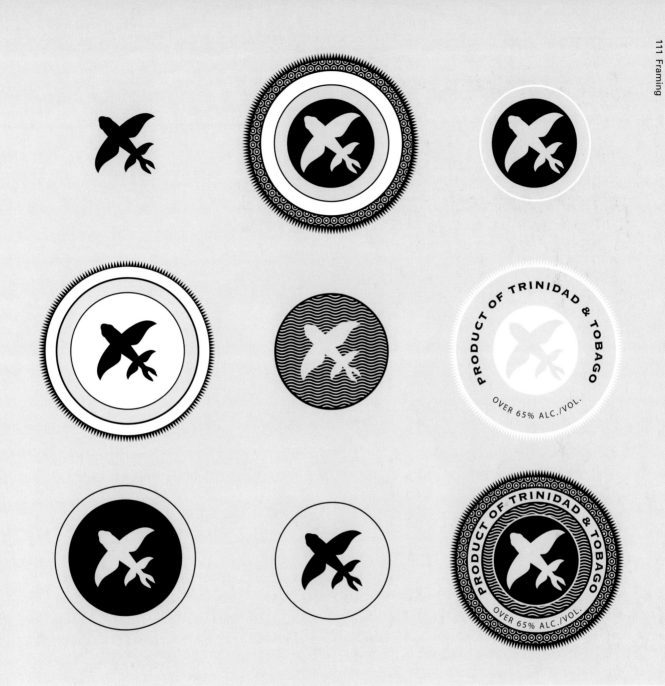

**Border Patrol** Frames interact with content
in different ways. In the examples shown here,
the border sometimes calls attention to the
icon, lending it stature; in other instances, the
border itself takes over, becoming the dominant
form. Robert Lewis, MFA Studio.

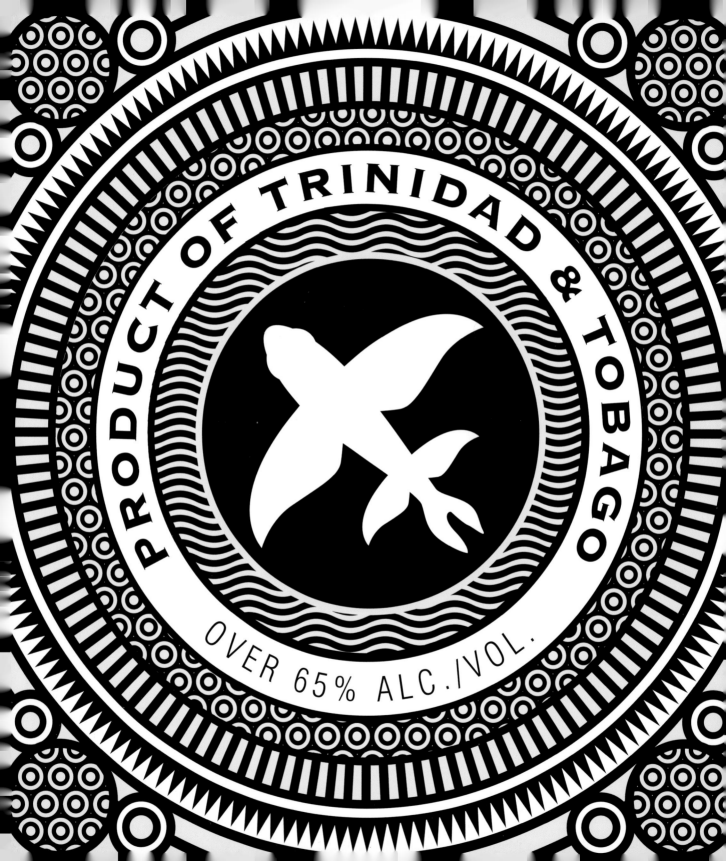

PRODUCT OF TRINIDAD & TOBAGO

OVER 65% ALC./VOL.

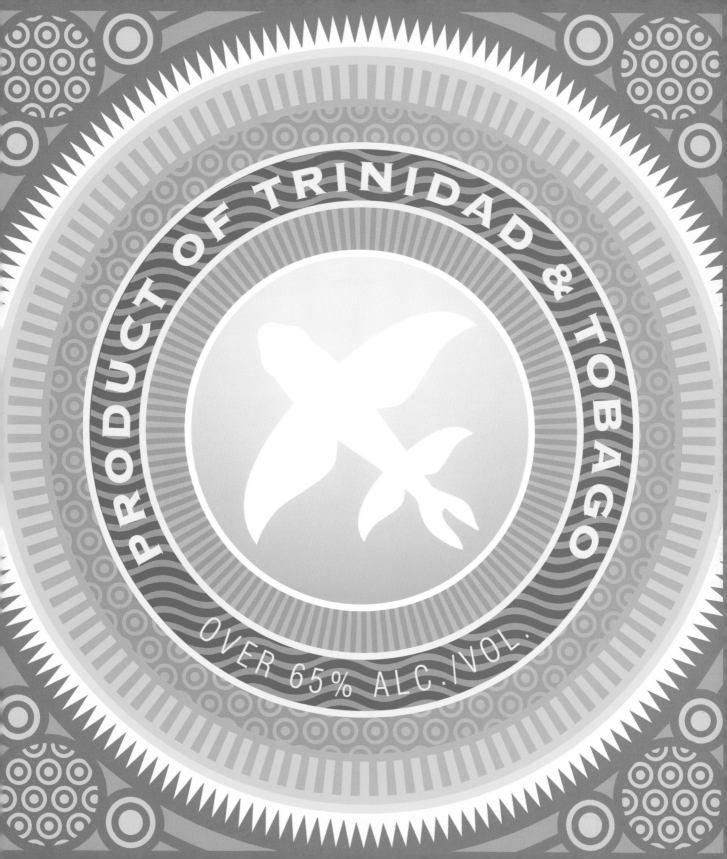

PRODUCT OF TRINIDAD & TOBAGO

OVER 65% ALC./VOL.

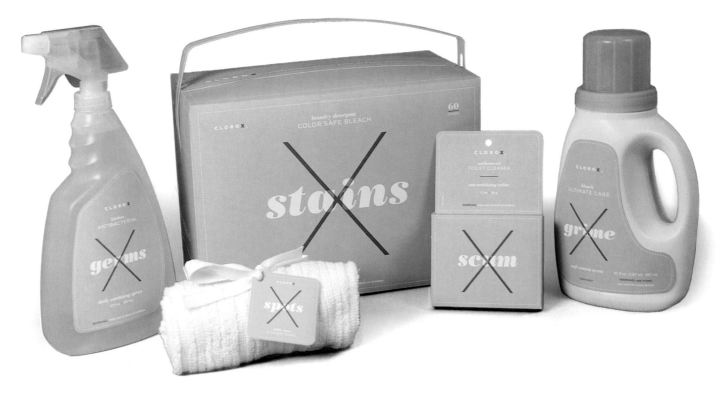

# Hierarchy

Design is the conscious effort to impose a **meaningful order**.
Victor Papanek

Hierarchy is the order of importance within a social group (such as the regiments of an army) or in a body of text (such as the sections and subsections of a book). Hierarchical order exists in nearly everything we know, including the family unit, the workplace, politics, and religion. Indeed, the ranking of order defines who we are as a culture.

Hierarchy is expressed through naming systems: general, colonel, corporal, private, and so on. Hierarchy is also conveyed visually, through variations in scale, value, color, spacing, placement, and other signals. Expressing order is a central task of the graphic designer. Visual hierarchy controls the delivery and impact of a message. Without hierarchy, graphic communication is dull and difficult to navigate.

Like fashion, graphic design cycles through periods of structure and chaos, ornament and austerity. A designer's approach to visual hierarchy reflects his or her personal style, methodology, and training as well as the zeitgeist of the period. Hierarchy can be simple or complex, rigorous or loose, flat or highly articulated. Regardless of approach, hierarchy employs clear marks of separation to signal a change from one level to another. As in music, the ability to articulate variation in tone, pitch, and melody in design requires careful delineation.

In interaction design, menus, texts, and images can be given visual order through placement and consistent styling, but the user often controls the order in which information is accessed. Unlike a linear book, interactive spaces feature multiple links and navigation options that parcel the content according to the user's actions. Cascading Style Sheets (CSS) articulate the structure of a document separately from its presentation so that information can be automatically reconfigured for different output devices, from desktop computer screens to mobile phones, PDAs, kiosks, and more. A different visual hierarchy might be used in each instance.

The average computer desktop supports a complex hierarchy of icons, applications, folders, menus, images, and palettes—empowering users, as never before, to arrange, access, edit, and order vast amounts of information—all managed through a flexible hierarchy controlled and customized by the user.

As technology allows ever greater access to information, the ability of the designer to distill and make sense of the data glut gains increasing value.

**Inverted Hierarchy** This package design project asks students to redirect a product line to an unexpected audience. This design for cleaning products reorders the hierarchy and voice to spark the interest of young, progressive consumers who may be new to housekeeping. The brand name is subtle and sits back, while the offending soil takes center stage. Oliver Munday, Advancd Design. Jennifer Cole Phillips, faculty.

**Basic Typographic Hierarchy**
The table of contents of a printed book—especially one with many parts—provides a structural picture of the text to follow. When books are marketed online, the table of contents is often reproduced to allow potential buyers to preview the book. A well-designed table of contents is thus not only functional but also visually exciting and memorable.

The basic function of a table of contents is to help readers locate relevant information and provide an image of how the book is organized. Does the text fall into a few main parts with various subdivisions, or does it consist of numerous small, parallel entries? The designer uses alignment, leading, indents, and type sizes and styles to construct a clear and descriptive hierarchy.

A poorly designed table of contents often employs conflicting and contradictory alignments, redundant numbering systems, and a clutter of graphic elements. Analyzing tables of contents—as well as restaurant menus and commercial catalogs—is a valuable exercise.

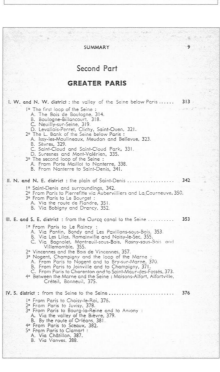

CONTENTS

**What's Wrong with this Picture?**
The function of a table of contents is to list the elements of a book and help readers locate them. In the table of contents shown here, the page numbers are stretched across the page from the chapter titles, and the word "Chapter" has been repeated twenty-four times. *Manners for the Millions*, 1932.

SUMMARY 9

Second Part
**GREATER PARIS**

**Lost in Paris** In this table of contents for a travel guide, the designer has used a muddled mix of centered, justified, and flush-left alignments. The desire to create an overall justified setting dominates the logic of the page—hence the long first lines and rows of dots at the top level of information. The three titling lines at the head of the page are centered (a traditional solution), but the result is awkward in relation to the irregular mass of subheads, which weight the page to the left. The whole affair is further confused by the elaborate system of indents, numerals, and letters used to outline the book's subsections. *Blue Guide to Paris*, 1957.

# CONTENTS

**Book as Billboard** This table of contents serves as a billboard for the book as well as a functional guide to its elements. The designer has approached the spread as a whole, with content stretching across it horizontally. The page numbers are aligned in columns next to the article titles, making it easy for readers to connect content with location. (No old-fashioned leader lines needed!) Chapter numbers aren't necessary because the sequential page numbers are sufficient to indicate the order of the pieces. The book has many contributors, a point made clear through the type styling. Nicholas Blechman, *Empire*, 2004.

Think with the Senses
Feel with the Mind.
Art in the Present Tense
Venice Biennale
52nd International Art Exhibition
10 June – 21 November
National and Regional Pavilions
and Presentations.
Parallel Exhibitions and Projects

No hierarchy

Think with the Senses
Feel with the Mind.
Art in the Present Tense
**Venice Biennale**
52nd International Art Exhibition
10 June – 21 November
National and Regional Pavilions
and Presentations.
Parallel Exhibitions and Projects

Contrasting weight

Think with the Senses
Feel with the Mind.
Art in the Present Tense
Venice Biennale
52nd International Art Exhibition
10 June – 21 November
National and Regional Pavilions
and Presentations.
Parallel Exhibitions and Projects

Contrasting color

Think with the Senses
Feel with the Mind.
Art in the Present Tense
Venice Biennale
52nd International Art Exhibition
10 June – 21 November
National and Regional Pavilions
and Presentations.
Parallel Exhibitions and Projects

Alignment

Think with the Senses
Feel with the Mind.
Art in the Present Tense

Venice Biennale

52nd International Art Exhibition
10 June – 21 November
National and Regional Pavilions
and Presentations.
Parallel Exhibitions and Projects

Spatial intervals

Think with the Senses
Feel with the Mind.
Art in the Present Tense

VENICE BIENNALE

52nd International Art Exhibition
10 June – 21 November

National and Regional Pavilions
and Presentations.
Parallel Exhibitions and Projects

Uppercase and spatial intervals

Think with the Senses
Feel with the Mind.
Art in the Present Tense

Venice Biennale

52nd International Art Exhibition
10 June – 21 November

National and Regional Pavilions
and Presentations.
Parallel Exhibitions and Projects

Weight, color, space, alignment

Think with the Senses
Feel with the Mind.
Art in the Present Tense

Venice Biennale

52nd International Art Exhibition
10 June – 21 November

National and Regional Pavilions
and Presentations.
Parallel Exhibitions and Projects

Scale, space, alignment

*Think with the Senses*
*Feel with the Mind.*
*Art in the Present Tense*

Venice Biennale

52nd International Art Exhibition
10 June – 21 November

National and Regional Pavilions
and Presentations.
Parallel Exhibitions and Projects

Italic, scale, color, alignment

**Hierarchy 101** A classic exercise is to work
with a basic chunk of information and explore
numerous simple variations, using just
one type family. The parts of a typographic
hierarchy can be signaled with one or more
cues: line break, type style, type size, rules,
and so on.

```
void setup()
{
        size(200, 200);
        frameRate(12);
        sx = width;
        sy = height;
        world = new int[sx][sy][2];
        stroke(255);

                for (int i = 0; i < sx * sy * density; i++)
                        {
                          world[(int)random(sx)][(int)random(sy)][1] = 1;
                        }
}

void draw()
{
        background(0);

        for (int x = 0; x < sx; x=x+1)
                {
                for (int y = 0; y < sy; y=y+1)
                        {
                        if ((world[x][y][1] == 1) || (world[x][y][1] == 0 &&
world[x][y][0] == 1))
                                {
                                world[x][y][0] = 1;
                                point(x, y);
                                }
                        if (world[x][y][1] == -1)
                                {
                                world[x][y][0] = 0;
                                }
                                world[x][y][1] = 0;
                        }
                }

        for (int x = 0; x < sx; x=x+1)
                {
                for (int y = 0; y < sy; y=y+1)
                        {
                        int count = neighbors(x, y);

                        if (count == 3 && world[x][y][0] == 0)
                                {
                                world[x][y][1] = 1;
                                }
                        if ((count < 2 || count > 3) && world[x][y][0] == 1)
                                {
                                world[x][y][1] = -1;
                                }
                        }
                }
}

int neighbors(int x, int y)
{
        return world[(x + 1) % sx][y][0] +
        world[x][(y + 1) % sy][0] +
        world[(x + sx - 1) % sx][y][0] +
        world[x][(y + sy - 1) % sy][0] +
        world[(x + 1) % sx][(y + 1) % sy][0] +
        world[(x + sx - 1) % sx][(y + 1) % sy][0] +
        world[(x + sx - 1) % sx][(y + sy - 1) % sy][0] +
        world[(x + 1) % sx][(y + sy - 1) % sy][0];
}
```

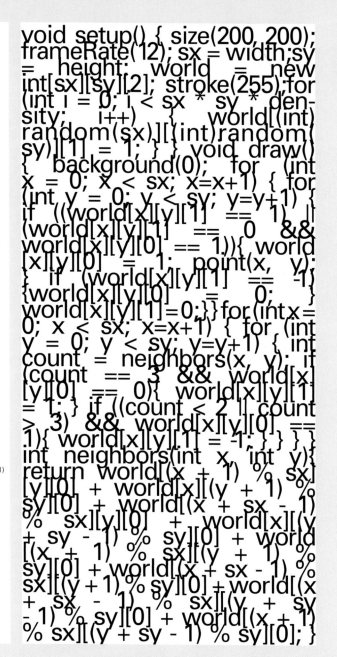

**Code Hierarchy** Computer code is written with a structural hierarchy; functions, routines, and subroutines are nested within each other in a way that determines the performance of the code. Indents and line breaks are used to make this hierarchy clear to the programmer.

**Flat Hierarchy** The visual hierarchy makes no difference, however, to the machine. All that matters from the software's point of view is the linear order of the code. Although the visually flat sequence shown here functions for the computer, it is confusing for the human programmer. Yeohyun Ahn, MFA Studio.

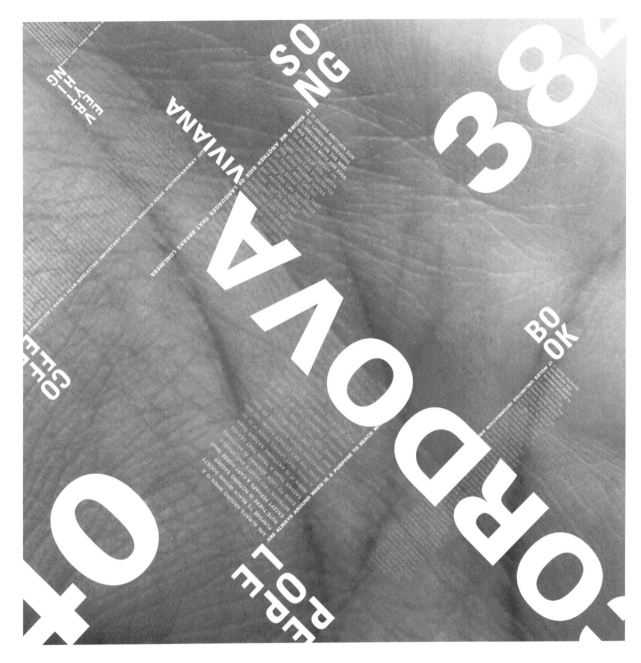

**Hierarchy through Contrast** The Russian constructivists discovered that the dramatic use of scale, photography, and color imbued their political messages with a powerful and provocative voice. These pioneers used contrast in the size, angle, and value of elements to create hierarchical separation.

This project asked designers to build a hierarchy by combining an image of their hand with a list of autobiographical facts. Elements were restricted to 30 or 45 degree angles; scale, position, color, and transparency were employed to control the transmission of information. Viviana Cordova, MFA Studio.

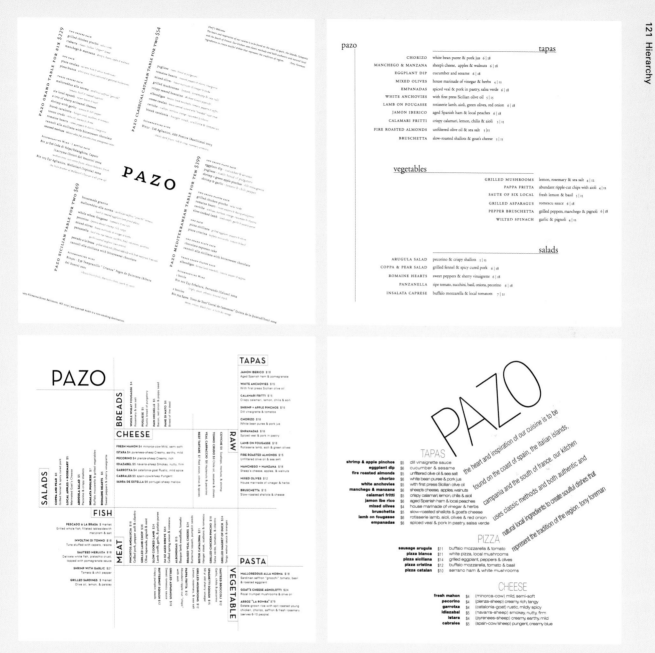

HyunSoo Lim
Katie MacLachlan

Claire Smalley
Anna Eshelman

**Menu of Options** Designers use scale, placement, alignment, type style, and other cues to bring visual order to a body of content. Expressing hierarchy is an active, inquisitive process that can yield dynamic visual results. Typography I. Jennifer Cole Phillips, faculty.

Robert Ferrell

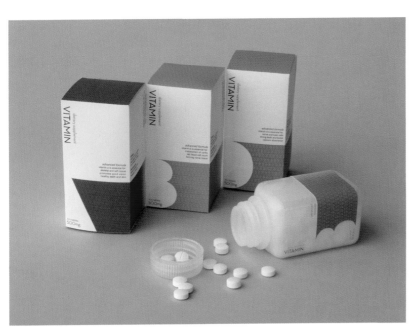

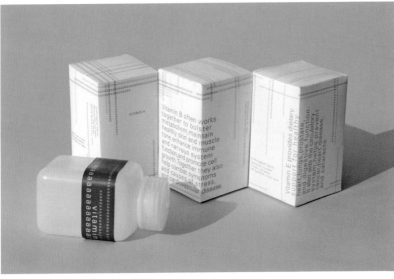

Emily Addis

## Dimensional Hierarchy

Messages applied to three-dimensional form have the added challenge of legibility across and around planes. Objects sitting in an environment are bathed in shadow and light. Unlike books that can conceal elaborate worlds inside their covers—automatically separated from exterior contexts—environmental messages must interact beyond their boundaries and become either a harmonious counterpart or poignant counterpoint to their neighbors.

Notice in these examples how type, color fields, and graphic elements carry the viewer's eye around the dimensional form, often making a visual if not verbal connection with neighboring packages when stacked side by side or vertically.

**Typography Across Three Dimensions**
A visual hierarchy is often necessary for objects in a series. In these designs for vitamin packaging, students have expressed the identity of the individual product as well as the overall brand. Typography II. Jennifer Cole Phillips, faculty.

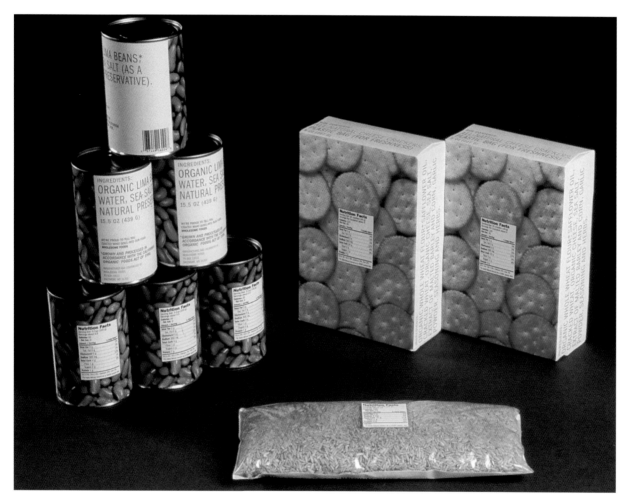

Bruce Willen

**Unexpected Hierarchy** This project takes existing brands and redirects them to unexpected audiences. Here, the designer focuses on a generic food line and reverses the usual order of emphasis by placing the nutrition facts front and center; instead of words, images of the actual product are used to promote what's inside. Advanced Graphic Design. Jennifer Cole Phillips, faculty.

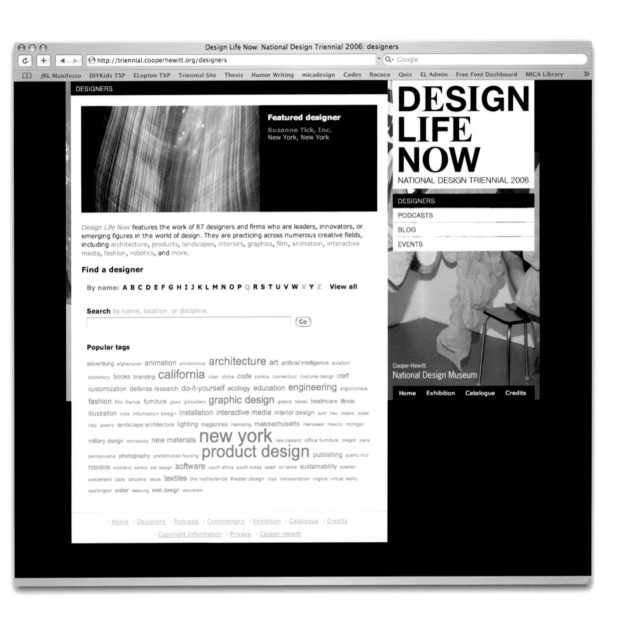

**Web Hierarchy** In a complex website, numerous systems of hierarchy are at work simultaneously. Here, the navigation consists of a global menu along the right edge as well as a more finely grained index positioned in the main content window.

A "data cloud" uses different sizes of type to automatically represent the frequency with which these tags occur. In many sites, such data clouds change in response to user-added content. The search feature allows users to cut through the hierarchy altogether. William Berry, Cooper-Hewitt, National Design Museum.

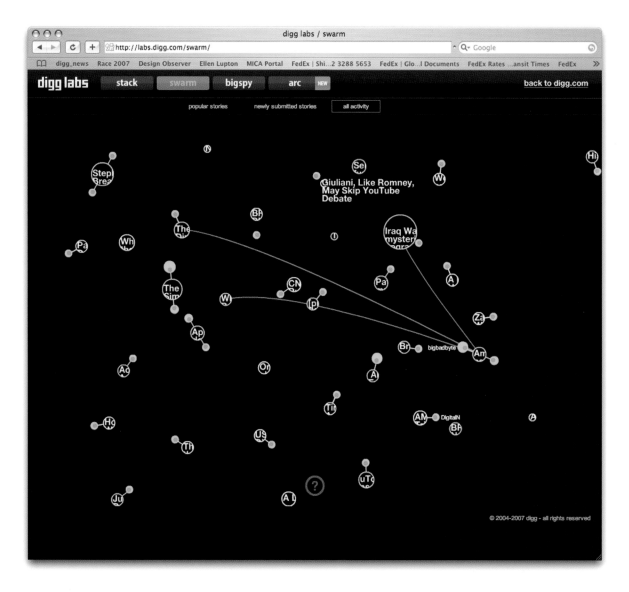

**Dynamic Hierarchy** This popular web portal
displays stories in swarms as authors submit
them in real time. The interface feels like a
computer game, where trigger-fast selections
are needed to engage the content. Elements
in the field grow and gain color according to
the number of "diggs," reflecting a changing
hierarchy. Stamen Design.

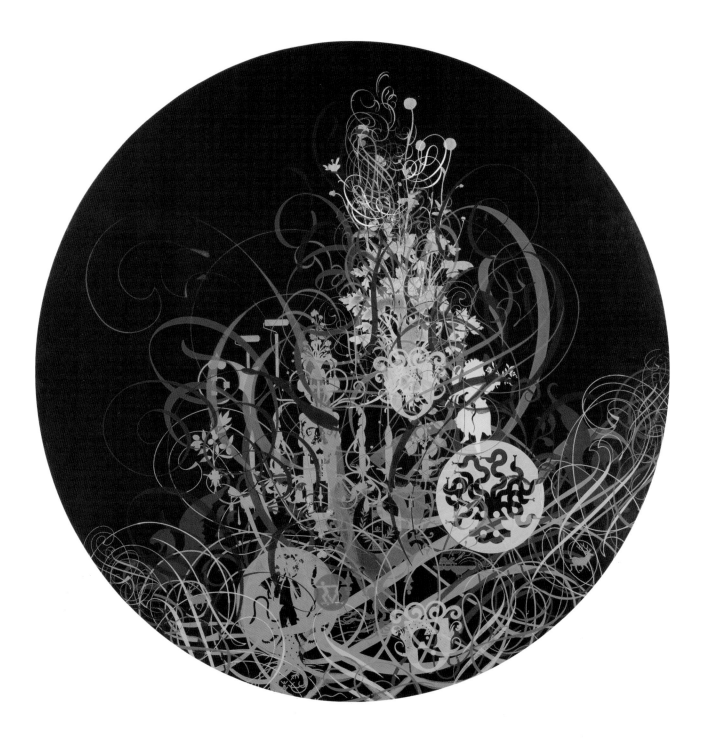

# Layers

Under cities you always find **other cities**; under churches other churches; and under houses other houses. Pablo Picasso

Layers are simultaneous, overlapping components of an image or sequence. They are at work in countless media software programs, from Photoshop and Illustrator to audio, video, and animation tools, where multiple layers of image and sound (tracks) unfold in time.

The concept of layers comes from the physical world, and it has a long history in the traditions of mapping and musical notation. Maps and time lines use overlapping layers to associate different levels of data, allowing them to contribute to the whole while maintaining their own identities.

Most printing techniques require that an image be split into layers before it can be reproduced. From ink-jet printing to silkscreen and commercial lithography, each color requires its own plate, film, screen, ink cartridge, or toner drum, depending on the process. Digital technologies automate this process, making it more or less invisible to the designer.

Before the early 1990s, designers created "mechanicals" consisting of precisely aligned layers of paper and acetate. The designer or paste-up artist adhered each element of the page—type, images, blocks of color—to a separate layer, placing any element that touches any other element on its own surface.

This same principle is at work in the digital layers we use today, mobilized in new and powerful ways. The layers feature in Photoshop creates a new layer whenever the user adds text or pastes an image. Each layer can be independently filtered, transformed, masked, or multiplied. Adjustment layers allow global changes such as levels and curves to be revised or discarded at any time. The image file becomes an archaeology of its own making, a stack of elements seen simultaneously in the main window, but represented as a vertical list in the layers palette.

Layers allow the designer to treat the image as a collection of assets, a database of possibilities. Working with a layered file, the designer quickly creates variations of a single design by turning layers on and off. Designers use layered files to generate storyboards for animations and interface elements such as buttons and rollovers.

Although the layered archeology of the printed page or digital file tends to disappear in the final piece, experimental work often uncovers visual possibilities by exposing layers. The Dutch designer Jan van Toorn has used cut-and-paste techniques to create images whose complex surfaces suggest political action and unrest.

Many designers have explored an off-register or misprinted look, seeking rawness and accidental effects by exposing the layers of the printing and production processes. Contemporary graphic artists Ryan McGinness and Joshua Davis create graphic images composed of enormous numbers of layers that overlap in arbitrary, seemingly uncoordinated ways.

Layers, always embedded in the process of mechanical reproduction, have become intuitive and universal. They are crucial to how we both read and produce graphic images today.

**Printed Layers** Artist and designer Ryan McGinness piles numerous layers on top of each other to yield composite images that celebrate both flatness and depth. Ryan McGinness, *Arab Cadillac Generator*, 2006. Acrylic on wood panel, 48 inches diameter. Collection of Charles Saatchi. Courtesy Deitch Projects, New York. Photo: Tom Powel Imaging, Inc.

## Cut and Paste

The cubist painters popularized collage in the early twentieth century. By combining bits of printed paper with their own drawn and painted surfaces, they created an artistic technique that profoundly influenced both design and the fine arts. Like the cubists, modern graphic designers use collage to juxtapose layers of content, yielding surfaces that oscillate between flatness and depth, positive and negative.

The cut-and-paste function used in nearly every software application today refers to the physical process of collage. Each time you copy or delete a picture or phrase and insert it into a new position, you reference the material act of cutting and pasting. The collaged history of an image or a document largely disappears in the final work, and designers often strive to create seamless, invisible transitions between elements. Foregrounding the cut-and-paste process can yield powerful results that indicate the designer's role in shaping meaning.

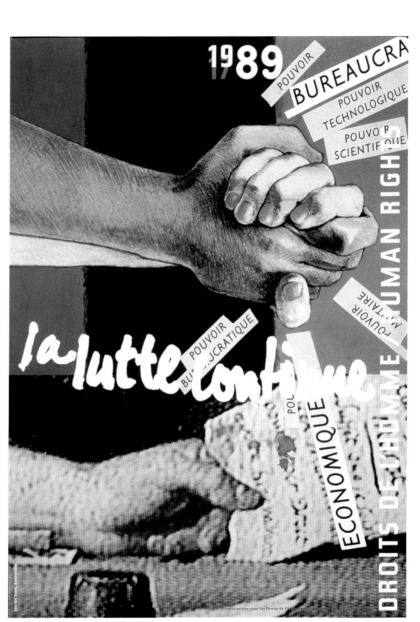

**Mixing Media** Published in 1989 to commemorate the Declaration of Human Rights a century earlier, this poster by Jan van Toorn used photomechanical processes to mix handmade and mass-media imagery. Scraps of paper radiate like energy from the central handshake. Jan van Toorn, *La Lutte Continue* (The Fight Continues), 1989.

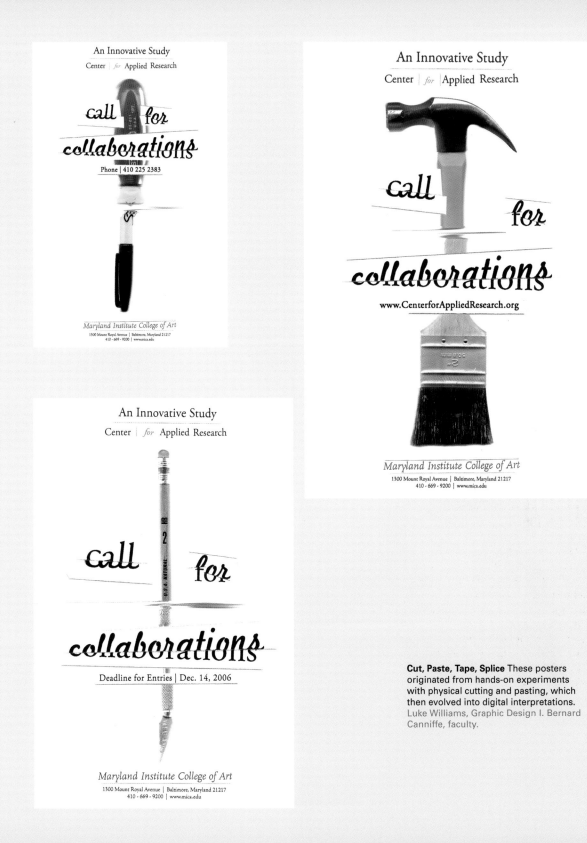

**Cut, Paste, Tape, Splice** These posters originated from hands-on experiments with physical cutting and pasting, which then evolved into digital interpretations. Luke Williams, Graphic Design I. Bernard Canniffe, faculty.

The many-sidedness of human experience is seriously threatened by the common denominator of mass communication. That is why designers who are concerned by the corporate take-over of expression must first allow themselves sufficient room to maneuver for a **dissident attitude** vis-a-vis the normative determination of the media culture. Jan van Toorn

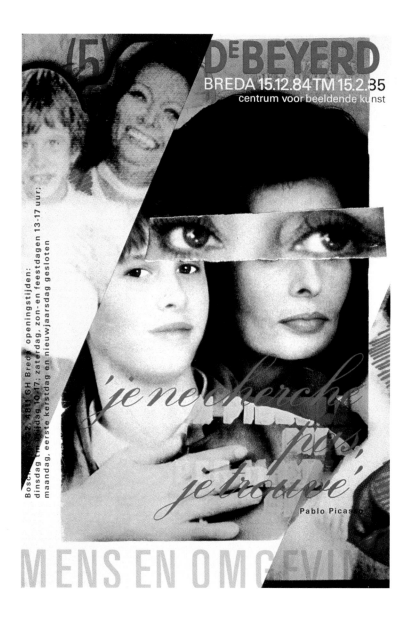

**Combine and Contrast**
In the project shown here, students were given two digital photographs and the quotation above by the legendary Dutch designer Jan van Toorn. The photographs depict two idealized visions of femininity: an industrially produced garden statue of the Madonna and a department-store mannequin. The quote by van Toorn calls on designers to manipulate creatively the global language of standardized images.

As part of the design process, students were asked to study van Toorn's work and consider the ways he splices and overlaps words and images. Seeking to express his own "dissident attitude" toward mass media, van Toorn generates surprise and tension by presenting fragments of words and images, working primarily with hands-on cut-and-paste techniques and photomechanical processes. He often cuts or places images at an angle to indicate informality and change. Graphic Design II. Jan van Toorn, visiting faculty.

**Cut, Crop, Paste** To create this museum poster, the Dutch designer Jan van Toorn cut and pasted elements, assembling them for photomechanical reproduction. Jan van Toorn. Je ne cherche pas, je trouve (I do not search, I find). Cultural centre De Beyerd, Breda, Netherlands, 1985.

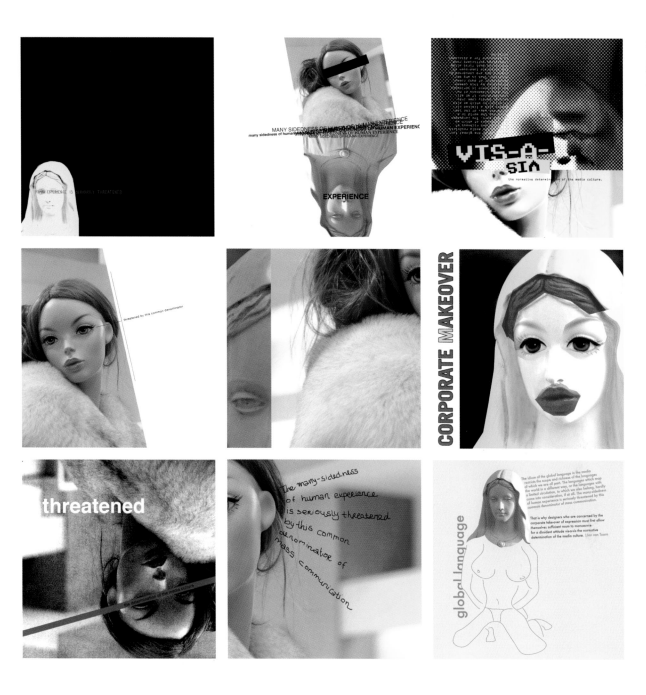

Claire Smalley
Grey Haas
Sisi Recht

Lindsey Sherman
Katie Evans
Marleen Kuijf

Giulia Marconi
Jonnie Hallman
Dani Bradford

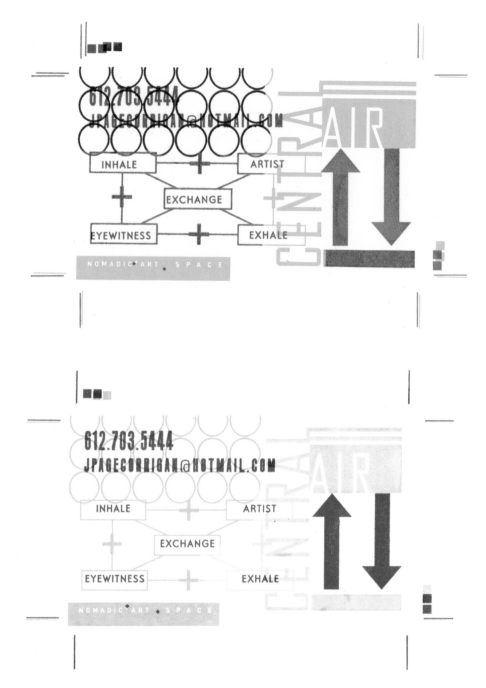

**Printed Layers** Nearly every color printing process uses layers of ink, but the layers are usually compiled to create the appearance of a seamless, singular surface. The screen prints above use overlapping and misaligned layers of ink to call attention to the structure of the surface. John P. Corrigan, MFA Studio.

**Makeready** To conserve materials, printers reuse old press sheets while getting their presses up to speed, testing ink flow and position before pulling their final prints. Called "makereadies," these layered surfaces are full of beautiful accidental effects, as seen in this screen-printed makeready. Paul Sahre and David Plunkert.

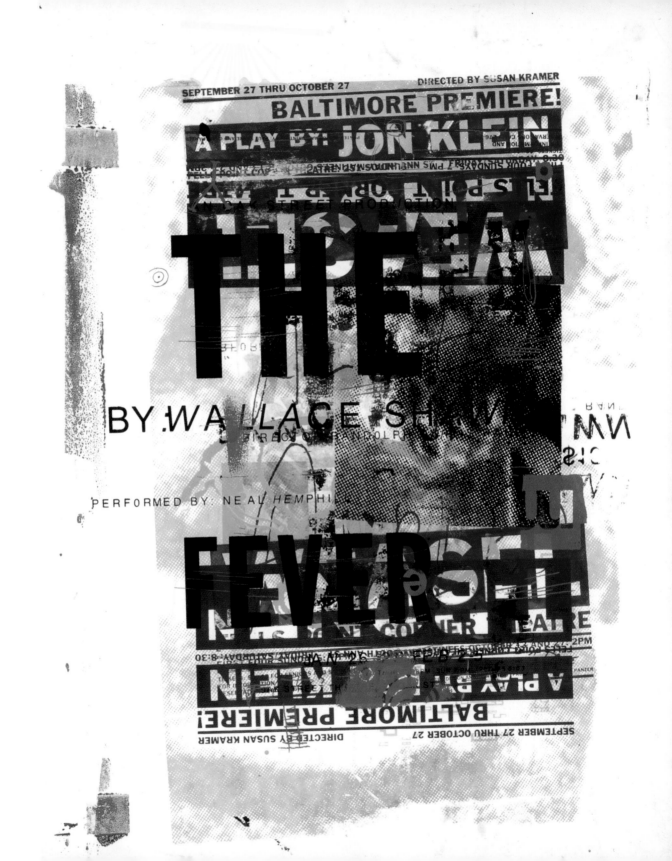

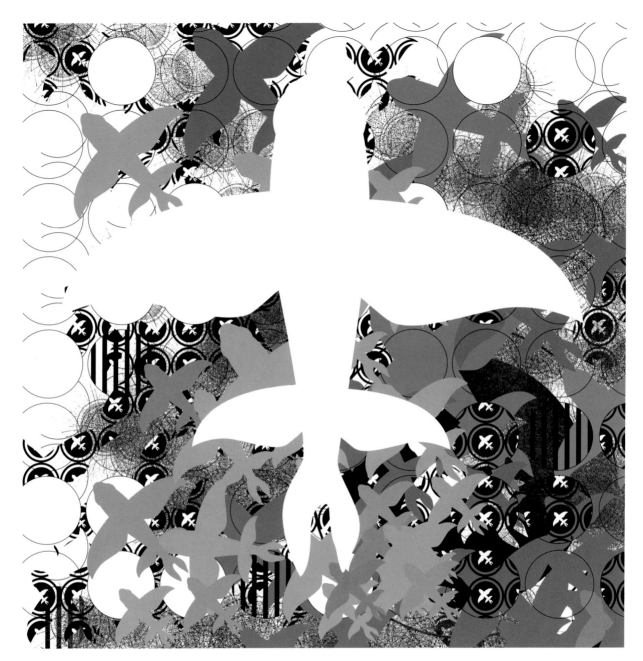

**Mixing Layers** The two compositions shown here were each made from the same set of digital images, layered together to create different designs. Various relationships are built by changing the scale, position, color, or transparency of elements. MFA Studio. Source images: Jason Okutake, photography; Robert Lewis, flying fish.

April Osmanof

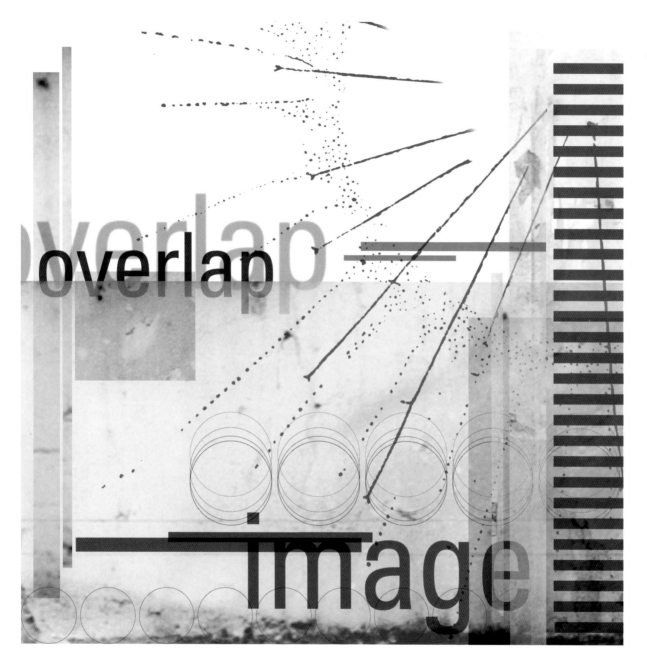

HyunSoo Lim

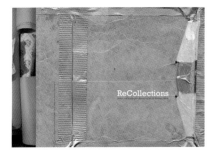

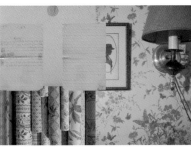

## Spatial Layers

Layered objects and surfaces exist throughout the visual environment. On the walls of an old farmhouse, layers—from wallpaper and works of art to ordinary electrical outlets—accumulate over time.

By layering scans of flat surfaces with photographs of three-dimensional space, the designer of the book shown here has created an interplay between surface and depth. Overlapping forms and optical alignments produce surprising spatial relationships. Even the shallow space of a scanned surface can reveal an element of depth through its texture, folds, transparency, and imperfections. The surface thus conveys a sense of time and history.

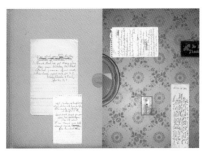

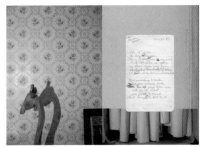

**Collage with Depth** The designer has combined a stack of poems written by his grandfather with photographs of the wallpaper in his farmhouse. The pages invite the viewer to read the texts against a complex spatial surface. Jeremy Botts, MFA Studio. Charles Bonner, handwritten poems.

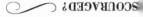

—Brother Robert

Remember the day you were
~~started~~ to drive? Nov 1977

The car on the front
made me think of the time
you were learning to drive
and it got out of line
you drove in the shed to
to learn how to do it
Were it not for the crates
you would have gone through it,

a crash, and a bang!
The splinters all flew.
William ran up & said
What in earth did you do?

"I smashed up the chicken crates,"
I think you replied,
your face was all red
and nervous smile

What pop gonna say?
Was all our concern.
But it all worked out
for the good, we did learn,

Now a few years past
since you first learned to drive
Your driving's much
better at ~~65~~ 60 and 5

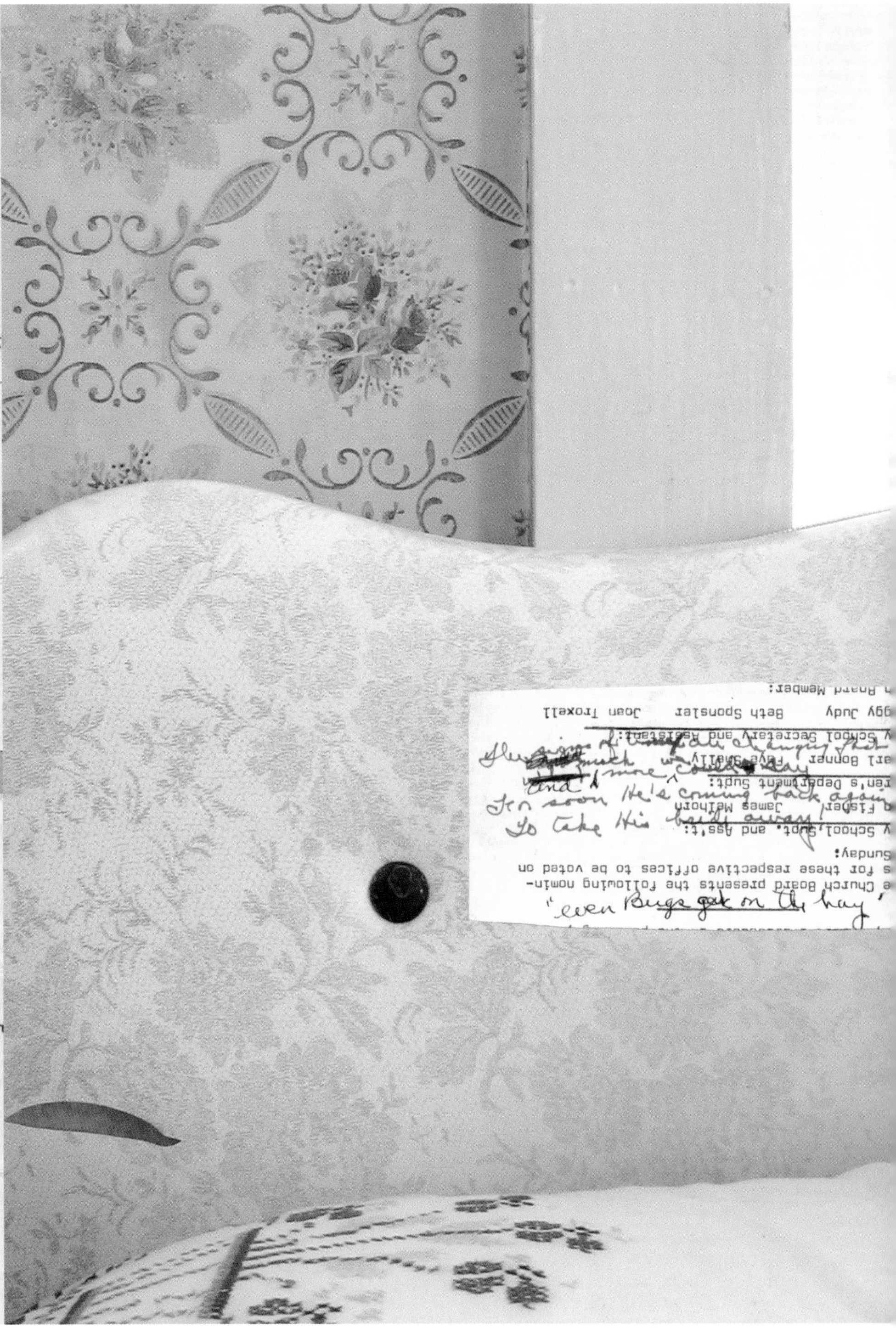

She ... much ... a laugh
and ... more ... day
It soon He's coming back again
To take His ...

"even Bugs get on the hay,"

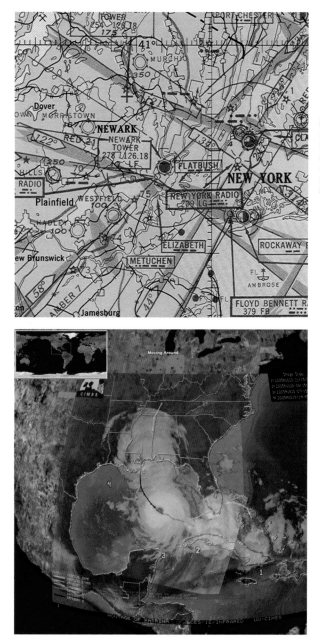

**Data Layers: Static** This map uses point, line, plane, and color to indicate geographic borders, topographical features, towns and cities, and points of interest, as well as radio systems used by pilots in the air. The purple lines indicating radio signals read as a separate layer. Aeronautical map, 1946.

## Data Layers

Maps compress various types of information—topography, water systems, roadways, cities, geographic borders, and so on—onto a single surface. Map designers use color, line, texture, symbols, icons, and typography to create different levels of information, allowing users to read levels independently (for example, learning what roads connect two destinations) as well as perceiving connections between levels (will the journey be mountainous or flat?).

Sophisticated map-making tools are now accessible to designers and general practitioners as well as to professional cartographers. Google Earth enables users to build personalized maps using satellite photography of the Earth's surface. The ability to layer information over a base image is a central feature of this immensely powerful yet widely available tool.

**Data Layers: Dynamic** An image of Hurricane Katrina has been layered over a satellite photograph of Earth. The end user of a Google Earth overlay can manipulate its transparency in order to control the degree of separation between the added layer and the ground image. Storm: University of Wisconsin, Madison Cooperative Institute for Meteorogical Satellite Studies, 2005. Composite: Jack Gondela.

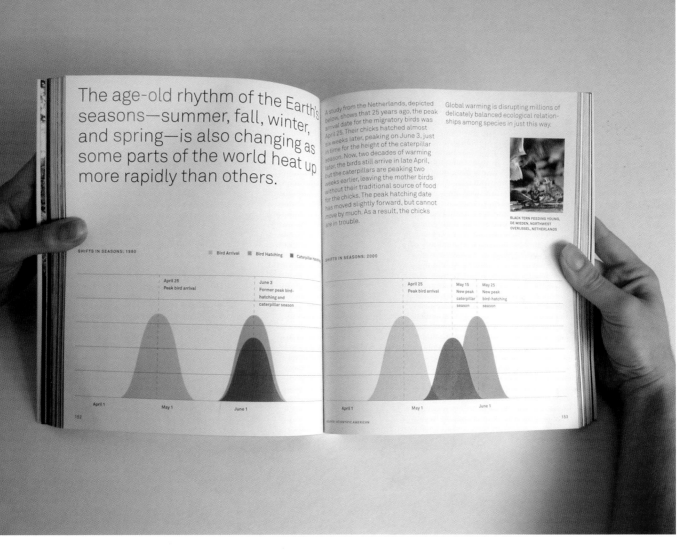

**Comparing Data Layers** In this graph from Al Gore's book *An Inconvenient Truth,* the designers have used color and transparency to make it easy for readers to compare two sets of data. The graphs show how climate change is affecting the life cycle of animals and their food supplies. Alicia Cheng, Stephanie Church, and Lisa Maione, MGMT Design, *An Inconvenient Truth,* 2006.

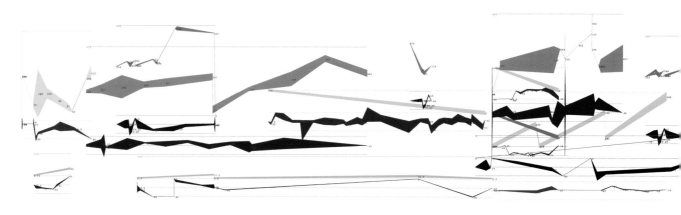

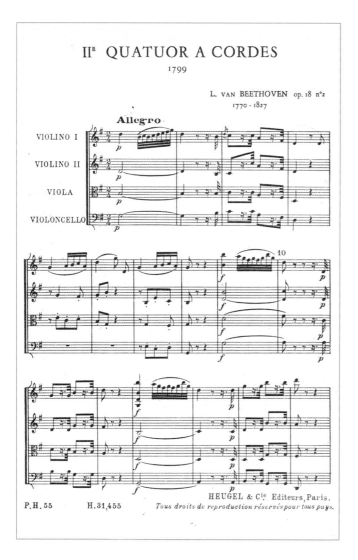

**Temporal Layers**

In musical notation, the notes for each instrument in a symphony or for each voice in a chorus appear on parallel staffs. The graphic timelines used in audio, video, and animation software follow this intuitive convention, using simultaneous tracks to create composite layers of image and sound.

In soap operas and television dramas, parallel threads unfold alongside each other and converge at key moments in the story. The split screens, inset panels, and text feeds commonly seen in news programming allow several visual tracks to play simultaneously.

From musical notation and computer interfaces to narrative plot lines, parallel linear tracks (layers in time) are a crucial means for describing simultaneous events.

**Musical Notation** This score shows the notes played by four different musicians simultaneously (first violin, second violin, viola, and cello). Each staff represents a separate instrument. Ludwig van Beethoven, musical score, *String Quartet No. 2 in G Major*, 1799.

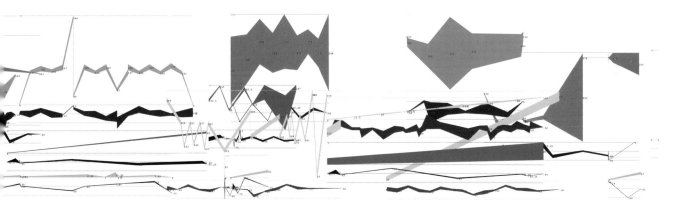

**Interactive Notation** Digital composer Hans-Christoph Steiner has devised his own graphic notation system to show how to manipulate digital samples. Time flows from left to right. Each color represents a sample.

Each sample controller has two arrays: the brighter, bigger one on top controls sample playback, and a smaller, darker one at the bottom controls amp and pan. The lowest point of the sample array is the beginning

of the sample, the highest is the end, and the height of the array is how much and what part of the sample to play, starting at that point in time. Hans-Christoph Steiner, interactive musical score, *Solitude*, 2004.

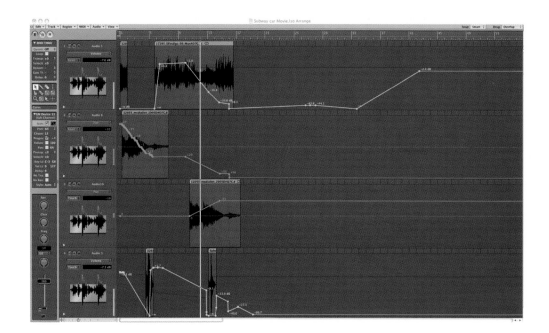

**Audio Software** Applications for editing digital audio tracks employ complex and varied graphics. Here, each track is represented by a separate timeline. The yellow lines indicate volume, and the green lines show panning left to right. Audio composed by Jason Okutake, MFA Studio. Software: Apple Logic Pro Audio.

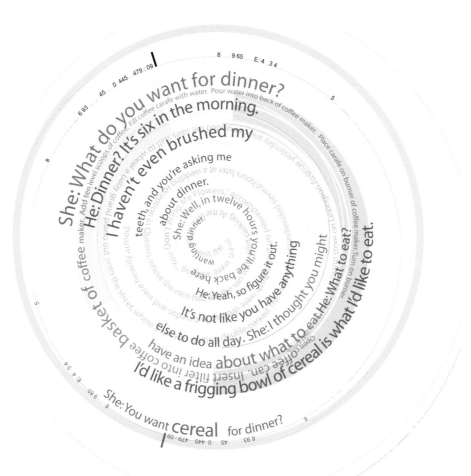

She: What do you want for dinner?
He: Dinner? It's six in the morning.
I haven't even brushed my teeth, and you're asking me about dinner.
She: Well, in twelve hours you'll be back here wanting dinner.
He: Yeah, so figure it out.
It's not like you have anything else to do all day. She: I thought you might have an idea about what to eat. He: What to eat?
I'd like a frigging bowl of cereal is what I'd like to eat.
She: You want cereal for dinner?

Yue Tuo

**Typographic Layers** In everyday life as well as in films and animations, multiple stories can unfold simultaneously. A person can talk on the phone while folding the laundry and hearing a song in the background. In films, characters often carry on a conversation while performing an action.

This typographic exercise presents three narratives taking place during a two-minute period: a news story broadcast on a radio, a conversation between a married couple, and the preparation of a pot of coffee. Typography, icons, lines, and other elements are used to present the three narratives within a shared space. The end result can be obvious or poetic. Whether the final piece is an easy-to-follow transcription or a painterly depiction, it is made up of narrative elements that define distinct layers or visual channels. Graphic Design MFA Studio.

Two men broke into a piano store on Lexington Avenue yesterday and demanded the sales staff to wheel a baby grand piano out onto the street, where a van was waiting double-parked. The man were apprehended several hours later at a wedding reception in Queens, where the men had left the van with valet parking. At the time of the arrest, the men were singing "You Don't Bring Me Flowers.", accompanied on piano. Both were dressed in tuxedos and were heavily armed.

Yong Seuk Lee

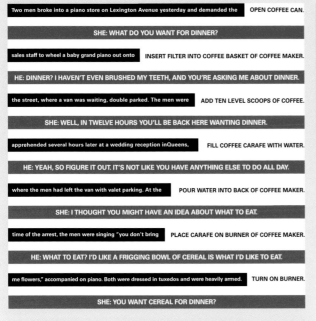

Robert Lewis

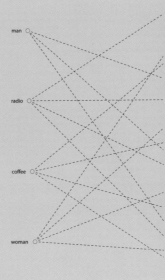

April Osmanof

HyunSoo Lim

Visakh Menon

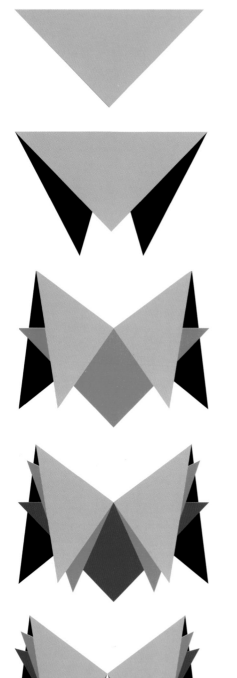

**Physical, Virtual, and Temporal Layers** In this project, designers began by creating a series of six-by-six-inch collages with four square sheets of colored paper. (We used origami paper). Each designer cut a square window into a larger sheet of paper so that they could move the colored sheets around and experiment with different designs.

In the second phase of the project, designers translated one of their physical collages into digital layers. Each physical layer became a separate layer in the digital file. They generated new compositions by digitally changing the color, scale, transparency, orientation, and position of the digital layers.

In the third phase, one digital composition became a style frame (the basis of a sequential animation). Each designer planned a sequence, approximately ten seconds long, that loops: that is, it begins and ends on an identical frame. They created nine-panel storyboards showing the sequence.

In the final phase, designers imported their style frames into a digital animation program (Flash), distributing each layer of the style frame to a layer in the timeline to create strata that change over time. Graphic Design II. Ellen Lupton, faculty.

Lauretta Dolch

**Physical Layers**     **Digital Layers**     **Temporal Layers**

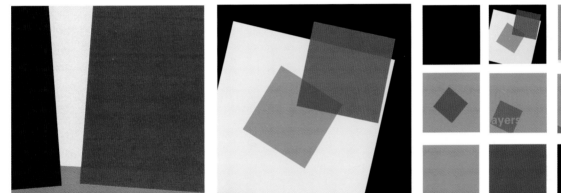

**Windows** Each layer is a window through which other layers are visible. Kelly Horigan.

**Squares** Complete, uncut squares move in and out of the frame. Doug Hucker.

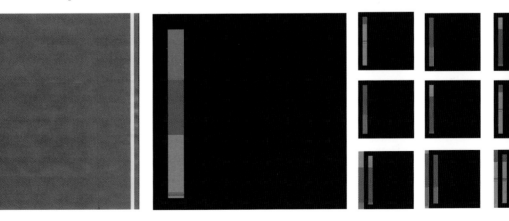

**Slit** Moving layers are glimpsed through a slit in the outer surface. Yuta Sakane.

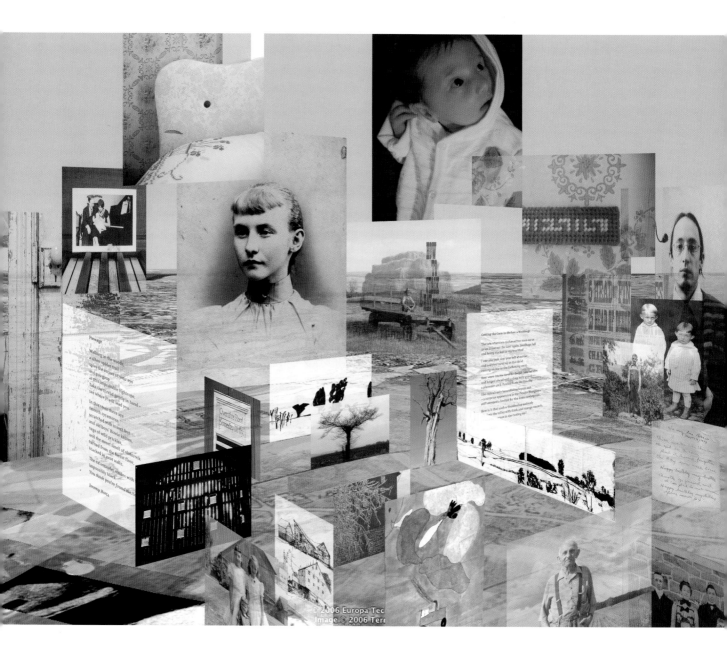

# Transparency

Transparency means a **simultaneous perception of different spatial locations**.... The position of the transparent figures has equivocal meaning as one sees each figure now as the closer, now as the farther one. Gyorgy Kepes

As a social value, transparency suggests clarity and directness. The idea of "transparent government" promotes processes that are open and understandable to the public, not hidden behind closed doors. Yet in design, transparency is often used not for the purposes of clarity, but to create dense, layered imagery built from veils of color and texture.

Any surface in the physical world is more or less transparent or opaque: a piece of wood has 100 percent opacity, while a room full of air has nearly zero. Image-editing software allows designers to adjust the opacity of any still or moving picture. Software lets you see through wood, or make air into a solid wall.

Transparency becomes an active design element when its value is somewhere between zero and 100 percent. In this chapter, we assume that a "transparent" image or surface is, generally, opaque to some degree. Indeed, you will discover that a surface built out of completely opaque elements can function in a transparent way.

Transparency and layers are related phenomena. A transparent square of color appears merely pale or faded until it passes over another shape or surface, allowing a second image to show through itself. A viewer thus perceives the transparency of one plane in relation to a second one. What is in front, and what is behind? What dominates, and what recedes?

Video and animation programs allow transparency to change over time. A fade is created by making a clip gradually become transparent. Dissolves occur when one clip fades out (becoming transparent) while a second clip fades in (becoming opaque).

This chapter begins by observing the properties of physical transparency, and then shows how to build transparent surfaces out of opaque graphic elements. We conclude by looking at the infinite malleability of digital transparency.

Transparency is a fascinating and seductive principle. How can it be used to build meaningful images? Transparency can serve to emphasize values of directness and clarity through adjustments and juxtapositions that maintain the wholeness or legibility of elements. Transparency also can serve to build complexity by allowing layers to mix and merge together. Transparency can be used thematically to combine or contrast ideas, linking levels of content. When used in a conscious and deliberate way, transparency contributes to the meaning and visual intrigue of a work of design.

**Life History** Historical and contemporary photographs and documents are layered over a satellite image from Google Earth of the land these people have inhabited. Transparency is used to separate the elements visually. Jeremy Botts, MFA Studio.

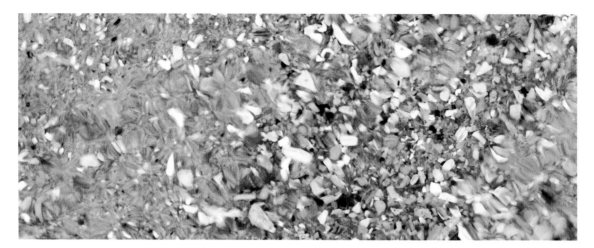

**Water** Jason Okutake

## Physical Transparency

No material is wholly transparent. Ripples disturb the transparency of water, while air becomes thick with smoke or haze. Glass can be tinted, mirrored, cracked, etched, scratched, frosted, or painted to diminish its transparency. The reflective character of glass makes it partially opaque, an attribute that changes depending on light conditions.

A solid material such as wood or metal becomes transparent when its surface is perforated or interrupted. Venetian blinds shift from opaque to transparent as the slats slant open. Adjusting the blinds changes their degree of transparency.

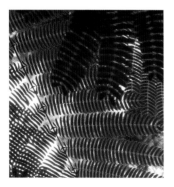

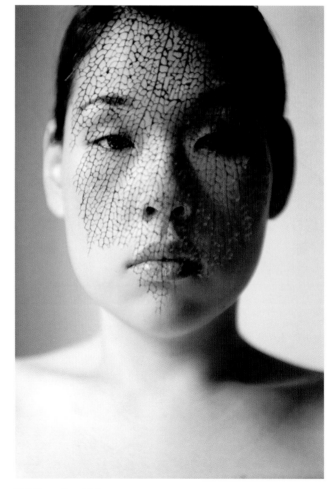

**Tree** Jeremy Botts

**Veil** Nancy Froehlich

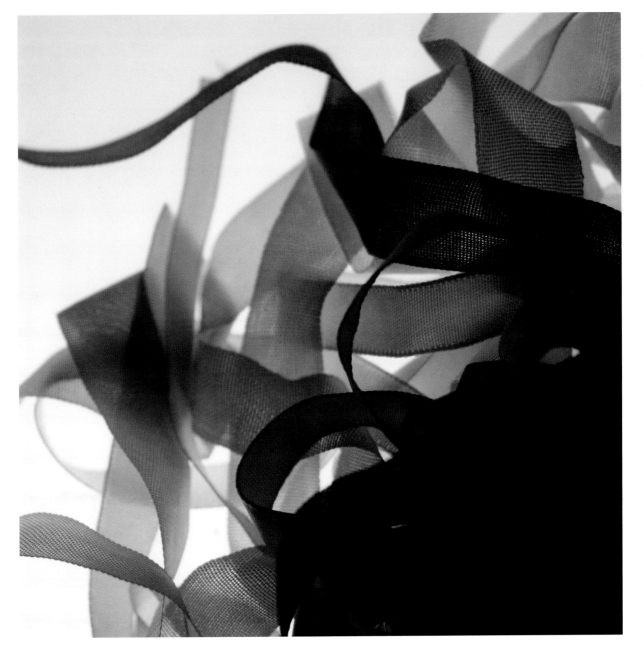

**Ribbon** Yue Tuo

**Materials and Substances** Observing
transparent objects and surfaces throughout
the physical environment yields countless
ideas for combining images and surfaces in
two-dimensional design. MFA Studio.

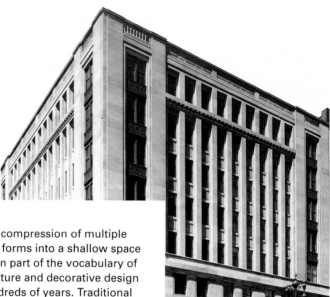

**Graphic Transparency**

Designers can translate the effects of physical transparency into overlapping layers of lines, shapes, textures, or letterforms. We call this phenomenon "graphic transparency." Just as in physical transparency, two or more surfaces are visible simultaneously, collapsed onto a single surface. A field of text placed over an image is transparent, revealing parts of the image through its open spaces.

The compression of multiple graphic forms into a shallow space has been part of the vocabulary of architecture and decorative design for hundreds of years. Traditional patterns such as plaid use colored thread to build up intersecting fields of color. Linear elements in classical and modern architecture, such as columns and moldings, often appear to pass through each other.[1]

**Macmillan Company Building**, New York, 1924. This early skyscraper employs vertical elements that span the upper stories of the building. The horizontal elements sit back behind the vertical surface, establishing a second plane that appears to pass continuously behind the front plane, like the threads in a plaid fabric. Architects: Carrère and Hastings with Shreve and Lamb. Vintage photograph.

1. On transparency in architecture, see Colin Rowe and Robert Slutzky, "Transparency: Literal and Phenomenal (Part 2)," in Joan Ockman, ed., *Architecture Culture, 1943–1968: A Documentary Anthology* (New York: Rizzoli, 1993), 205–25.

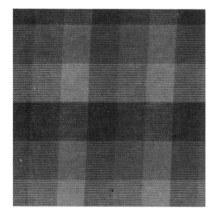

**Plaid Fabric** Traditional plaid fabrics are made by weaving together bands of colored thread over and under each other. Where contrasting colors mix, a new color appears. The horizontal and vertical stripes literally pass through each other on the same plane. Lee Jofa, *Carousel*, plaid fabric, cotton and rayon.

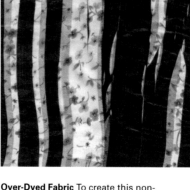

**Over-Dyed Fabric** To create this non-traditional print, fashion designer Han Feng bunched and folded a delicate floral print and then dyed it, creating long irregular stripes that sit on top of the floral pattern. The result is two competing planes of imagery compressed onto a single surface. Han Feng, polyester fabric.

If one sees two or more figures partly overlapping one another, and each of them claims for itself the common overlapped part, then one is confronted with a contradiction of spatial dimensions.

**Typographic Plaid** Layers of lines pass in front of a base text. The lines are like a slatted or perforated surface through which the text remains visible. Alissa Faden, MFA Studio.

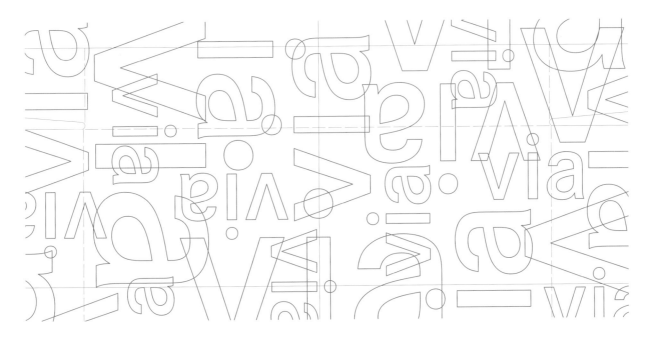

**Linear Transparency** The letterforms in this pattern have been reduced to outlines, rendering them functionally transparent even as they overlap each other. Abbott Miller and Jeremy Hoffman, Pentagram, packaging for Mohawk Paper.

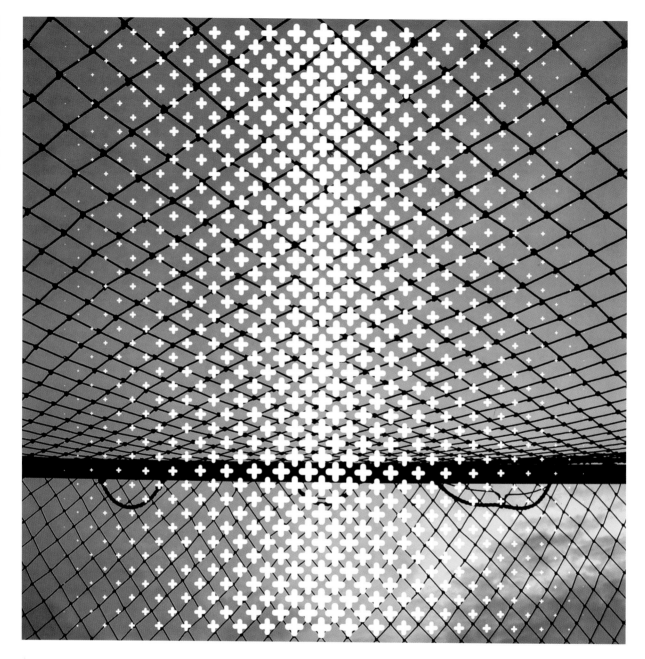

**Graphic Transparency** In each of these compositions, a photograph has been overlaid with a field of graphic elements. The graphic layer becomes an abstracted commentary on the image underneath. MFA Studio.

Jeremy Botts

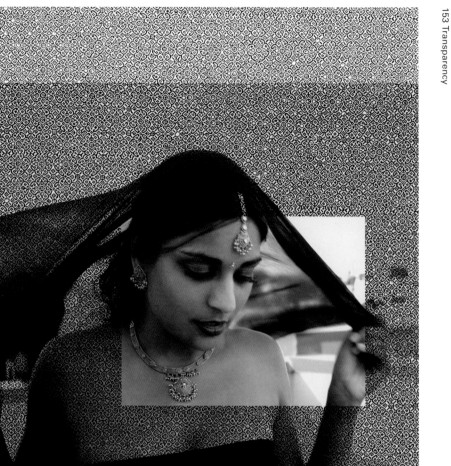

Jason Okutake

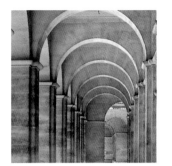

100 percent opacity

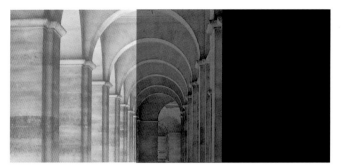

50 percent opacity. Fade-to-black is a standard transition in film and video.

## Digital Transparency

Imaging software allows designers to alter the opacity of nearly any graphic element, including type, photographs, and moving images. To do this, the software employs an algorithm that multiplies the tonal values of one layer against those of another, generating a mix between the two layers. To make any image transparent involves compromising its intensity, lowering its overall contrast.

Transparency is used not only to mix two visual elements, but also to make one image fade out against its background. In video and animation, such fades occur over time. The most common technique is the fade-to-black, which employs the default black background. The resulting clip gradually loses intensity while becoming darker. Video editors create a fade-to-white by placing a white background behind the clip. The same effects are used in print graphics to change the relationship between an image and its background.

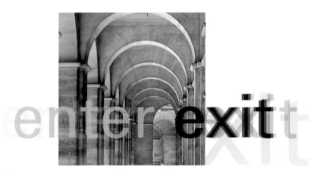

Transparent type, opaque image

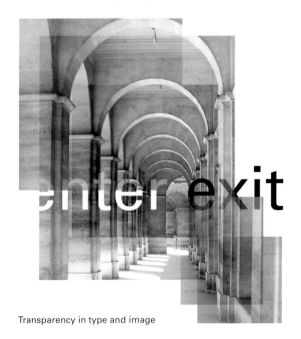

Transparency in type and image

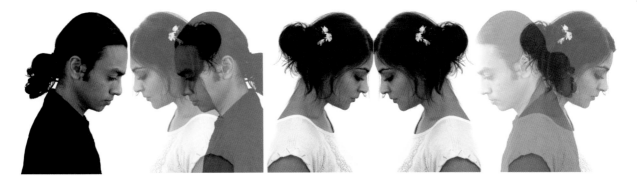

**Opposites Attract** Transparency serves
to build relationships between images.
Here, male and female mix and overlap.
Jason Okutake, MFA Studio.

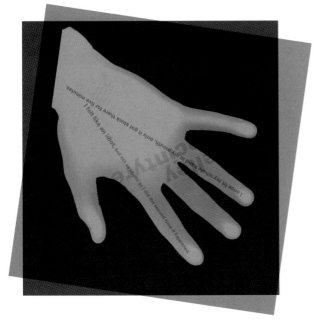

**Life Lines** Transparent layers of text and image
intersect. Kelley McIntyre, MFA Studio.

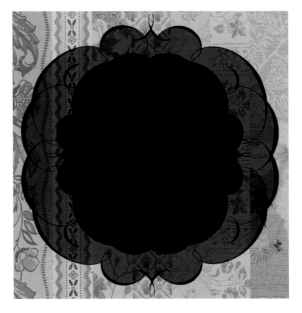

**Wall Flowers** Transparent layers build
up to make a dense frame or cartouche.
Jeremy Botts, MFA Studio.

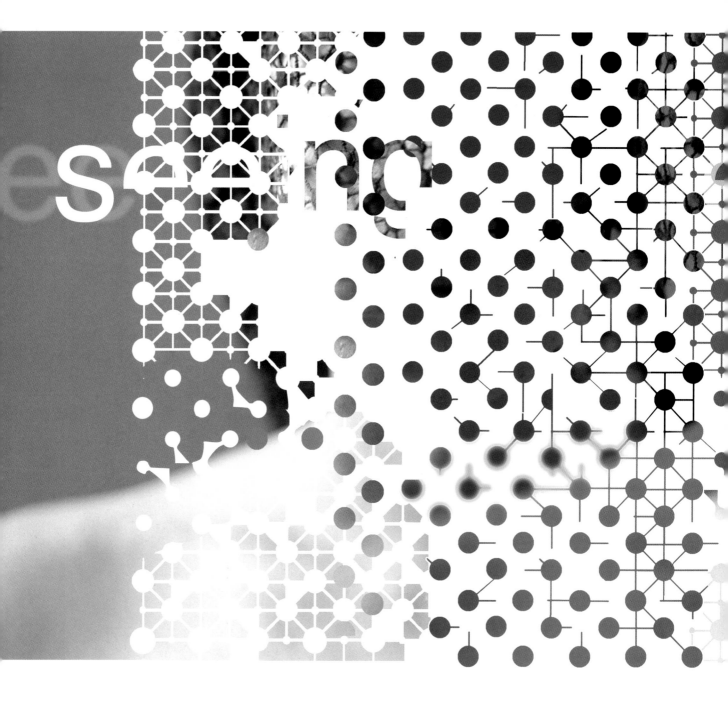

**Seeing Through** This composition builds
relationships between layers of graphic
elements and an underlying photograph.
The designer has manipulated the elements
graphically as well as changing their
digital transparency. Yue Tuo, MFA Studio.
Photography: Nancy Froehlich.

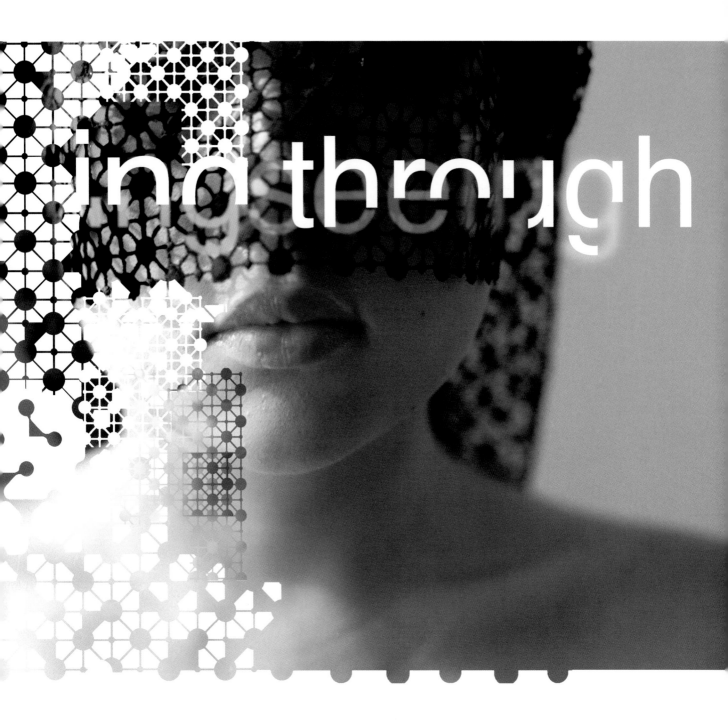

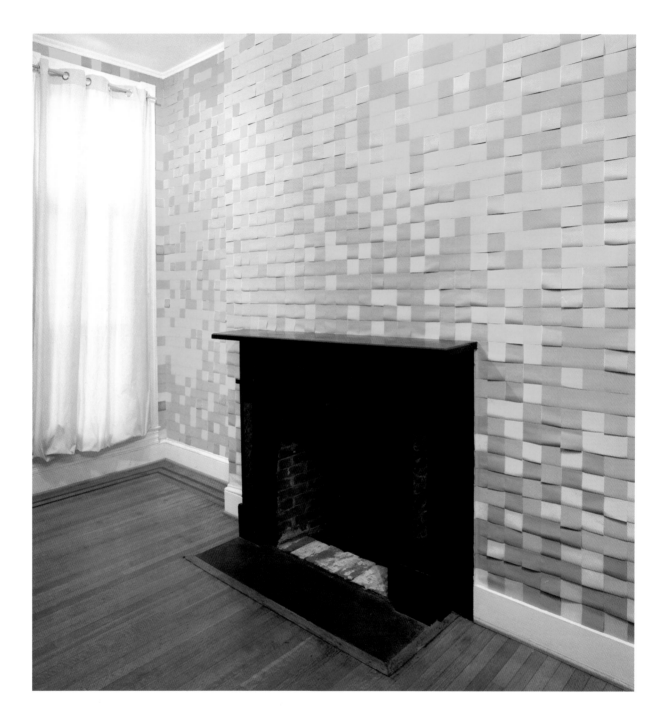

# Modularity

Two eight-stud LEGO bricks can be combined in twenty-four ways.
Three eight-stud LEGO bricks can be combined in 1,060 ways.
**Six eight-stud LEGO bricks can be combined in 102,981,500 ways.**
With eight bricks the possibilities are virtually endless.

*The Ultimate LEGO Book*

Every design problem is completed within a set of constraints or limitations. These limits can be as broad as "design a logo," as generic as "print on standard letter paper," or as narrow as "arrange six circles in a square space." Working within the constraints of a problem is part of the fun and challenge of design.

Modularity is a special kind of constraint. A module is a fixed element used within a larger system or structure. For example, a pixel is a module that builds a digital image. A pixel is so small, we rarely stop to notice it, but when designers create pixel-based typefaces, they use a grid of pixels to invent letterforms that are consistent from one to the next while giving each one a distinctive shape.

A nine-by-nine grid of pixels can yield an infinite number of different typefaces. Likewise, a tiny handful of LEGO bricks contains an astonishing number of possible combinations.[1] The endless variety of forms occurs, however, within the strict parameters of the system, which permits just one basic kind of connection.

Building materials—from bricks to lumber to plumbing parts— are manufactured in standard sizes. By working with ready-made materials, an architect helps control construction costs while also streamlining the design process.

Designers are constantly making decisions about size, color, placement, proportion, relationships, and materials as well as about subject matter, style, and imagery. Sometimes, the decision-making process can be so overwhelming, it's hard to know how to begin and when to stop. When a few factors are determined in advance, the designer is free to think about other parts of the problem. A well-defined constraint can free up the thought process by taking some decisions off the table. In creating a page of typography, for example, a designer can choose to work within the constraints of one or two type families, and then explore different combinations of size, weight, and placement within that family of elements.

The book you are reading is organized around a typographic grid whose basic module is a square. By accepting the square unit as a given, we were able to mix and match images while creating a feeling of continuity across the book. The square units vary in size, however (keeping the layouts from getting dull), and some pictures stretch across more than one module (or ignore the grid altogether). Rules are helpful, but it's fun to break them.

1. *The Ultimate LEGO Book* (New York: DK Publishing, 1999).

**Post-it Wallpaper** This wall installation was built solely from three colors of Post-it neon note sheets, creating the optical effect of an enlarged halftone image or modular supergraphic. Nolen Strals and Bruce Willen, Post Typography.

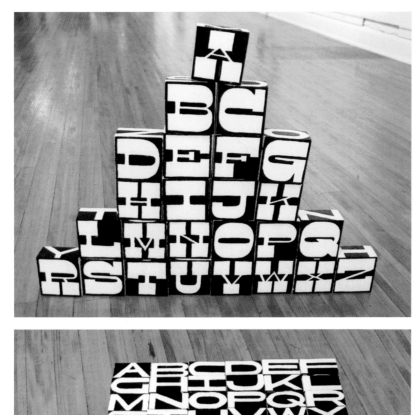

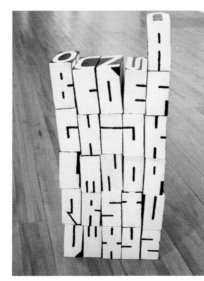

**Alphabet Blocks** These rectangular wooden blocks have a different alphabet painted on each side. Nolen Strals and Bruce Willen, Post Typography.

### Working with Constraints

In the projects shown here, graphic designers have used modular elements to produce unpredictable results. Try looking at familiar systems from a fresh angle. Given the constraints of any system, how can you play with the rules to make something new?

A child's set of alphabet blocks looks a certain way, for example, because the blocks are made from perfect cubes. But what if alphabet blocks were made from rectangles instead of cubes? The oddly proportioned faces of the blocks at left provided a framework for designing new letterforms in response to the constraints provided by the blocks of wood.

Standard materials such as laser paper are often used in generic ways. A standard sheet of office paper can be very dull indeed. Yet with creative thinking, an ordinary piece of paper can be used for dramatic effect. The temporary signage program shown on the opposite page employs economical processes and everyday materials to produce graphics at a lavish scale— at a very low cost.

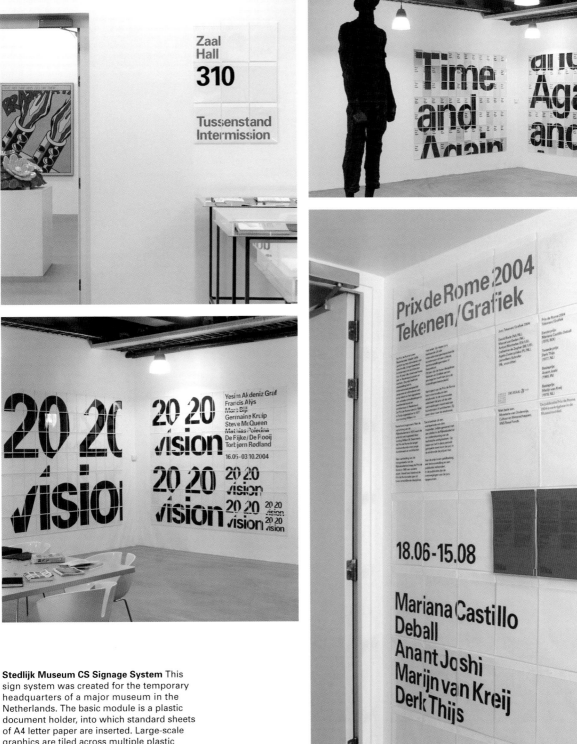

**Stedlijk Museum CS Signage System** This sign system was created for the temporary headquarters of a major museum in the Netherlands. The basic module is a plastic document holder, into which standard sheets of A4 letter paper are inserted. Large-scale graphics are tiled across multiple plastic envelopes. Experimental Jetset.

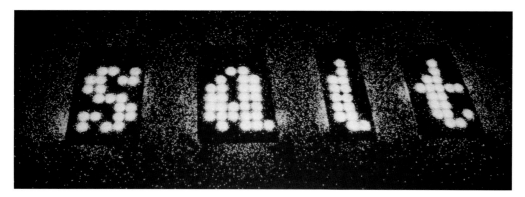

salt

Colin Ford

**Clean and Dirty Systems** Working with a nine-by-nine-square grid of circles, students created four letterforms with common characteristics such as weight, proportion, and density.

After creating a consistent and well-structured set of characters, the students introduced decay, degradation, distortion, randomness, or physicality into the design. The underlying structure becomes an armature for new and unexpected processes.

Approaches to making the clean system dirty include graphic techniques such as applying a filter to the source image or systematically varying the elements, as well as using physical techniques such as painting, stitching, or assembling. Typography I. Ellen Lupton, faculty.

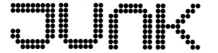

Kristen Bennett

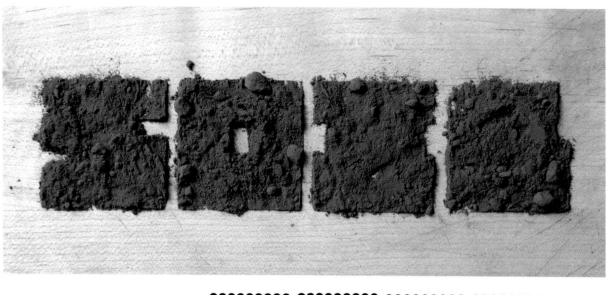

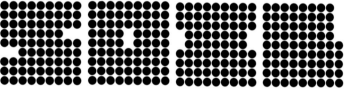

Emily Goldfarb

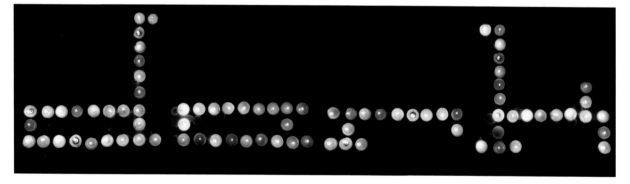

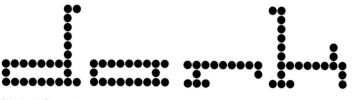

Nicolette Cornelius

ABCDEFGHIJKLM
NOPQRSTUVWXYZ

Austin Roesberg

ABCDEFGHIJ
KLMNOPQRS
TUVWXYZ!?..

Andy Bonner

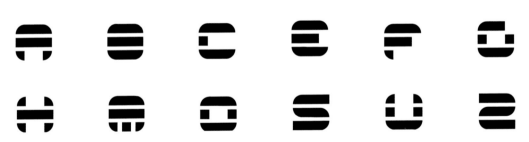

METEOR
ABCDEFGHIJ
KLMNOPQRS
TUVWXYZ!?..

Zachary Richter

**Modular Alphabet** In these examples, designers created systems of characters using three basic shapes: a square (each side equals one unit), a rectangle (one unit by two units), and a quarter-circle (radius equals one unit). Shapes could be assembled in any way, but their relative scale could not change.

Some forms are dense and solid, while others are split apart. Some use the curved elements to shape the outer edge, while others use curves to cut away the interior. Most have a simple profile, but it is also possible to build a detailed texture out of smaller-scaled elements. Experimental Typography. Nolen Strals and Bruce Willen, faculty.

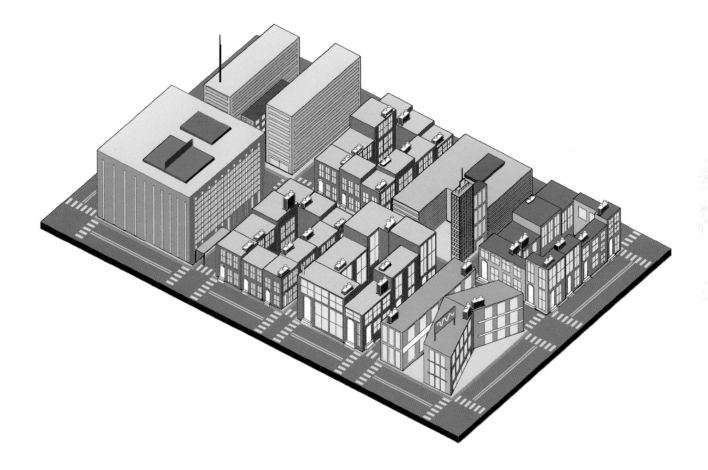

**Architectural Alphabet** The three-dimensional design software AutoCAD has been used to spell out the phrase "word book" in buildings. The rectilinear modules of architecture become the building blocks for letterforms. Johanna Barthmaier, Typography I. Ellen Lupton, faculty.

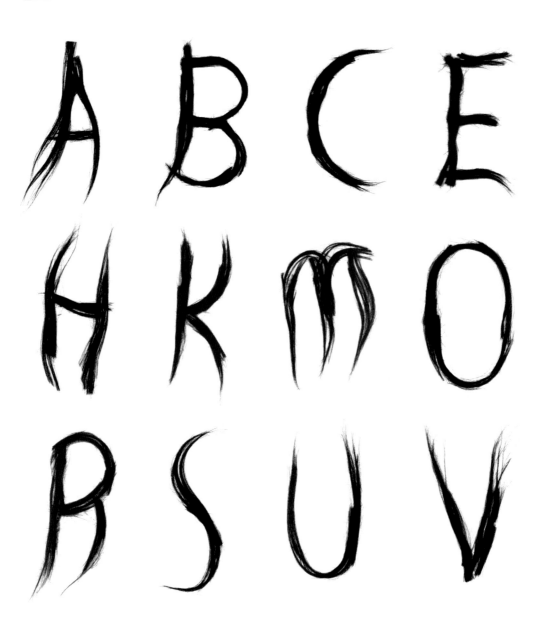

**Ready-made Alphabet** The challenge here was to create a set of characters using objects from the environment rather than drawing them digitally or by hand. The designers discovered letterforms hidden in the things around them. Experimental Typography. Nolen Strals and Bruce Willen, faculty.

Jennifer Baghieri

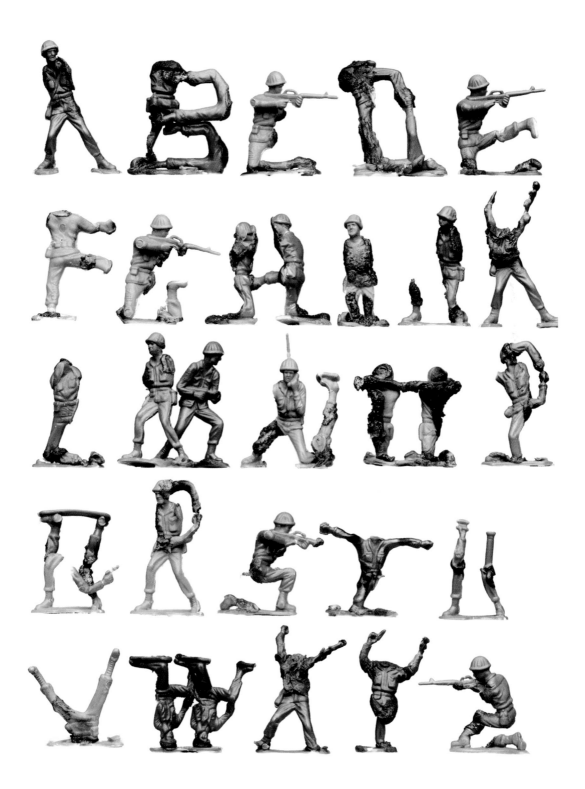

Oliver Munday

## Symbol Systems

A symbol stands for or represents objects, functions, and processes. Many familiar symbols, such as McDonald's golden arches, are highly distilled, stripped of extraneous detail, delivering just enough information to convey meaning. Symbol systems are often based on geometric modules that come together to create myriad forms and functions.

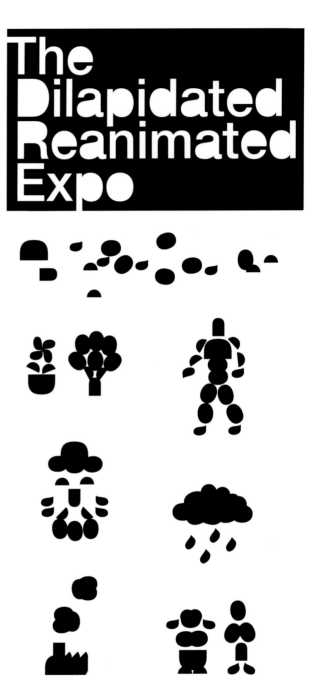

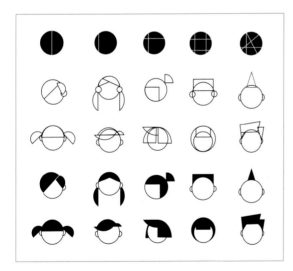

**Modular Hairdos** Geometrically derived forms combine to shape myriad hair styles. Yue Tuo, MFA Studio.

**Counterform Pictures** Counters extracted from letters in a title cohere into visual narratives. Nolen Strals and Bruce Willen, Post Typography.

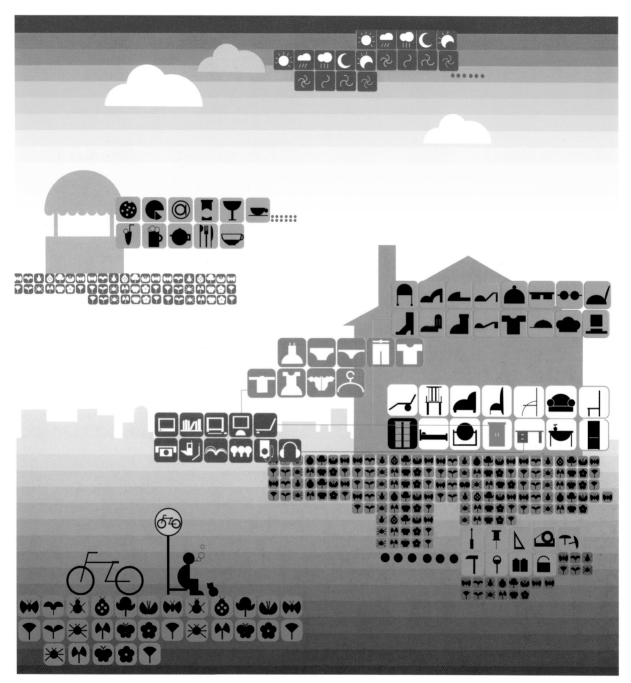

**Symbolscape** This landscape is built and described by a series of modularly structured symbols stacked and layered to denote fauna, flora, and form. Yue Tuo, MFA Studio.

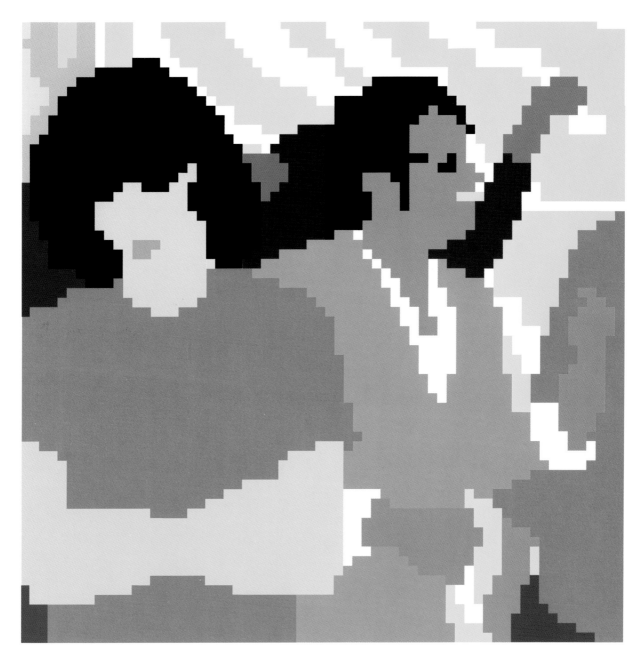

**Pixel Art** The image above is built from a modular grid of squares, colored and combined to make a highly pixilated social scene. Pixels are the building block of any digital image. Here, they become an expressive element. April Osmanof, MFA Studio.

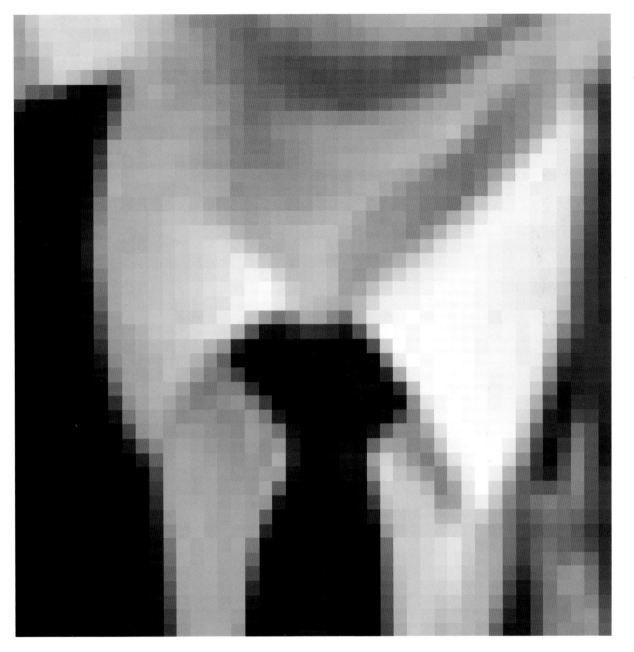

**Pixel Effects** Like a Chuck Close painting, this photographic detail takes on an abstract quality when enlarged—smooth, graduated, tonal hues divide into elemental square segments. April Osmanof, MFA Studio. Photograph: Marc Alain.

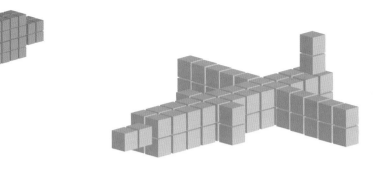

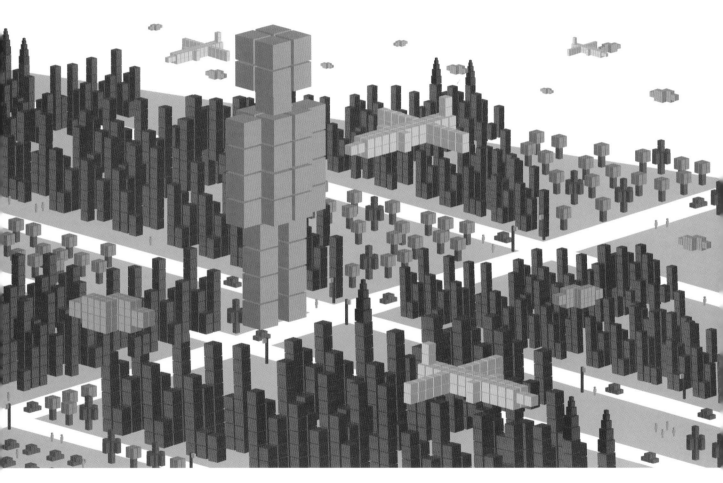

**A City of Cubes** An urban landscape teems with people, planes, clouds, automobiles, skyscrapers, and trees—all built from cubes in Adobe Illustrator. Yong Seuk Lee, MFA Studio.

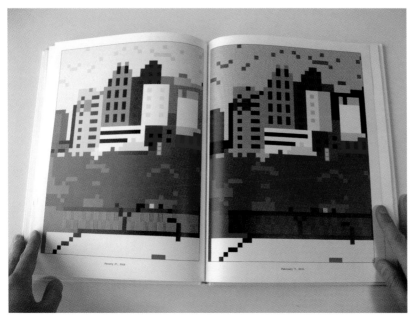

**Extrapolations in Excel** These elaborate
drawings utilize the gridded compartments
of an Excel spreadsheet as a catalyst and a
constraint. Danielle Aubert, MFA thesis, Yale
University School of Art.

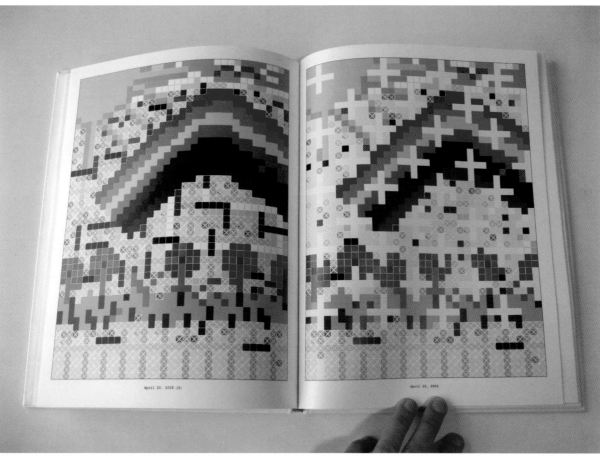

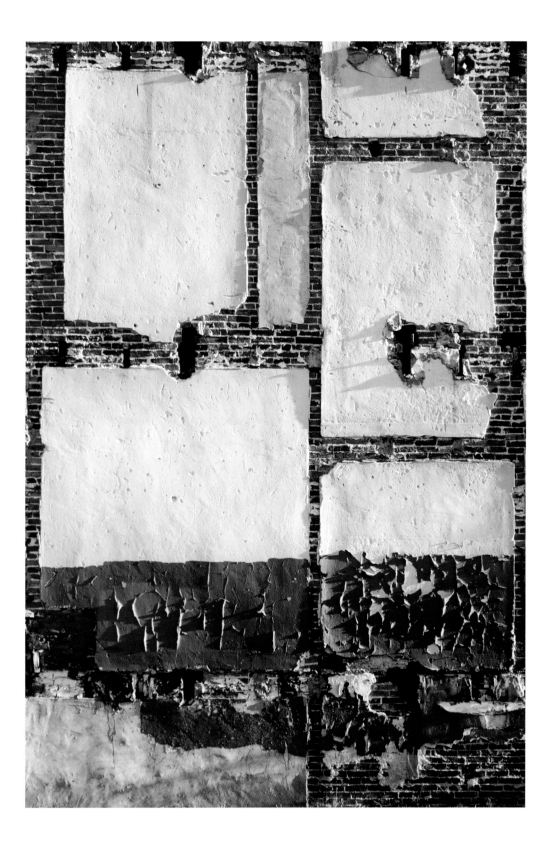

# Grid

Typography is mostly an act of **dividing** a limited surface. Willi Baumeister

A grid is a network of lines. The lines in a grid typically run horizontally and vertically in evenly paced increments, but grids can be angled, irregular, or even circular as well.

When you write notes on a pad of lined paper, or sketch out a floor plan on graph paper, or practice handwriting or calligraphy on ruled pages, the lines serve to guide the hand and eye as you work.

Grids function similarly in the design of printed matter. Guidelines help the designer align elements in relation to each other. Consistent margins and columns create an underlying structure that unifies the pages of a document and makes the layout process more efficient. In addition to organizing the active content of the page (text and images), the grid lends structure to the white spaces, which cease to be merely blank and passive voids but participate in the rhythm of the overall system.

A well-made grid encourages the designer to vary the scale and placement of elements without relying wholly on arbitrary or whimsical judgments. The grid offers a rationale and a starting point for each composition, converting a blank area into a structured field.

**Flag Wall** Grids appear throughout the built environment, revealing both order and decay. Jason Okutake, MFA Studio.

Many artists have embraced the grid as a rational, universal form that exists outside of the individual producer. At the same time, the grid is culturally associated with modern urbanism, architecture, and technology. The facades of many glass high rises and other modern buildings consist of uniform ribbons of metal and glass that wrap the building's volume in a continuous skin. In contrast with the symmetrical hierarchy of a classical building, with its strong entranceway and tiered pattern of windows, a gridded facade expresses a democracy of elements.

Grids function throughout society. The street grids used in many modern cities around the globe promote circulation among neighborhoods and the flow of traffic, in contrast with the suburban cul de sac, a dead-end road that keeps neighborhoods closed off and private.

The grid imparts a similarly democratic character to the printed page. By marking space into numerous equal units, the grid makes the entire page available for use; the edges become as important as the center. Grids help designers create active, asymmetrical compositions in place of static, centered ones. By breaking down space into smaller units, grids encourage designers to leave some areas open rather than filling up the whole page.

Software interfaces encourage the use of grids by making it easy to establish margins, columns, and page templates. Guidelines can be quickly dragged, dropped, and deleted and made visible or invisible at will. (Indeed, it is a good idea when working on screen to switch off the guidelines from time to time, as they can create a false sense of fullness and structure as well as clutter one's view.)

This chapter looks at the grid as a means of generating form, arranging images, and organizing information. The grid can work quietly in the background, or it can assert itself as an active element. The grid becomes visible as objects come into alignment with it. Some designers use grids in a strict, absolute way, while others see them as a starting point in an evolving process. This book is designed with a strong grid, but when an image or layout needs to break step with the regiment, it is allowed to do so.

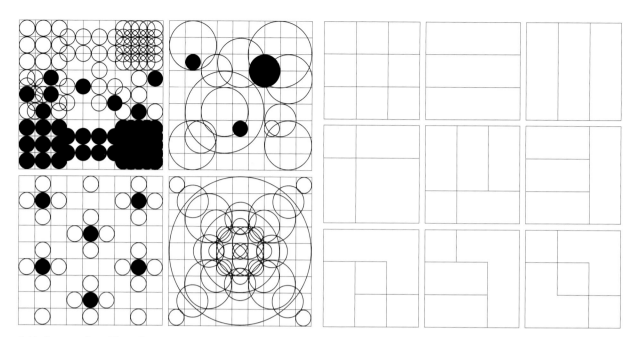

**Grids Generate Form** The cells and nodes of a grid can be used to generate complex pattern designs as well as simple rectangles. Dividing a square into nine identical units is a classic design problem. Numerous simple forms and relationships can be built against this simple matrix. Jason Okutake and John P. Corrigan, MFA Studio.

## Form and Content

The grid has a long history within modern art and design as a means for generating form. You can construct compositions, layouts, and patterns by dividing a space into fields and filling in or delineating its cells in different ways. Try building irregular and asymmetric compositions against the neutral, ready-made backdrop of a grid. The same formal principles apply to organizing text and images in a publication design.

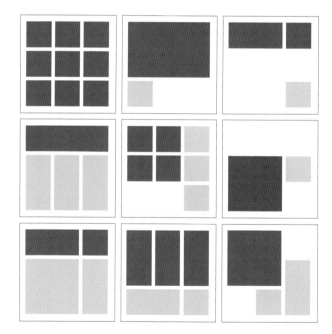

**Grids Organize Content** The nine-square grid divides the page into spaces for images and text. Although each layout has its own rhythm and scale, the pages are unified by the grid's underlying structure. The book you are reading is built around a similar nine-square grid. John P. Corrigan, MFA Studio.

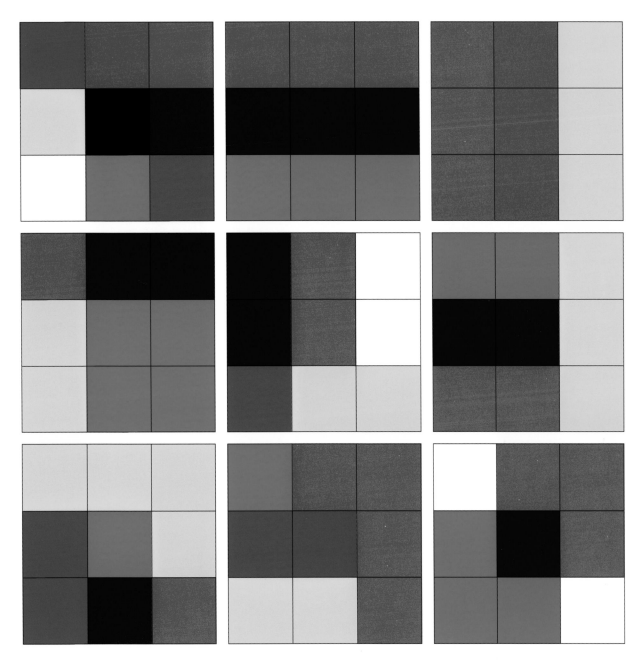

**Nine-square Grid: Color Fields** The grid
provides a structure for organizing fields
of color that frame and overlap each other.
Complexity emerges against a simple
armature. John P. Corrigan, MFA Studio.

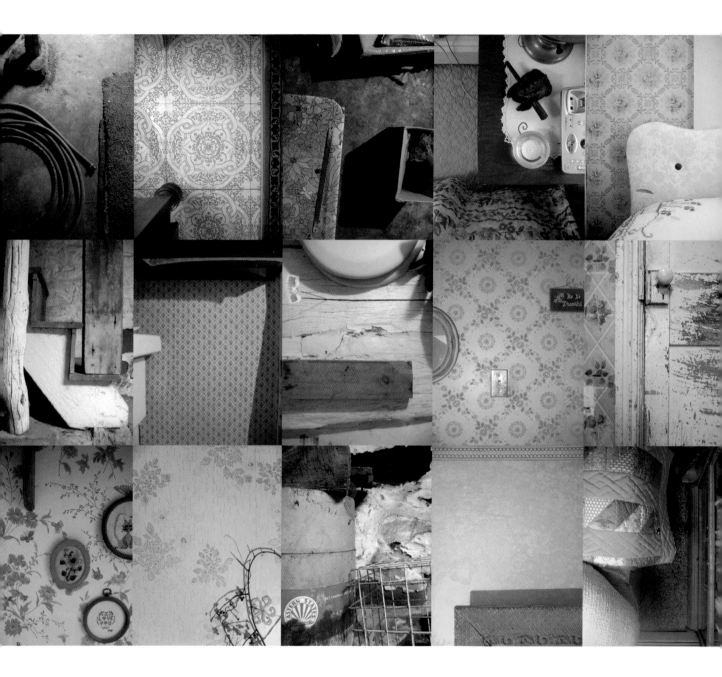

**Strict Grid** Here, the rigidly imposed grid emphasizes the flat, graphic character and head-on viewpoint of the photographs.
Jeremy Botts, MFA Studio.

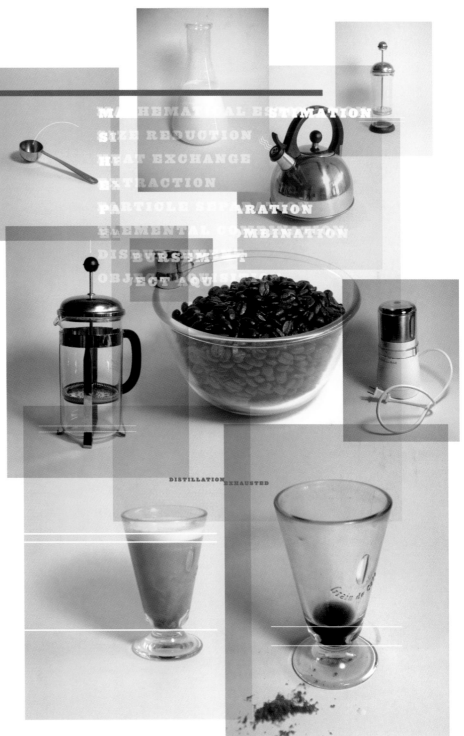

**Broken Grid** The rectilinear photographs overlap and misalign to create a sense of movement and depth. Individually, each image is static, but together, they convey action and change. John P. Corrigan, MFA Studio.

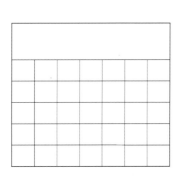

**Monthly Calendar** The column and row structure of the familiar monthly calendar is open to reinterpretation. Graphic Design I. Kim Bost, faculty.

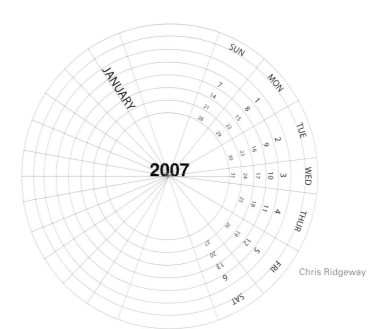

Chris Ridgeway

## Calendar Grid

Standard calendar designs use columns and rows to organize the weeks and days that make up a month. The days of the week align in vertical columns, while each week occupies a horizontal row. This form has become standard and universal, as have various templates used in day planners.

Developing alternate ways to structure a calendar is a good design challenge. The underlying problem in any calendar design is to use two-dimensional space to represent a sequence in time. The grid can be circular, diagonal, or freeform.

Jessica Neil

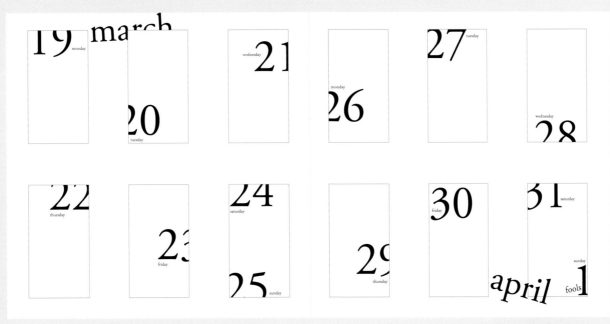

April Osmanof

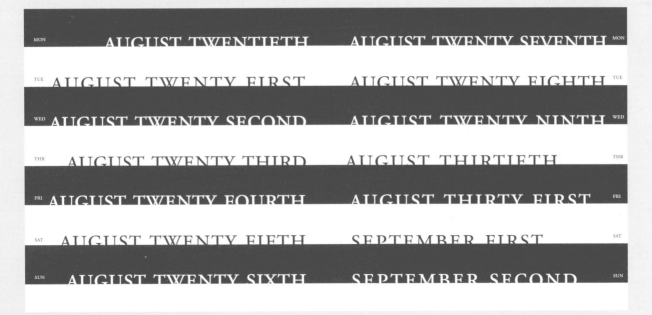

**Weekly Calendar** These pages and spreads from a day planner organize the days of the week and provide space for users to record notes. Typography I. Ellen Lupton, faculty.

Lindsey Sherman

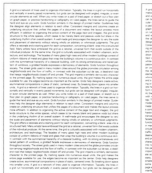

**One column**

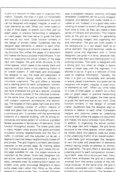

**Two columns**

**Three columns**

**Four columns**

## Page Grids

A standard textbook is designed with a one-column grid: a single block of body copy is surrounded by margins that function as a simple frame for the content. For hundreds of years, Bibles have been designed with pages divided into two columns. Textbooks, dictionaries, reference manuals, and other books containing large amounts of text often use a two-column grid, breaking up space and making the pages less overwhelming for readers.

Magazines typically use grids with three or more vertical divisions. Multiple columns guide the placement of text, headlines, captions, images, and other page elements. One or more horizontal "hang lines" provide additional structure. A skilled designer uses a grid actively, not passively, allowing the modules to suggest intriguing shapes and surprising placements for elements.

**Multicolumn Grid** This complex design is built around a four-column grid structure. It comments on medieval book design traditions. Charles Calixto, Typography I. Ellen Lupton, faculty.

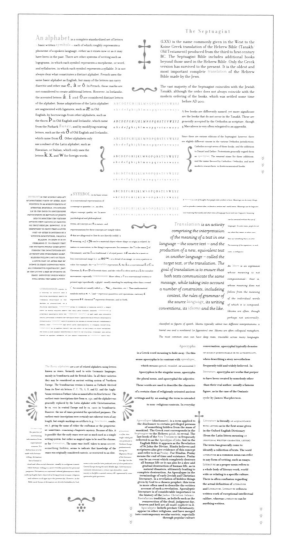

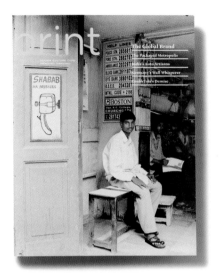
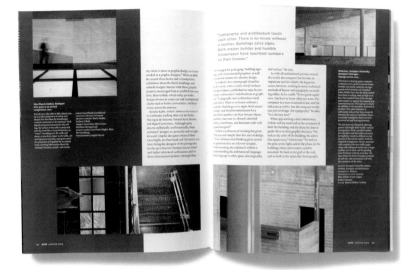

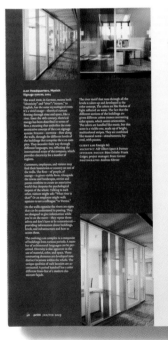
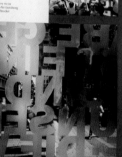

**Many Columns, Many Choices** The page layouts shown here from *Print* magazine, designed by Pentagram, employ a complex, multicolumn grid. The column structure gives the pages their vertical grain, while horizontal hang lines anchor each spread, bringing elements into taut alignment. The grid helps the layout designer create active, varied pages that are held together by an underlying structure. The grid accommodates a mix of sizes and proportions in both image and text blocks. And, where appropriate, the designer breaks the grid altogether.
Abbott Miller and John Kudos, Pentagram. *Print* magazine.

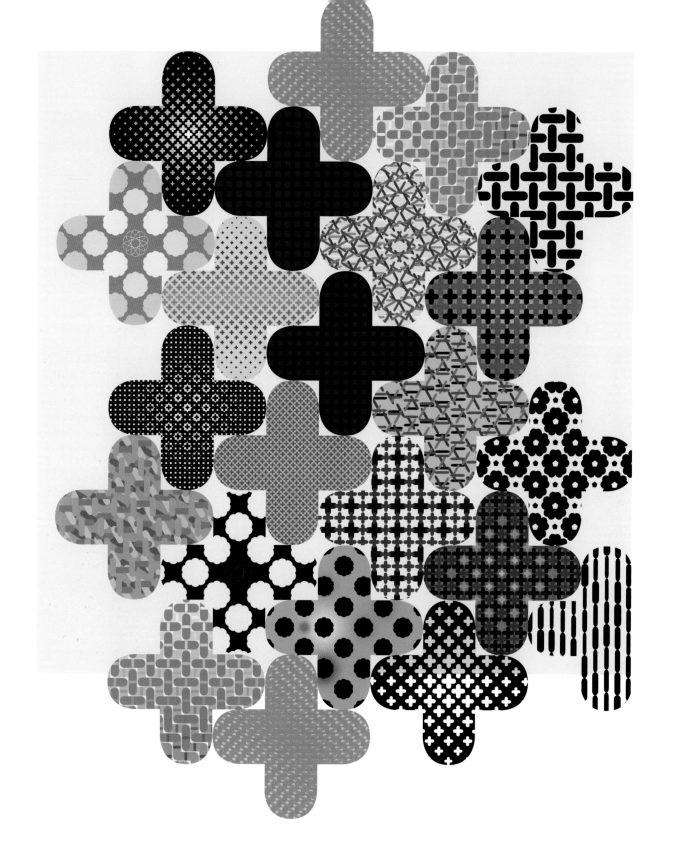

# Pattern

The **principles** discoverable in the works
of the past belong to us; not so the **results**.

Owen Jones

The creative evolution of ornament spans all of human history. Shared ways to generate pattern are found in cultures around the world. Universal principles underlie diverse styles and icons that speak to particular times and traditions.

This chapter shows how to build complex patterns around core concepts. Dots, stripes, and grids provide the architecture behind an infinite range of designs. By composing a single element in different schemes, the designer can create endless variations, building complexity around a logical core.

Styles and motifs of pattern-making evolve within and among cultures, and they move in and out of fashion. They travel from place to place and time to time, carried along like viruses by the forces of commerce and the restless desire for variety.

In the twentieth century, modern designers avoided ornate detail in favor of minimal adornment. In 1908, the Viennese design critic Adolf Loos famously conflated "Ornament and Crime." He linked the human lust for decoration with primitive tattoos and criminal behavior.[1]

Yet despite the modern distaste for ornament, the structural analysis of pattern is central to modern design theory. In 1856, Owen Jones created his monumental *Grammar of Ornament*, documenting decorative vocabularies from around the world.[2] Jones's book encouraged Western designers to copy and reinterpret "exotic" motifs from Asia and Africa, but it also helped them recognize principles that unite an endless diversity of forms.

Today, surface pattern is creating a vibrant discourse. The rebirth of ornament is linked to the revival of craft in architecture, products, and interiors, as well as to scientific views of how life emerges from the interaction of simple rules.

The decorative forms presented in this chapter embrace a mix of formal structure and organic irregularity. They meld individual authorship with rule-based systems, and they merge formal abstraction with personal narrative. By understanding how to produce patterns, designers learn how to weave complexity out of elementary structures, participating in the world's most ancient and prevalent artistic practice.

**Crazy Quilt** Mixing and matching patterns is an ancient enterprise. Here, a mix is made with a palette of digital elements that communicate with each other. Jeremy Botts, MFA Studio.

1. Adolf Loos, *Ornament and Crime: Selected Essays* (Riverside, CA: Ariadne Press, 1998).
2. Owen Jones, *The Grammar of Ornament* (London: Day and Son, 1856).

The secret to success in all ornament is the production of a broad general effect by the repetition of **a few simple elements**.

Owen Jones

### Dots, Stripes, and Grids

In the nineteenth century, designers began analyzing how patterns are made. They found that nearly any pattern arises from three basic forms: isolated elements, linear elements, and the criss-crossing or interaction of the two.[1] Various terms have been used to name these elementary conditions, but we will call them dots, stripes, and grids.

Any isolated form can be considered a dot, from a simple circle to an ornate flower. A stripe, in contrast, is a linear path. It can consist of a straight, solid line, or it can be built up from smaller elements (dots) that link together visually to form a line.

These two basic structures, dots and stripes, interact to form grids. As a grid takes shape, it subverts the identity of the separate elements in favor of a larger texture. Indeed, creating that larger texture is what pattern design is all about. Imagine a field of wildflowers. It is filled with spectacular individual organisms that contribute to an overall system.

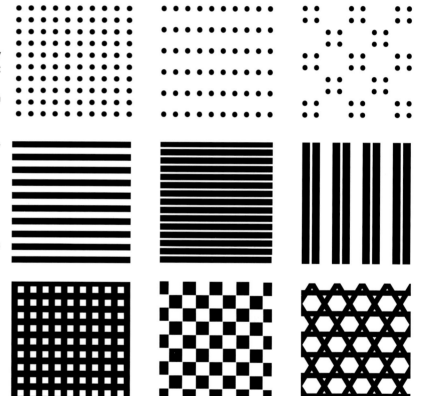

1. Our scheme for classifying ornament is adapted from Archibald Christie, *Traditional Methods of Pattern Designing; An Introduction to the Study of the Decorative Art* (Oxford: Clarendon Press, 1910).

**From Point to Line to Grid** As dots move together, they form into lines and other shapes (while still being dots). As stripes cross over each other and become grids, they cut up the field into new figures, which function like new dots or new stripes.

Some of the most visually fascinating patterns result from figure/ground ambiguity. The identity of a form can oscillate between being a figure (dot, stripe) to being a ground or support for another, opposing figure.

## Repeating Elements

How does a simple form—a dot, a square, a flower, a cross—populate a surface to create a pattern that calms, pleases, or surprises us?

Whether rendered by hand, machine, or code, a pattern results from repetition. An army of dots can be regulated by a rigid geometric grid, or it can randomly swarm across a surface via irregular handmade marks. It can spread out in a continuous veil or concentrate its forces in pockets of intensity.

In every instance, however, patterns follow some repetitive principle, whether dictated by a mechanical grid, a digital algorithm, or the physical rhythm of a craftsperson's tool as it works along a surface.

In the series of pattern studies developed here and on the following pages, a simple lozenge form is used to build designs of varying complexity. Experiments of this kind can be performed with countless base shapes, yielding an endless range of individual results.

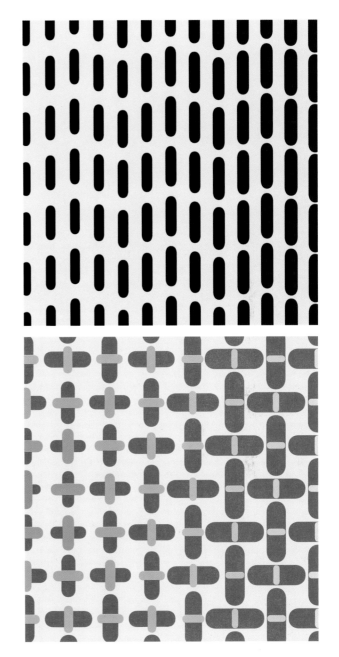

**One Element, Many Patterns** The basic element in these patterns is a lozenge shape. Based on the orientation, proximity, scale, and color of the lozenges, they group into overlapping lines, forming a nascent grid. Jeremy Botts, MFA Studio.

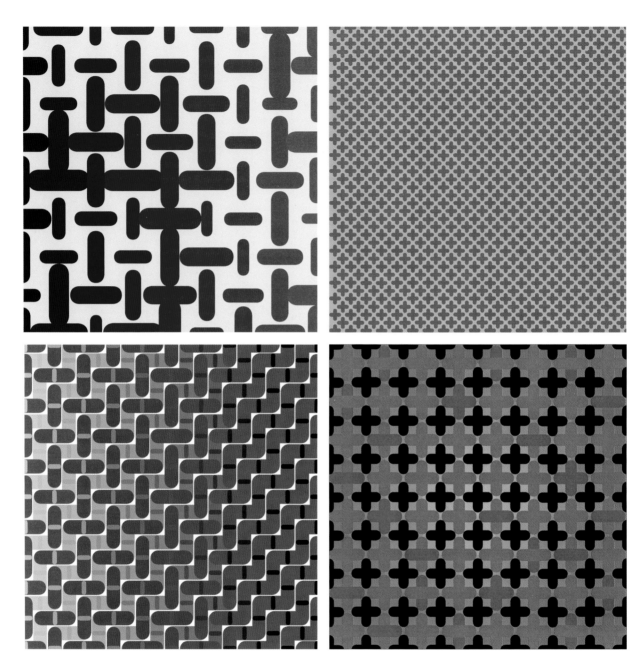

**One Element, Many Patterns** In this series of designs, the lozenge shape functions as a dot, the primitive element at the core of numerous variations. This oblong dot combines with other dots to form quatrefoils (a new super-dot) as well as lines.

As lozenges of common color or orientation begin to associate with each other visually, additional figures take shape across the surface. Jeremy Botts, MFA Studio.

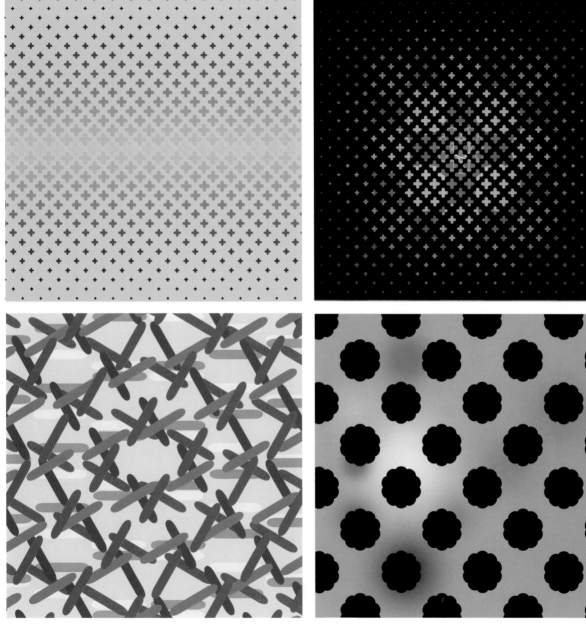

**Changing Color, Scale, and Orientation**
Altering the color contrast between elements or changing the overall scale of the pattern transforms its visual impact. Color shifts can be uniform across the surface, or they can take place in gradients or steps.

Turning elements on an angle or changing their scale also creates a sense of depth and motion. New figures emerge as the lonzenge rotates and repeats. Jeremy Botts, MFA Studio.

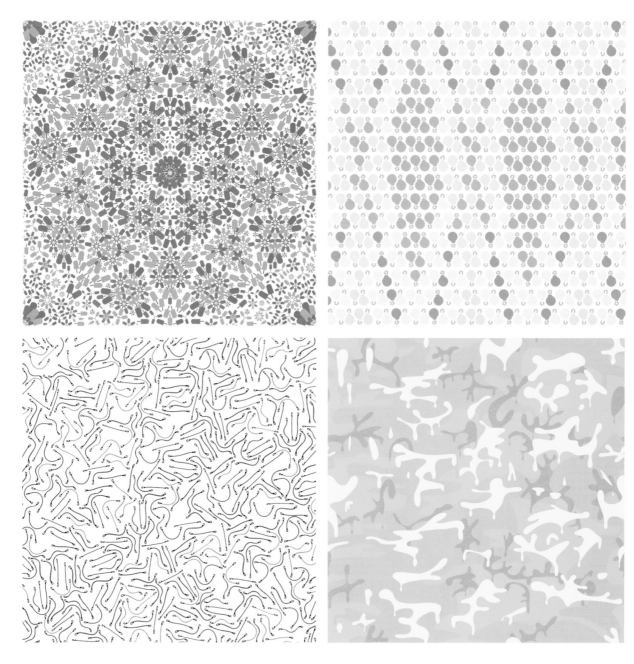

**Iconic Patterns** Here, traditional pattern structures have been populated with images that have personal significance for the designer: popsicles, bombs, bungee cords, yellow camouflage, and slices of bright green cake. The single tiles above can be repeated into larger patterns, as shown opposite. Spence Holman, MFA Studio.

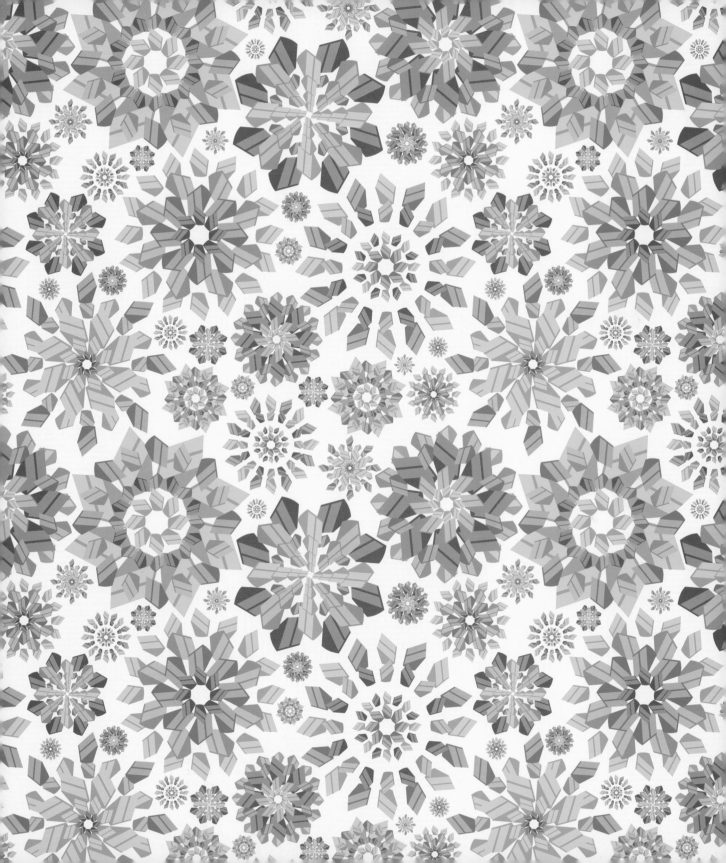

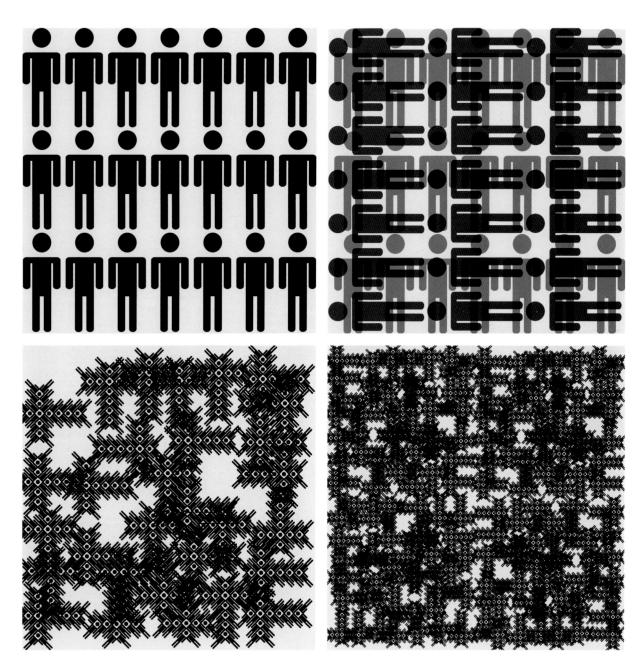

**Regular and Irregular** Interesting pattern designs often result from a mix of regular and irregular forces as well as abstract and recognizable imagery. Here, regimented rows of icons overlap to create dense crowds as well as orderly battalions. Yong Seuk Lee, MFA Studio.

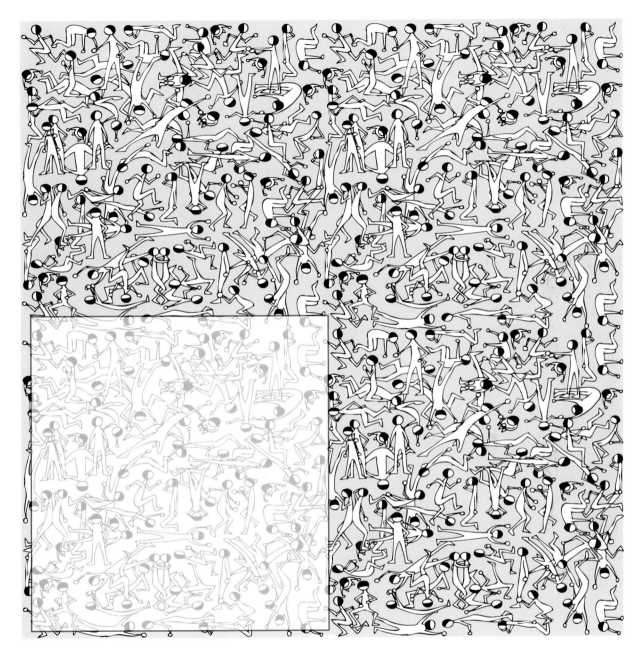

**Random Repeat** These patterns appear highly irregular, yet they are composed of repeating tiles. To make this kind of pattern, the designer needs to make the left and right edges and the top and bottom edges match up with those of an identical tile. Anything can take place in the middle of the tile.

The tiles shown here are square, but they could be rectangles, diamonds, or any other interlocking shape. Yong Seuk Lee, MFA Studio.

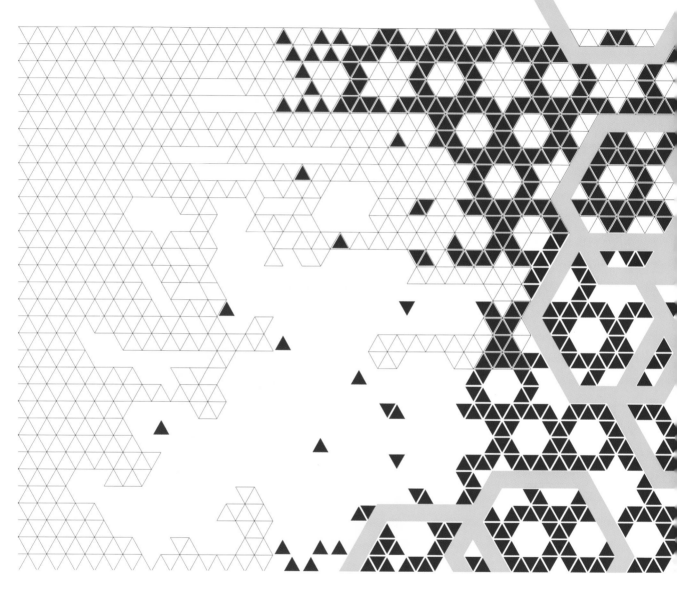

**Grid as Matrix** An infinite number of patterns can be created from a common grid. In the simplest patterns, each cell is turned on or off. Larger figures take shape as neighboring clusters fill in.

More complex patterns occur when the grid serves to locate forms without dictating their outlines or borders. Jason Okutake, MFA Studio.

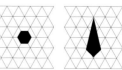

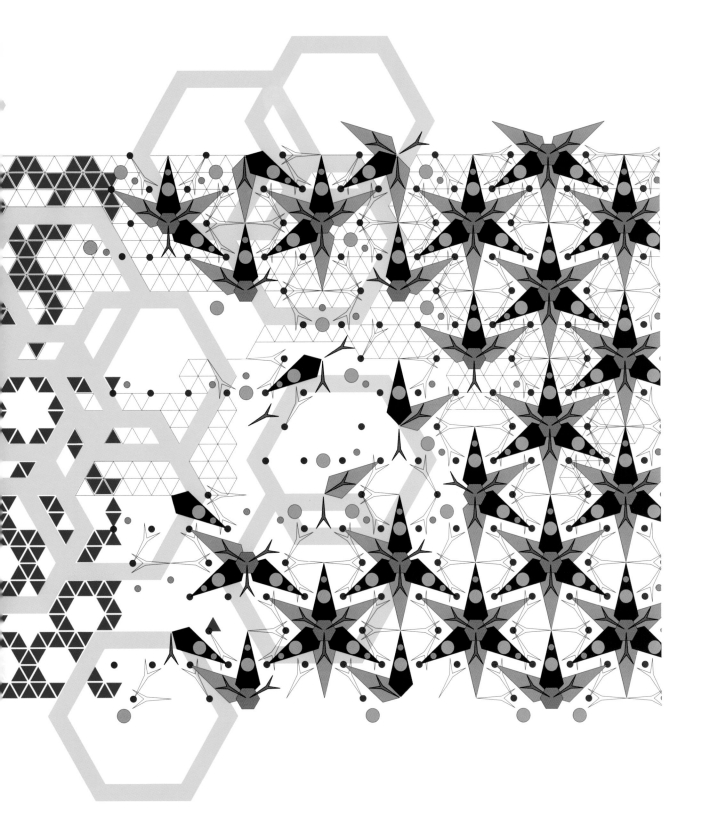

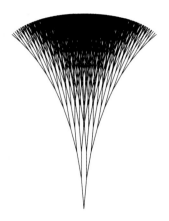

## Code-Based Patterns

Every pattern follows a rule. Defining rules with computer code allows the designer to create variations by changing the input to the system. The designer creates the rule, but the end result may be unexpected.

The patterns shown here were designed using Processing, the open-source computer language created for designers and visual artists. All the patterns are built around the basic form of a binary tree, a structure in which every node yields no more than two offspring. New branches appear with each iteration of the program.

The binary tree form has been repeated, rotated, inverted, connected, and overlapped to generate a variety of pattern elements, equivalent to "tiles" in a traditional design. By varying the inputs to the code, the designer created four different tiles, which she joined together in Photoshop to produce a larger repeating pattern. The principle is no different from that used in many traditional ornamental designs, but the process has been automated, yielding a different kind of density.

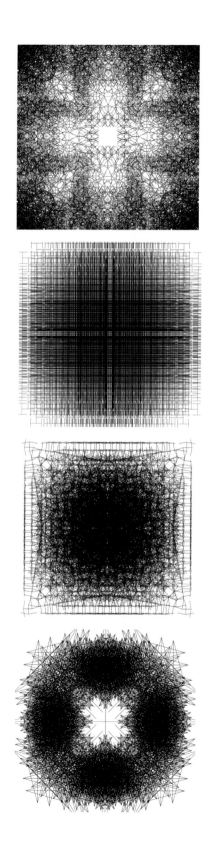

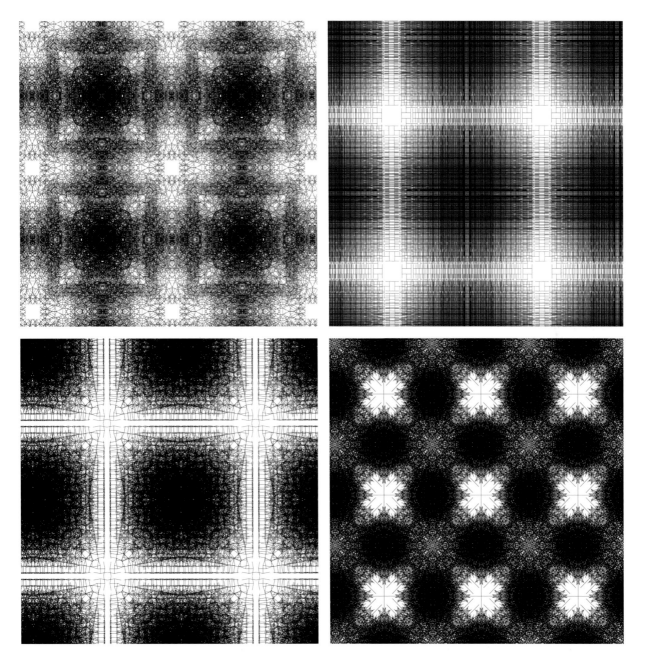

**Vary the Input** Four different base elements were created by varying the input to the code. The base "tiles" are joined together to create a repeat pattern; new figures emerge where the tiles come together, just as in traditional ornament. Yeohyun Ahn, Interactive Media II. James Ravel, faculty.

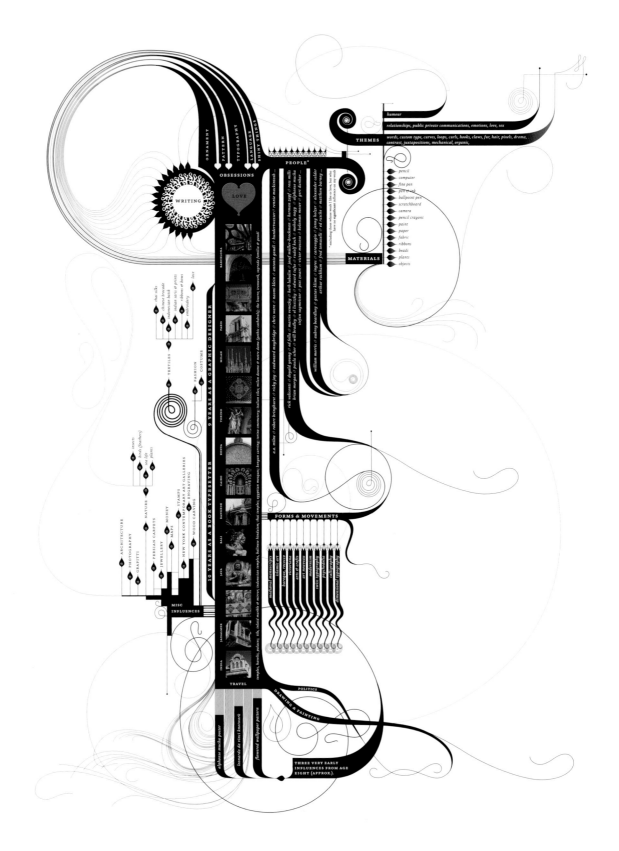

# Diagram

In emphasizing evidential quality and beauty, I also want to move the practices of **analytical design** far away from the practices of propaganda, marketing, graphic design, and commercial art.

Edward R. Tufte

A diagram is a graphic representation of a structure, situation, or process. Diagrams can depict the anatomy of a creature, the hierarchy of a corporation, or the flow of ideas. Diagrams allow us to see relationships that would not come forward in a straight list of numbers or a verbal description.

Many of the visual elements and phenomena described in this book— from point, line, and plane to scale, color, hierarchy, layers, and more— converge in the design of diagrams. In the realm of information graphics, the aesthetic role of these elements remains important, but something else occurs as well. Graphic marks and visual relationships take on specific meanings, coded within the diagram to depict numerical increments, relative size, temporal change, structural links, and other conditions.

The great theorist of information design is Edward R. Tufte, who has been publishing books on this subject since 1983. Tufte finds a certain kind of beauty in the visual display of data—a universal beauty grounded in the laws of nature and the mind's ability to comprehend them.[1]

Tufte has called for removing the practice of information design from the distorting grasp of propaganda and graphic design. He argues that a chart or diagram should employ no metaphoric distractions or excessive flourishes (what he has called "chart junk"), but should stay within the realm of objective observation.

Tufte's purist point of view is profound and compelling, but it may be overly restrictive. Information graphics do have a role to play in the realm of expressive and editorial graphics. The language of diagrams has yielded a rich and evocative repertoire within contemporary design. In editorial contexts, diagrams often function to illuminate and explain complex ideas. They can be clean and reductive or richly expressive, creating evocative pictures that reveal surprising relationships and impress the eye with the sublime density and grandeur of a body of data.

Many of the examples developed in this chapter are rigorous but not pure. Some pieces use diagrams to depict personal histories, a process that forces the designer to develop systematic ways to represent subjective experience. Such an approach is seen in the extravagant autobiographical diagram presented on the page opposite, by Marian Bantjes. Her map does not aim to convey evidence in a strictly scientific way, but rather uses analytical thinking to unleash a language that is both personal and universal, building complexity around basic structures.

1. Edward R. Tufte, *Beautiful Evidence* (Cheshire, CT: Graphics Press, 2006).

**Map of Influences** This alluring diagram by designer and artist Marian Bantjes describes her visual influences, which range from medieval and Celtic lettering, to baroque and rococo ornament, to Swiss typography and American psychedelia. Those diverse influences come alive in the flowing, filigreed lines of the piece. Marian Bantjes.

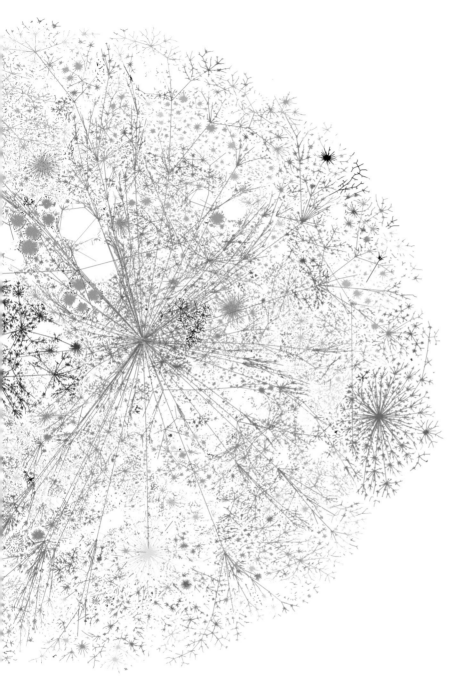

## Making Connections

A network, also called a graph, is a set of connections among nodes or points.[1] There are various ways to connect the nodes in a network, resulting in different kinds of organization. Centralized networks include pyramids and trees, where all power issues from a common point. A decentralized network has a spine with radiating elements, as in an interstate highway system. A distributed network has node-to-node relationships with no spine and no center. The Internet is a distributed network peppered with concentrated nodes of connectivity.

Networks are everywhere—not just in technology, but throughout nature and society. A food chain, a city plan, and the pathway of a disease are all networks that can be described graphically with points and lines.

**Decentralized Network** This snapshot of the World Wide Web (detail) shows the connections among servers. A relatively small number of hubs dominate global traffic. Courtesy Lumeta Corp. © 2005 Lumeta Corp.

1. On network theory, see Alexander Galloway and Eugene Thacker, "Protocol, Control and Networks," *Grey Room* 12 (Fall 2004): 6–29. See also Christopher Alexander, "The City is Not a Tree," in Joan Ockman, ed., *Architecture Culture, 1943–1968: A Documentary Anthology* (New York: Rizzoli, 1993), 379–88.

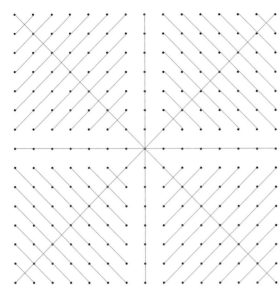

**Centralized** Kelly Horigan

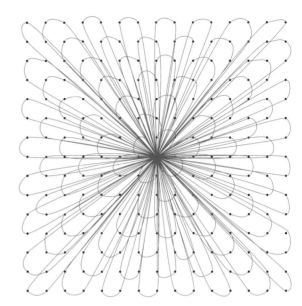

**Centralized** Lindsay Orlowski

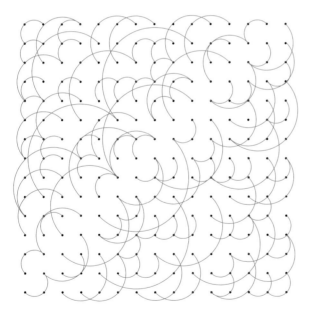

**Decentralized** Lindsay Orlowski

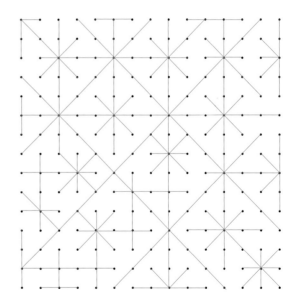

**Distributed** Kelly Horigan

**Designing Networks** In this project, designers connect a grid of dots with lines, producing designs that reflect different types of networks: centralized, decentralized, and distributed. Graphic Design II. Ellen Lupton, faculty.

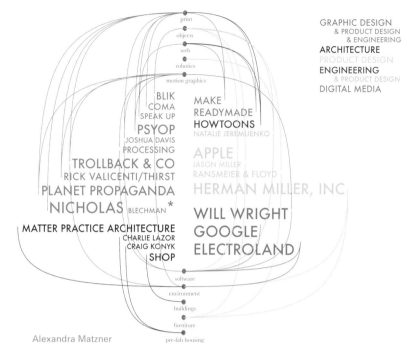

GRAPHIC DESIGN
& PRODUCT DESIGN
& ENGINEERING
ARCHITECTURE
PRODUCT DESIGN
ENGINEERING
& PRODUCT DESIGN
DIGITAL MEDIA

print
objects
web
robotics
motion graphics

BLIK
COMA
SPEAK UP
PSYOP
JOSHUA DAVIS
PROCESSING
TROLLBACK & CO
RICK VALICENTI/THIRST
PLANET PROPAGANDA
NICHOLAS BLECHMAN *
MATTER PRACTICE ARCHITECTURE
CHARLIE LAZOR
CRAIG KONYK
ShOP

MAKE
READYMADE
HOWTOONS
NATALIE JEREMIJENKO
APPLE
JASON MILLER
RANSMEIER & FLOYD
HERMAN MILLER, INC
WILL WRIGHT
GOOGLE
ELECTROLAND

software
environment
buildings
furniture
pre-fab housing

Alexandra Matzner

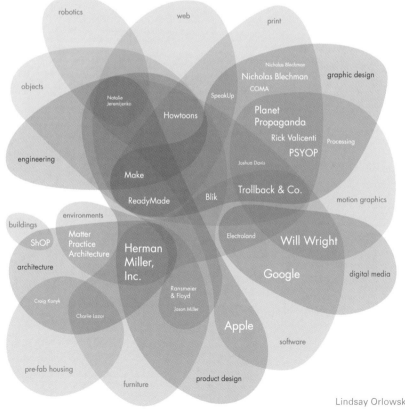

Lindsay Orlowski

**Overlapping Relationships** People don't fall into tidy categories. Any individual can have many identities: parent, child, professional, fan, taxpayer, and so on.

In the project shown here, students were given a list of designers and design firms who work in different fields (graphic design, architecture, and new media) and who produce different kinds of projects (buildings, websites, products, print, and so on). The list also ranked people according to the size of their firms (from single practitioners to large corporations). The design challenge was to represent these overlapping categories visually, using typography, scale, color, line, and other cues to indicate connections and differences.

Some of the solutions use dots of varying size to indicate scale or to mark points on a conceptual map. Others change the size of the typography to indicate the scale. Overlapping planes or crossing lines were used to indicate areas of overlap. This problem can be applied to any collection of objects, from a grocery list to categories of music or art. Graphic Design II. Ellen Lupton, faculty.

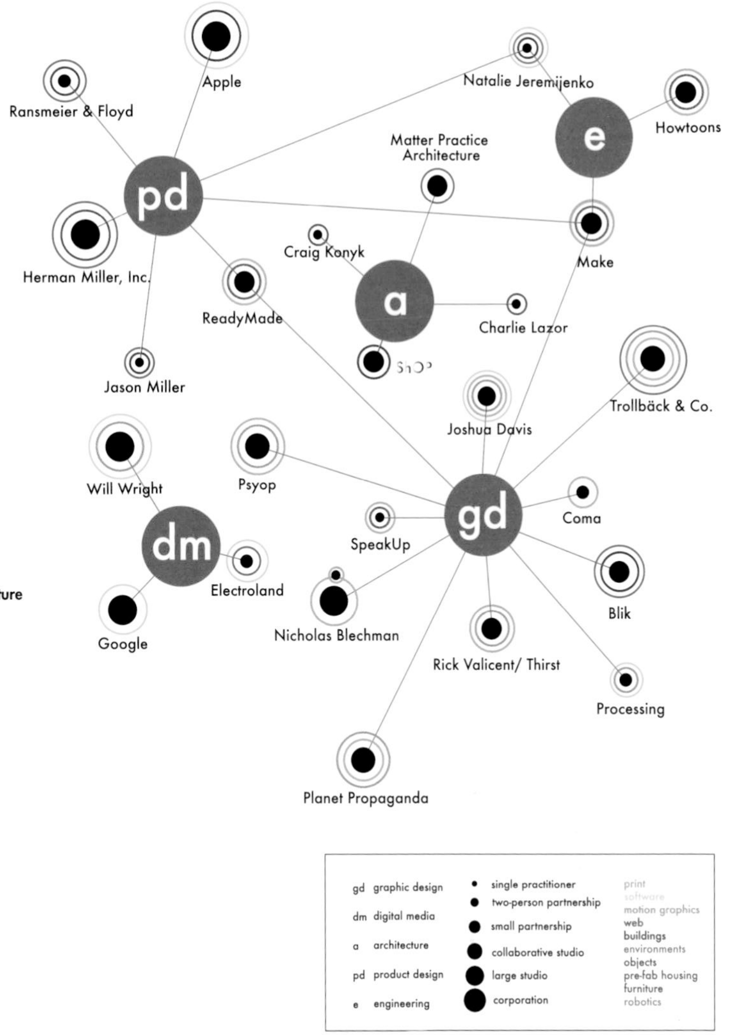

Network diagram labels:
- Apple
- Ransmeier & Floyd
- Natalie Jeremijenko
- Howtoons
- **e** (engineering)
- Matter Practice Architecture
- **pd** (product design)
- Make
- Craig Konyk
- Herman Miller, Inc.
- **a** (architecture)
- Charlie Lazor
- ReadyMade
- ShOP
- Jason Miller
- Trollbäck & Co.
- Joshua Davis
- Will Wright
- Psyop
- Coma
- **gd** (graphic design)
- **dm** (digital media)
- SpeakUp
- Blik
- Electroland
- Nicholas Blechman
- Rick Valicent/ Thirst
- Google
- Processing
- Planet Propaganda

Row labels (left chart):
- COMA
- Will Wright
- SpeakUp
- Nicholas Blechman
- Rick Valicenti/Thirst
- ShOP
- Matter Practice Architecture
- Blik
- Craig Konyk
- Charlie Lazar
- Jason Miller
- Ransmeier & Floyd
- Trollbäck & Co.
- ReadyMade
- Howtoons
- Make
- Natalie jeremijenko
- Processing
- Joshua Davis
- Google
- PSYOP
- Planet Propaganda
- Apple
- Electroland
- Herman Miller, Inc

Legend:
| gd | graphic design | • | single practitioner | print |
| dm | digital media | • | two-person partnership | software |
| a | architecture | • | small partnership | motion graphics |
| | | • | collaborative studio | web |
| pd | product design | • | large studio | buildings |
| | | | | environments |
| e | engineering | • | corporation | objects |
| | | | | pre-fab housing |
| | | | | furniture |
| | | | | robotics |

Kelly Horigan

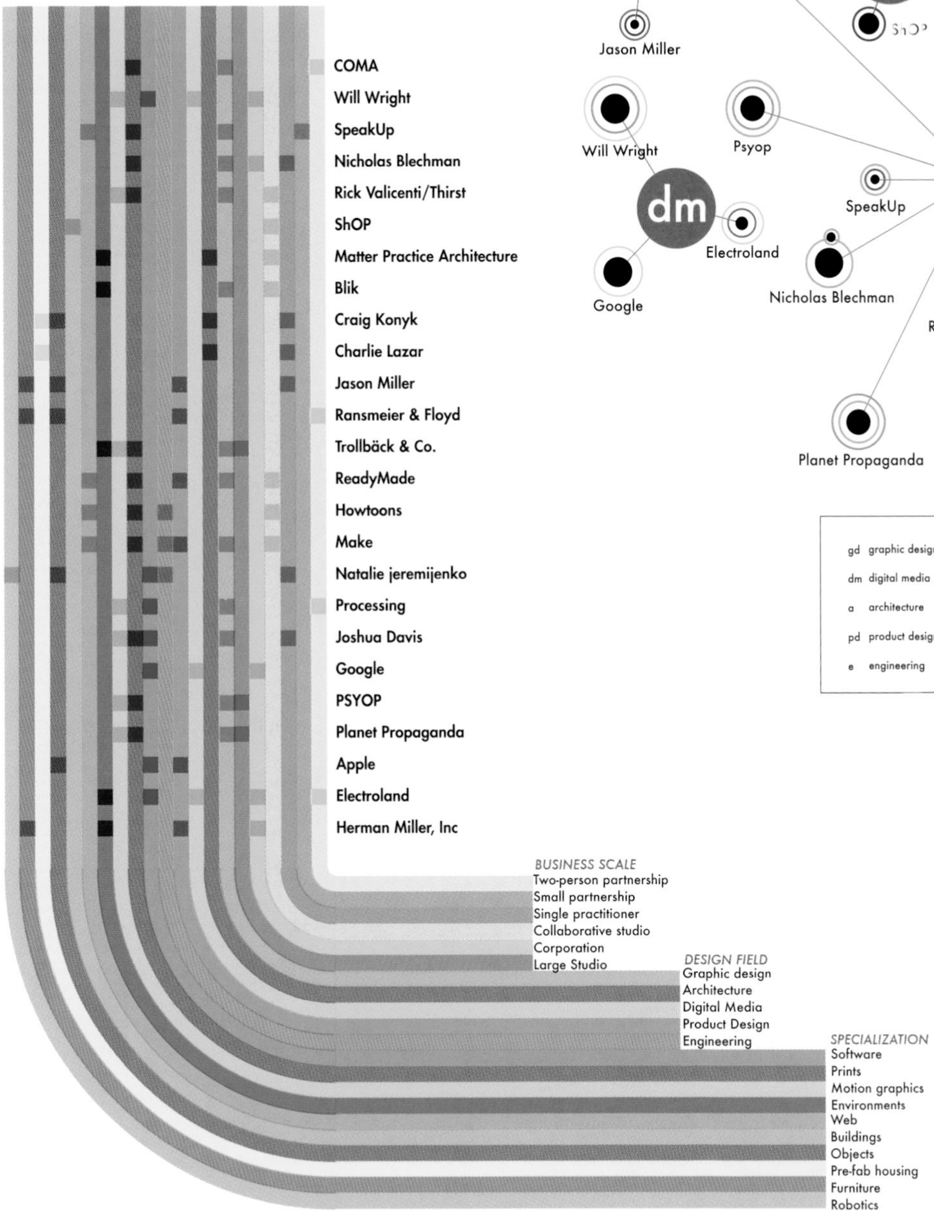

BUSINESS SCALE
Two-person partnership
Small partnership
Single practitioner
Collaborative studio
Corporation
Large Studio

DESIGN FIELD
Graphic design
Architecture
Digital Media
Product Design
Engineering

SPECIALIZATION
Software
Prints
Motion graphics
Environments
Web
Buildings
Objects
Pre-fab housing
Furniture
Robotics

Yuta Sakane

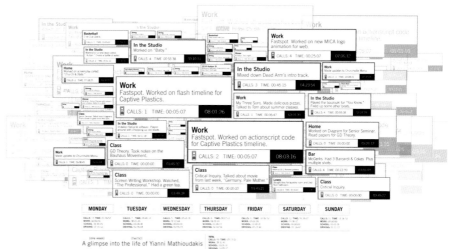

A glimpse into the life of Yianni Mathioudakis

**Biodiagram** This project asks designers to represent one facet of their lives according to a clear conceptual and visual framework. Form, color, and configuration must grow out of the hierarchy and nature of the content. Advanced Graphic Design. Jennifer Cole Phillips, faculty.

**Overworked** This diagram reflects the harried schedule of a self-supporting college student, showing his daily routines and errands. Yianni Mathioudakis.

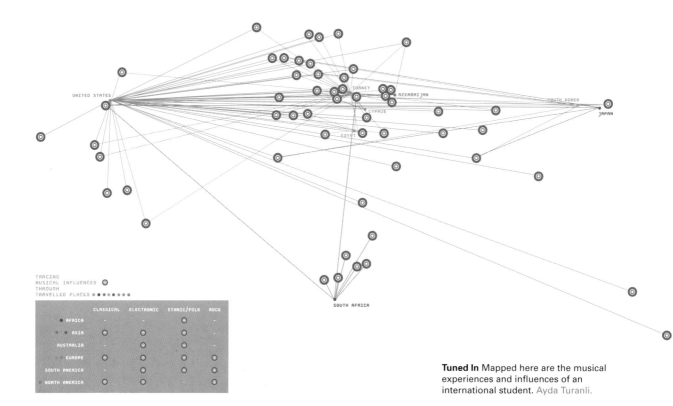

**Tuned In** Mapped here are the musical experiences and influences of an international student. Ayda Turanli.

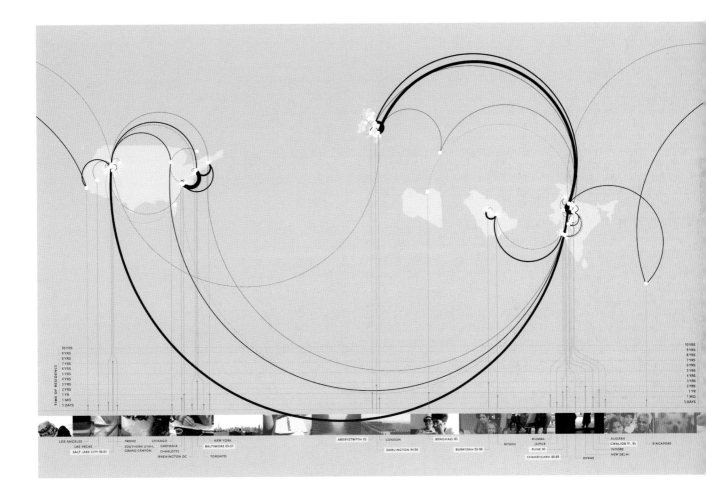

**Cosmopolitan** This diagram charts the number of days, months, and years a designer spent residing in places around the globe, illuminated with photographic, typographic, and diagrammatic details.
Meghana Khandekar.

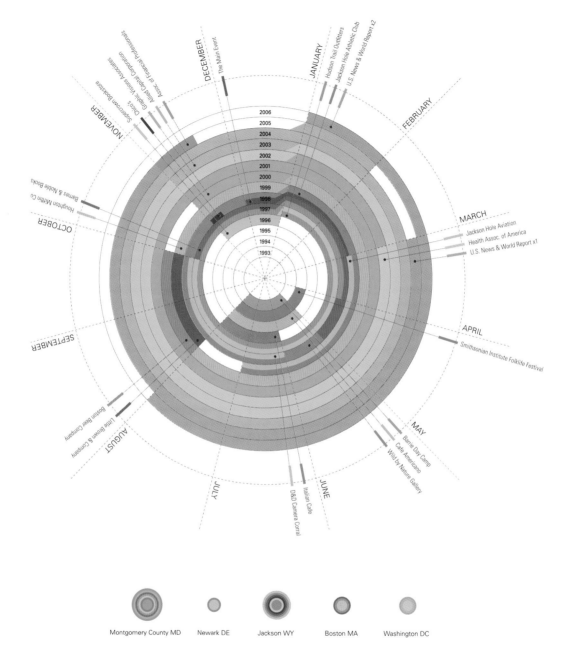

2006
2005
2004
2003
2002
2001
2000
1999
1998
1997
1996
1995
1994
1993

DECEMBER — The Main Event

JANUARY — Hudson Trail Outfitters / Jackson Hole Athletic Club / U.S. News & World Report x2

NOVEMBER — Chico's / Superctrown Bookstore / Graphic Visions Associates / Allied Capital Corporation / Assoc. of Financial Professionals

FEBRUARY

MARCH — Jackson Hole Aviation / Health Assoc. of America / U.S. News & World Report x1

OCTOBER — Houghton Mifflin Co / Barnes & Noble Books

APRIL — Smithsonian Institute Folklife Festival

SEPTEMBER

MAY — Barrie Day Camp / Cafe Americano / Wild by Nature Gallery

AUGUST — Little Brown & Company / Boston Beer Company

JULY

JUNE — Italian Cafe / D&D Camera Corral

Montgomery County MD    Newark DE    Jackson WY    Boston MA    Washington DC

**Work History** This circular diagram catalogs a designer's employment history by time and location. Kim Bentley, MFA Studio.

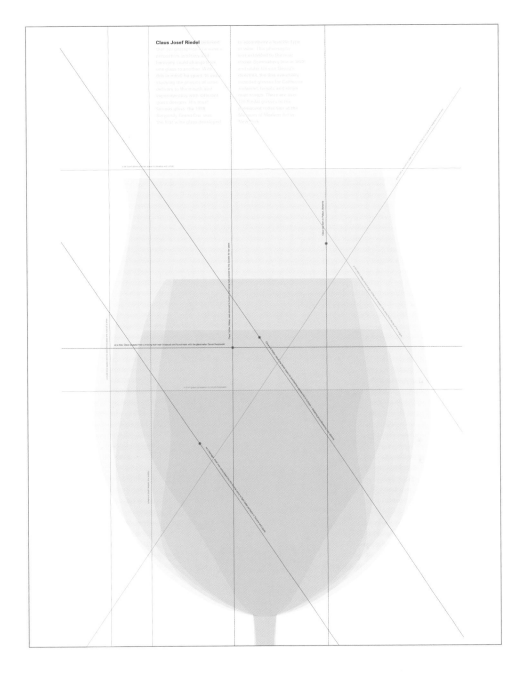

**Crystal Clear** Claus Josef Riedel was a
pioneering designer of wine glasses.
This poster illustrates Riedel's life work,
using transparent layers to represent
different shapes of stemware. Gregory May,
MFA Studio. Alicia Cheng, visiting faculty.

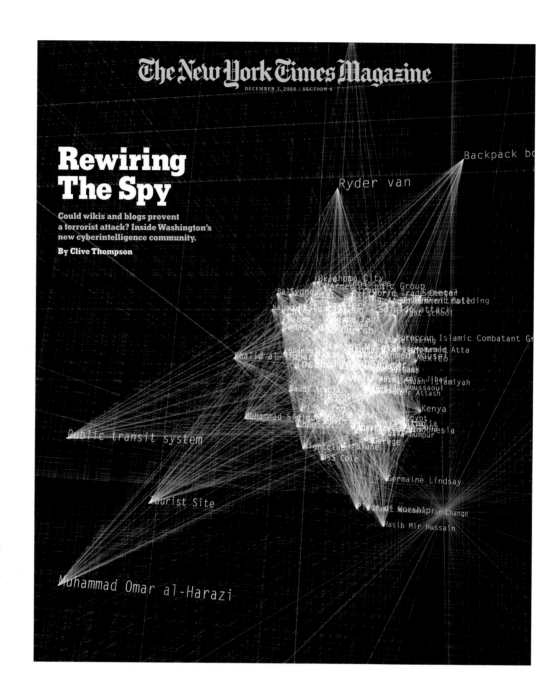

**Underground Networks** Created for the *New York Times Magazine* by media designer Lisa Strausfeld, this diagram visualizes complex relationships surrounding worldwide terrorist groups.

Produced using the computer language Processing, Strausfeld's diagram conveys the maddening difficulty involved in keeping track of countless potential links and dangers. Lisa Strausfeld, Pentagram.

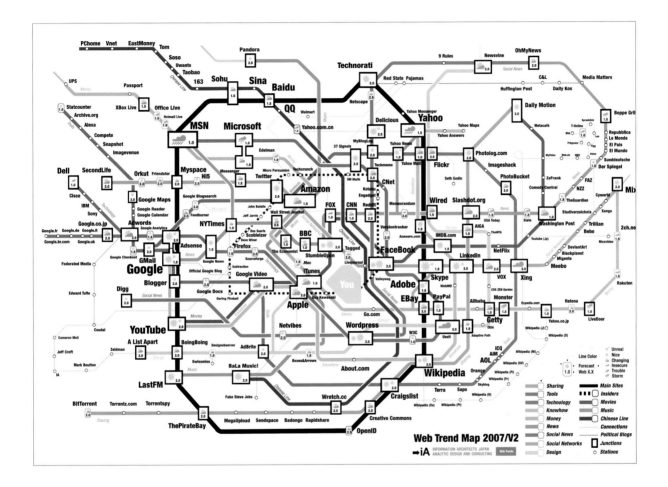

**Charting Trends** This seductive map selects and situates the world's two hundred most popular websites and classifies them according to categories such as design, music, moneymaking, and much more. The graphic is reminiscent of the subway map used in Tokyo, where this piece was designed. Information Architects.

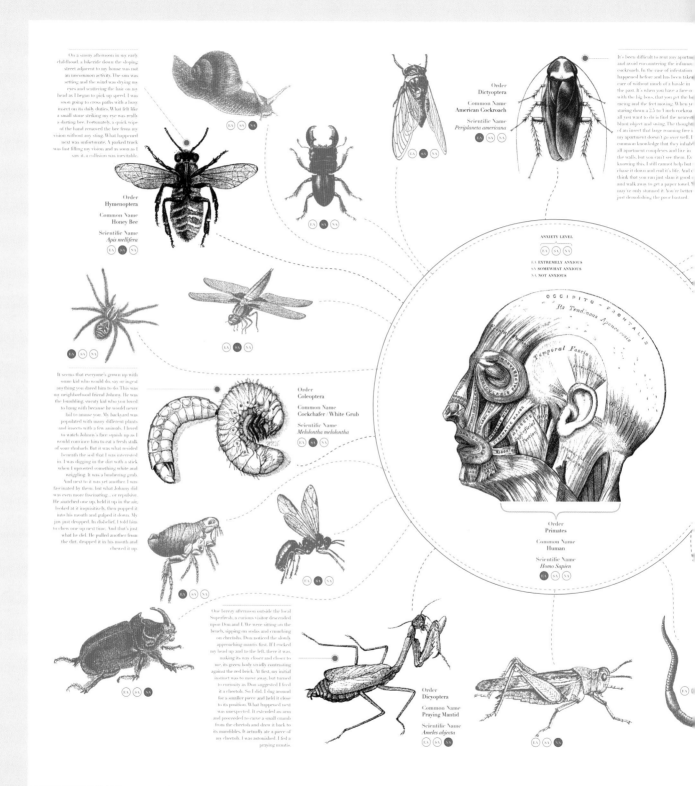

On a sunny afternoon in my early childhood, a bike ride down the sloping street adjacent to my house was not an uncommon activity. The sun was setting and the wind was drying my eyes and scattering the hair on my head as I began to pick up speed. I was soon going to cross paths with a busy insect on its daily duties. What felt like a small stone striking my eye was really a darting bee. Fortunately, a quick wipe of the hand removed the bee from my vision without any sting. What happened next was unfortunate. A parked truck was fast filling my vision and as soon as I saw it, a collision was inevitable.

It's been difficult to rent any apartment and avoid encountering the infamous cockroach. In the case of infestation happened before and has been taken care of without much of a hassle in the past. It's when you have a face-off with the big boys, that you get the heart racing and the feet moving. When you're staring down a 2.5 to 3 inch cockroach all you want to do is find the nearest blunt object and swing. The thought of an insect that large roaming free in my apartment doesn't go over well. It's common knowledge that they inhabit all apartment complexes and live in the walls, but you can't see them. Even knowing this, I still cannot help but chase it down and end it's life. And don't think that you can just slam it good and walk away to get a paper towel. It may've only stunned it. You're better just demolishing the poor bastard.

It seems that everyone's grown up with some kid who would do, say or ingest anything you dared him to do. This was my neighborhood friend Johnny. He was the bumbling, sweaty kid who you loved to hang with because he would never fail to amuse you. My backyard was populated with many different plants and insects with a few animals. I loved to watch Johnny's face squish up as I would convince him to eat a fresh stalk of sour rhubarb. But it was what resided beneath the soil that I was interested in. I was digging in the dirt with a stick when I uncovered something white and wriggling. It was a lumbering grub. And next to it was yet another. I was fascinated by them, but what Johnny did was even more fascinating... or repulsive. He snatched one up, held it up in the air, looked at it inquisitively, then popped it into his mouth and gulped it down. My jaw just dropped. In disbelief, I told him to chew one up next time. And that's just what he did. He pulled another from the dirt, dropped it in his mouth and chewed it up.

One breezy afternoon outside the local Superfresh, a curious visitor descended upon Don and I. We were sitting on the bench, sipping on sodas and crunching on cheetohs. Don noticed the slowly approaching mantis first. If I cocked my head up and to the left, there it was, making its way closer and closer to me, its green body vividly contrasting against the red brick. At first, my initial instinct was to move away, but turned to curiosity as Don suggested I feed it a cheetoh. So I did. I dug around for a smaller piece and held it close to its position. What happened next was unexpected. It extended an arm and proceeded to carve a small crumb from the cheetoh and drew it back to its mandibles. It actually ate a piece of my cheetoh. I was astonished. I fed a praying mantis.

Order
Hymenoptera

Common Name
Honey Bee

Scientific Name
*Apis mellifera*

Order
Dictyoptera

Common Name
American Cockroach

Scientific Name
*Periplaneta americana*

Order
Coleoptera

Common Name
Cockchafer / White Grub

Scientific Name
*Melolontha melolontha*

ANXIETY LEVEL

EA EXTREMELY ANXIOUS
SA SOMEWHAT ANXIOUS
NA NOT ANXIOUS

Order
Primates

Common Name
Human

Scientific Name
*Homo Sapien*

Order
Dicyoptera

Common Name
Praying Mantid

Scientific Name
*Ameles abjecta*

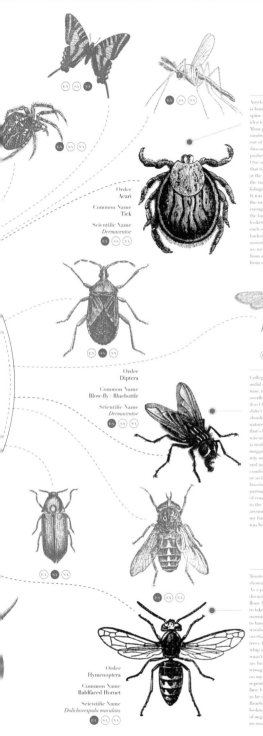

Order
Acari

Common Name
Tick

Scientific Name
*Dermacentor*

Order
Diptera

Common Name
Blow-fly / Bluebottle

Scientific Name
*Dermacentor*

Order
Hymenoptera

Common Name
Baldfaced Hornet

Scientific Name
*Dolichovespula maculata*

Anything tiny, mobile and blood-sucking is bound to send a shiver down my spine. It always seemed like a great idea to go to the park when I was a kid. Mom packed up the wagon and bologna sandwiches while Dad drug our asses out of bed. I laced up my awesome dinosaur converse sneaks as my brother pushed me over on his way out the door. One small detail we failed to realize was that tick season was in full force. Once at the park, we made our way around the trails, up and over rocks, roots and foliage when we began to feel the itch. It was as if they were raining from the trees. As I stood and stared long enough, I could watch as one landed on the back of my sister's leg. We must've looked like monkeys's fingering through each other's hair and examining our backsides, pulling off the little parasitic monstrosities. It wasn't long at all until we were back in the car, headed away from anything that could extract fluids from our bodies.

College dorms can breed some pretty awful situations with pests. Word to the wise, it's a huge mistake to let the trash overflow. When you are on trash duty, don't hesitate to dispose. My roommates didn't handle the trash as often as they should've. The result was Biblical in nature. A plague if you will. At least that's how it felt. How it really happened was unknown, but a high probability is resting on the fact that somehow maggots slithered and wriggled their way underneath the carpet lining and under the molding, making a comfortable home in the walls. A day or so later and you wake to a horrible buzzing sound at your balcony windows, parting the curtains to reveal a mass of confused and hungry flies, clinging to the windows. I could literally walk around the apartment with a vacuum in my hands, sucking them from the air. It was hell in a dorm.

Territorial insects are persistent in showing you where you shouldn't be. As a piece of advice, stay away from decaying coniferous trees on the forest floor. My friend Don and I decided to take a long walk one early summer morning, in exploration of new places to hang out. Veering from a path in the woods, we decided to check out a rocky overhang and took a rest on some fallen trees. I noticed a decidedly irrated fly whip around my head over and over. It wasn't long until I noticed it land on my head, swatting it away. That was the wrong thing to do. It proceeded to land on my upper lip, forehead and cheeks, repeatedly drilling it's stinger into my face. I shot up and ran. Don following as he quickly became a target as well. Reaching the roadside, we ran and ran, looking behind us in horror as a cloud of angry, buzzing pain was gathering for an assault.

## Diagramming Editorial Content

Contemporary magazine design often breaks up content, dispersing elements across the page and integrating words and images to create engaging, nonlinear experiences for readers. Principles of diagramming and mapping are thus used to organize narrative in a spatial way. Information graphics typically combine visual and verbal information, requiring mastery of both typography and composition. The literate human mind has no difficulty switching between seeing and reading.

**Insect Phobia** This map studies the designer's fear of various insects. The bugs with the most potent negative associations are denoted in black; lesser ones are green. An additional system calls out degrees of fear with circled letters, from extremely anxious (EA) to somewhat anxious (SA) and not anxious (NA). Memorable insect stories are recounted via warm, well-written narratives.
Jacob Lockard, Advanced Graphic Design.
Jennifer Cole Phillips, faculty.

# THE
# SORDID
## UNDERBELLY
### OF ONE GIRL'S
# FILTHY
## APARTMENT

**A TRAGIC TALE TOLD IN 4 PARTS**
13 SECTIONS, 8 SUBSECTIONS, & 1 SUBSET

**UNDER THE BATHROOM SINK:**
2 bobby pins
1 ponytail elastic
1 cottonball
1 #2 pencil
1 cotton swab
$.06

**UNDER THE NIGHTSTAND:**
1 pair of down slippers
1 CD walkman
1 fuzzy pink knit hat
1 drimmel tool, with
   sander attachment
1 cough drop
3 dust bunnies
$.35

**UNDER THE DRESSER:**
1 pair of ugly tall black boots
1 pair of pretty tall brown boots
1 cordless phone
1 box of old photos
3 ponytail elastics
2 straw wrappers
1 dead leaf
1 dead beetle
$.51

12 BLACK-AND-WHITE FAMILY PHOTOS
20 FROM MY TRIP TO IRELAND
15 FROM MY FIRST 5 YEARS IN NYC
5 OF ME AND MY BROTHER AS KIDS
10 FROM MY CHUBBY YEARS

**UNDER THE BED:**
1 air mattress pump
2 flat air mattresses
2 glass bead garlands
1 pair of dark green wellies
1 coffee-stained issue of *Vogue*
1 storage bin of winter clothing
1 leopard-print slipper
1 holey sock
1 tube of cherry lip gloss
1 dead cricket
5 dust bunnies
$1.13

1 PAIR OF CORDUROYS
3 HEAVY SWEATERS
3 LONG-SLEEVE T-SHIRTS
2 PAIRS OF THERMAL UNDIES
8 PAIRS OF WOOL KNEE SOCKS
3 PAIRS OF GRAY KNIT TIGHTS

**BEHIND THE BED:**
2 rolling suitcases
1 military issue
   sleeping bag
1 box of tax records
3 argyle socks
1 black bikini
1 large beach towel
1 dusty cough drop
$.67

**UNDER THE BOOKCASE:**
1 paperback of *Jane Eyre*
3 tangled extension cords
1 pair of unflattering sunglasses
$.87

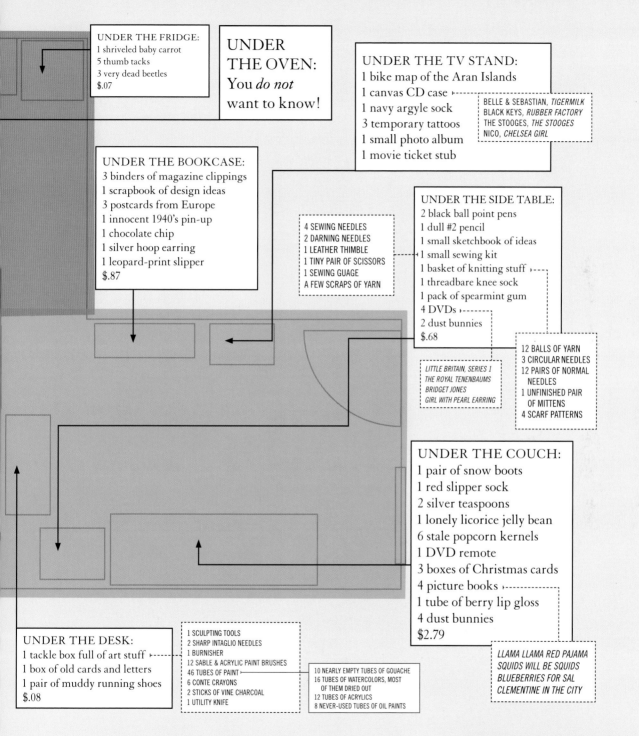

**UNDER THE FRIDGE:**
1 shriveled baby carrot
5 thumb tacks
3 very dead beetles
$.07

**UNDER THE OVEN:**
You *do not*
want to know!

**UNDER THE TV STAND:**
1 bike map of the Aran Islands
1 canvas CD case
1 navy argyle sock
3 temporary tattoos
1 small photo album
1 movie ticket stub

BELLE & SEBASTIAN, *TIGERMILK*
BLACK KEYS, *RUBBER FACTORY*
THE STOOGES, *THE STOOGES*
NICO, *CHELSEA GIRL*

**UNDER THE BOOKCASE:**
3 binders of magazine clippings
1 scrapbook of design ideas
3 postcards from Europe
1 innocent 1940's pin-up
1 chocolate chip
1 silver hoop earring
1 leopard-print slipper
$.87

4 SEWING NEEDLES
2 DARNING NEEDLES
1 LEATHER THIMBLE
1 TINY PAIR OF SCISSORS
1 SEWING GUAGE
A FEW SCRAPS OF YARN

**UNDER THE SIDE TABLE:**
2 black ball point pens
1 dull #2 pencil
1 small sketchbook of ideas
1 small sewing kit
1 basket of knitting stuff
1 threadbare knee sock
1 pack of spearmint gum
4 DVDs
2 dust bunnies
$.68

*LITTLE BRITAIN, SERIES 1*
*THE ROYAL TENENBAUMS*
*BRIDGET JONES*
*GIRL WITH PEARL EARRING*

12 BALLS OF YARN
3 CIRCULAR NEEDLES
12 PAIRS OF NORMAL
   NEEDLES
1 UNFINISHED PAIR
   OF MITTENS
4 SCARF PATTERNS

**UNDER THE COUCH:**
1 pair of snow boots
1 red slipper sock
2 silver teaspoons
1 lonely licorice jelly bean
6 stale popcorn kernels
1 DVD remote
3 boxes of Christmas cards
4 picture books
1 tube of berry lip gloss
4 dust bunnies
$2.79

*LLAMA LLAMA RED PAJAMA*
*SQUIDS WILL BE SQUIDS*
*BLUEBERRIES FOR SAL*
*CLEMENTINE IN THE CITY*

**UNDER THE DESK:**
1 tackle box full of art stuff
1 box of old cards and letters
1 pair of muddy running shoes
$.08

1 SCULPTING TOOLS
2 SHARP INTAGLIO NEEDLES
1 BURNISHER
12 SABLE & ACRYLIC PAINT BRUSHES
46 TUBES OF PAINT
6 CONTE CRAYONS
2 STICKS OF VINE CHARCOAL
1 UTILITY KNIFE

10 NEARLY EMPTY TUBES OF GOUACHE
16 TUBES OF WATERCOLORS, MOST
   OF THEM DRIED OUT
12 TUBES OF ACRYLICS
8 NEVER-USED TUBES OF OIL PAINTS

**List Mania** This clever editorial layout
recounts every object found underneath
the furniture in a designer's apartment.
Elements are keyed to locations in the
apartment. Kelley McIntyre, MFA Studio.

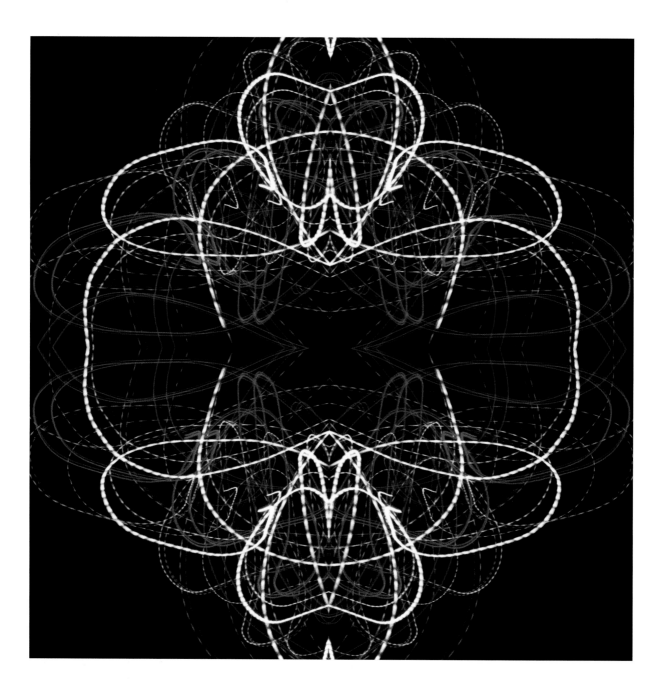

# Time and Motion

**Long Exposure Photography** A camera can capture a path of lights moving over time. The oscillations of AC currents are not visible to the eye, but, when recorded through a camera lens, the oscillations create a dashed line. DC currents generate smooth lines. Here, a single long-exposure photograph has been repeated and rotated to create a larger visual shape. Sarah Joy Jordahl Verville, MFA Studio.

Time and motion are closely related principles. Any word or image that moves functions both spatially and temporally. Motion is a kind of change, and change takes place in time. Motion can be implied as well as literal, however. Artists have long sought ways to represent the movement of bodies and the passage of time within the realm of static, two-dimensional space. Time and motion are considerations for all design work, from a multipage printed book, whose pages follow each other in time, to animations for film and television, which have literal duration.

Any still image has implied motion (or implied stasis), while motion graphics share compositional principles with print. Designers today routinely work in time-based media as well as print, and a design campaign often must function across multiple media simultaneously.

Animation encompasses diverse modes of visible change, including the literal movement of elements that fly on or off the screen as well as changes in scale, transparency, color, layer, and more. These alternative modes of change are especially useful for designing animated text on the web, where gratuitous movement can be more distracting than pleasing or informative.

It can be useful to think about the screen as an active, changing surface as well as a neutral stage or support onto which characters rush on and off. Thus a fixed field of dots, for example, can light up sequentially to spell out a message, or objects can become visible or invisible as the background behind them changes color or transparency. A word or design element can stay still while the environment around it changes.

Film is a visual art. Designers of motion graphics must think both like painters and typographers and like animators and filmmakers. A motion sequence is developed through a series of storyboards, which convey the main phases and movements of an animation. A style frame serves to establish the visual elements of a project, such as its colors, typefaces, illustrative components, and more. Such frames must be designed with the same attentiveness to composition, scale, color, and other principles as any work of design. In addition, the motion designer thinks about how all these components will change and interact with each other over time.

This chapter introduces some basic principles for conveying temporal change and motion, both in still and time-based media.

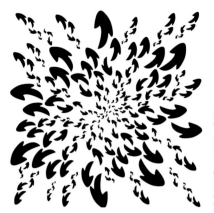

**Eruption of Form**
These shapes as well as their explosive arrangement suggest movement and change. Sasha Funk, Graphic Design I. Zvezdana Rogic, faculty.

## Implied Motion

Graphic designers use numerous techniques to suggest change and movement on the printed page. Diagonal compositions evoke motion, while rectilinear arrangements appear static. Cropping a shape can suggest motion, as does a sinuous line or a pointed, triangular shape.

**Static** A centered object sitting parallel to the edges of the frame appears stable and unmoving.

**Diagonal** An object placed on a diagonal appears dynamic.

**Cropped** An object that is partly cut off appears to be moving into or out of the frame.

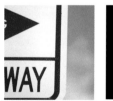

**Point the Way** The shape of an arrow indicates movement. Robert Ferrell and Geoff Hanssler, Digital Imaging. Nancy Froehlich, faculty.

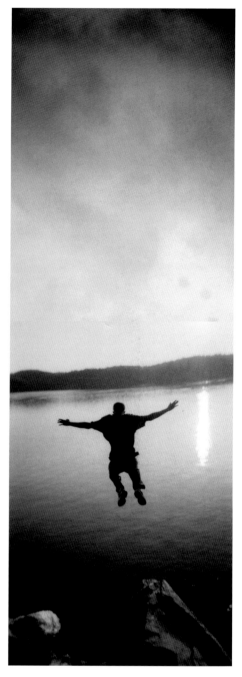

**Moment in Time** A skilled photographer can capture a moving object at a dramatic instant. Steve Sheets, Digital Imaging. Nancy Froehlich, faculty.

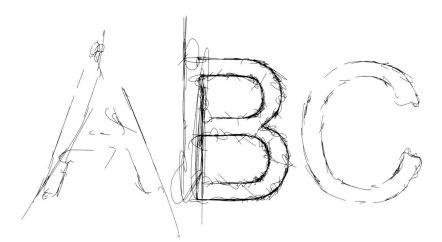

**Restless Line** These scratchy, sketchy lines contrast with the static letterforms they describe. The letters were drawn with Processing code. Ahn Yeohyun, MFA Studio.

**Dimensional Line** The dimensionality of these curving lines gives them movement in depth. The letters were manipulated in Adobe Illustrator. Ryan Gladhill, MFA Studio.

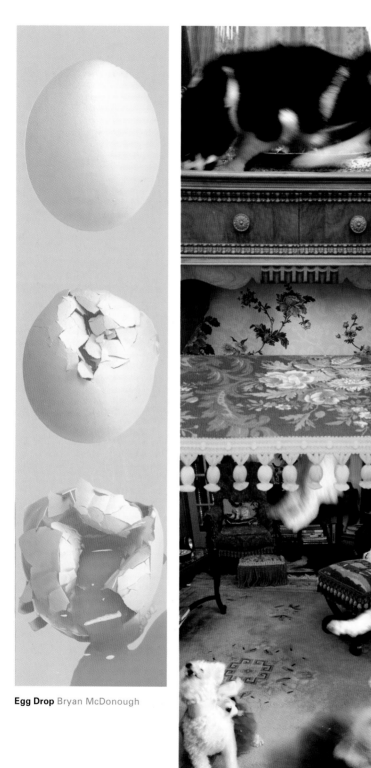

**Egg Drop** Bryan McDonough

**Sequential Time** Showing images in a row is an accepted way to represent time or movement on a two-dimensional surface. Drawings or photographs become like words in a sentence, linked together to tell a story. The designs shown here use cropping, sequence, and placement to suggest time and movement. Digital Imaging. Nancy Froehlich, faculty.

**Cat Walk** Sam Trapkin

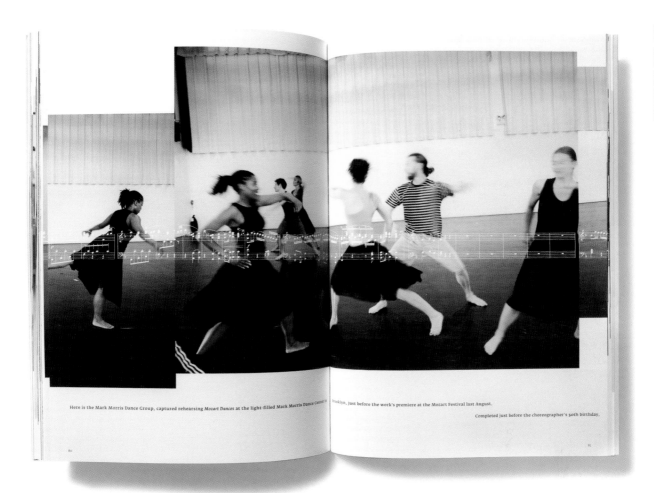

Here is the Mark Morris Dance Group, captured rehearsing *Mozart Dances* at the light-filled Mark Morris Dance Center in Brooklyn, just before the work's premiere at the Mozart Festival last August.

Completed just before the choreographer's 50th birthday.

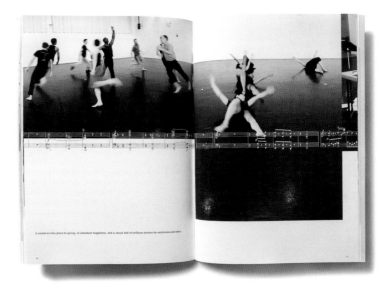

It seems to take place in spring, in abundant happiness, and is chock full of brilliant devices for entrances and exits.

**Connecting Time and Space** In these layouts for a photo essay documenting a piece by choreographer Mark Morris, the floor line becomes a point of connection, bringing together numerous shots taken over time. Abbott Miller and Kristen Spilman, Pentagram. *2wice* magazine. Photography: Katherine Wolkoff.

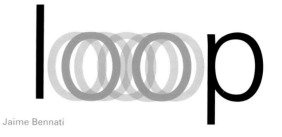

Jaime Bennati

**Implied Time and Motion** An effective logotype can be applied to anything from a tiny business card to a large-scale architectural sign to a computer screen or digital projection. The logotypes shown here use a variety of graphic strategies to imply motion.

In this project, designers created a graphic identity for a conference about contemporary media art and theory called "Loop." Each solution explores the concept of the loop as a continuous, repeating sequence. The designers applied each logo to a banner in an architectural setting and to a screen-based looping animation. (Photoshop was used to simulate the installation of the banners in a real physical space.)

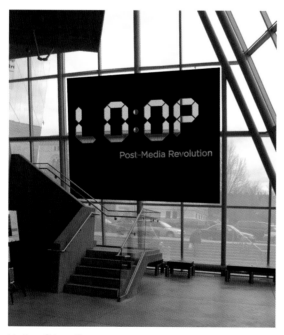

Lindsay Orlowski

**Loop Logo** Numerous techniques are used in these studies of the word "loop" to imply movement and repetition. Some designs suggest the duration of the design process itself by exposing the interface or by drawing the logo with an endless, looping line. Above, transparency is used to create an onion-skin effect; cropping the logo on the banner further implies movement. Graphic Design II. Ellen Lupton, faculty.

loop

LOOP

loop

88:88

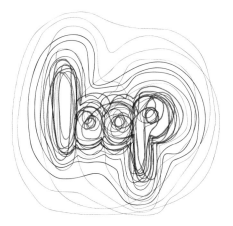

LOOP

May Yang
Sueyun Choi
Lauretta Dolch

Alexandra Matzner
Lindsay Orlowski
Yuta Sakane

**Key Frames** Depicted here are important moments within a dancer's continuous leap. Sarah Joy Jordahl Verville, MFA Studio.

## Animation Basics

Like film and other "motion pictures,"animation uses sequences of still images to create the optical illusion of movement. The brain retains images for a split-second longer than the images are actually before us, resulting in the illusion of movement when numerous images appear in rapid succession. This phenomenon is called "persistence of vision." As images appear to move and come alive, the illusion is powerful and fascinating. Images for animation can be created via software, photography, and drawing.

The smallest unit of animation is the frame, a single still image. In the technique of frame-by-frame animation, a series of still images are drawn or digitally created. These still images differ from frame to frame by successive deviations in scale, orientation, color, shape, layer, and/or transparency.

In producing animation, the most important frames, called "key frames," are the fixed states that a lead designer draws or creates. In both hand-drawn and digital animation, these key frames are normally the first and last frames of each short sequence of action, indicating the start and conclusion of one or more important changes in movement. For example, the key animator may create the frame of a person about to do a cartwheel and another key frame of that same person landing at the completion of the cartwheel. Assistant artists, known as "inbetweeners," then fill in the gap by drawing the missing in-between frames, which are called "tweens." The tweens can also be generated automatically by digital animation software, which automates the time-consuming production process while making a smooth transition over time between the key frames. The process of developing these in-between frames is called "tweening."

Some professional designers and animators prefer drawing all their images using the frame-by-frame animation process, rather than by automated tweening, because it provides cleaner edges, better quality of motion, more accurate details, and greater control of subtle elements such as facial expressions. However, frame-by-frame animation is more time-consuming to produce than computer-generated motion and can result in inconsistent images. Computer-generated tweening can cause jerky lines and unwanted shadows, but it has several advantages as well. The computer's memory can provide access to databases that store previously rendered people, landscapes, buildings, and other objects, and these renderings can be used repeatedly, saving time and production costs. In addition, with computer-generated frames designers can easily adjust such variables as timing, orientation, color, layering, and scale.

In general, typography and abstract graphic elements are easily animated via automatic tweening, as compared to facial expressions or complex bodily movements.

Research and writing assistance: Sarah Joy Jordahl Verville

**Composite Time and Motion** Nine frames are compressed into one image. Color moves from warm to cool, and layers accumulate from back to front, depicting change over time. The assets of animation are thus used here to compose a still image. Sarah Joy Jordahl Verville, MFA Studio.

**Change in Position** Every object on a two-dimensional surface has a pair of x/y coordinates. Changing the coordinates moves the object. (3-D animation includes the z axis.) In this sequence, the object's x position is changing, while the y position is fixed, yielding a horizontal movement.

## Change Over Time

All animation consists of change over time. The most obvious form of change consists of an element moving around on the screen—the Road Runner approach. The Road Runner can "walk" onto the screen like a character in a play, or it can appear there suddenly as in a cut in a film.

Changing the position of an object is just one way to make it change. Other modes of change include shifting its scale, color, shape, and transparency. By altering the degree of change and the speed with which the change takes place, the animator produces different qualities of movement. Complex and subtle behaviors are created by using different modes of change simultaneously. For example, an object can fade slowly onto the screen (changing transparency) while also getting bigger (changing in scale).

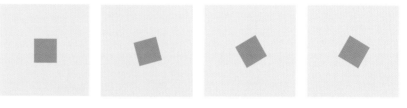

**Change in Rotation** Continuously altering the angle of an object creates the appearance of spinning, shaking, and other behaviors.

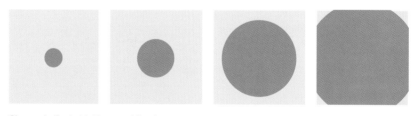

**Change in Scale** Making an object larger or smaller creates the impression of it moving backward or forward in space. Here, the object is not moving (changing its position); only its size is changing.

**Change in Shape** Letting a line wander can produce all types of shapes: abstract, amorphous, representational.

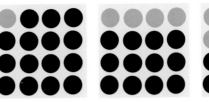
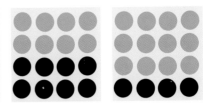

**Change in Color** Like a theater marquee that creates the appearance of movement by sequentially turning light bulbs on and off, color animation creates motion by sequentially illuminating or changing the color of predefined areas or objects.

Here, a wave of color appears to pass over a field of static objects. Countless variations are possible.

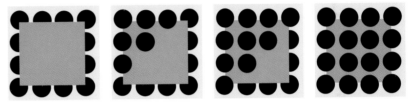

**Change in Depth** Many image-editing programs allow the designer to divide an image into layers, which are comparable to the sheets of transparent acetate used in traditional cell animation.

Layers can be duplicated, deleted, altered to support new image elements, merged into a single image, and hidden. Here, objects on back layers gradually move forward.

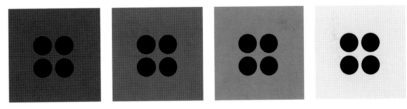

**Change in Transparency** Animators alter the transparency of an image to give it the appearance of fading in or out of view. Here, the top layer gradually becomes more transparent, revealing an image behind it.

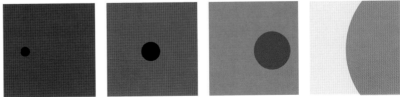
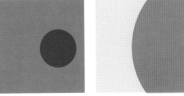

**Multiple Modes of Change** Most animations combine several modes of change at once.

This sequence incorporates changes in position, scale, color, and transparency.

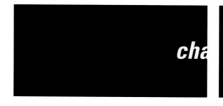

**Change in Position** Moving text around the screen is the most basic means of animating type. Commonly, type enters from the right side of the screen and moves left to support the normal direction of reading. Ticker or leader text also tends to move in this direction.

## Animating Type

In film and television and on the web, text is often in motion. Animating type is like animating other graphic elements, but the designer must pay special attention to legibility and reading order.

The most elementary technique is to shift the position of a word so that it appears to move around like a character or other object. Animated words do not have to literally move, however: they can fade in or fade out; they can flicker on or off the screen letter by letter; or they can change scale, color, layer, and so on.

When animating text, the designer adjusts the timing to make sure the words change slowly enough to be legible, but not so slowly that they become a drag to read. Context also is important. A constantly changing logo in a web banner, for example, will quickly become irritating, whereas sudden and constant motion in the title sequence of a film can help set the tone for the action to come.

**Change in Color** In the sequence shown here, the type itself is static, but a color change moves across the text letter by letter. Endless variations of this basic kind of change are possible.

**Change in Transparency** White type appears gradually on screen by gradually becoming opaque.

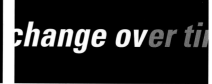

**Multiple Modes of Change** Many animations combine several techniques at once.

This sequence features change in position, scale, and transparency.

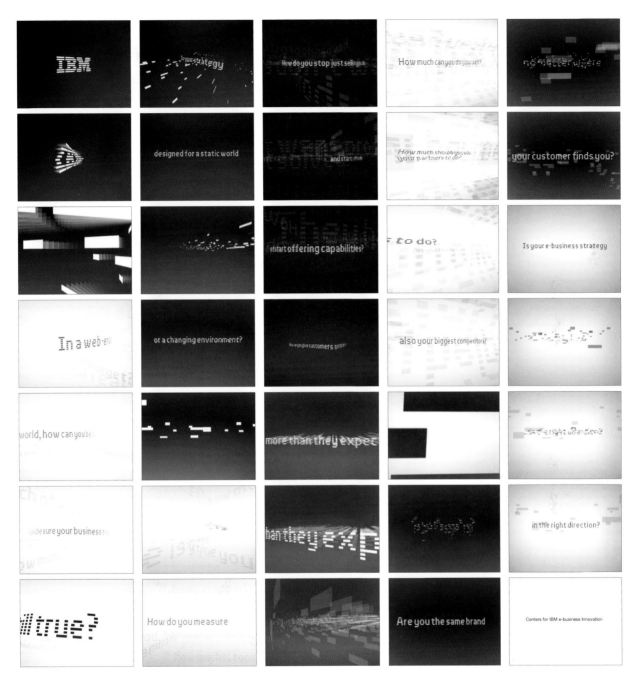

**Animated Typography** In this animation by Peter Cho, each letter is built from pixel-like units. The individual units as well as complete letters, words, and phrases are subject to change. Elements move in three-dimensional space and they change scale, color, and transparency.

All these complex and simultaneous changes serve to emphasize the text and make the message readable over time. Peter Cho, Imaginary Forces, 2000, for the Centers for IBM e-Business Innovation.

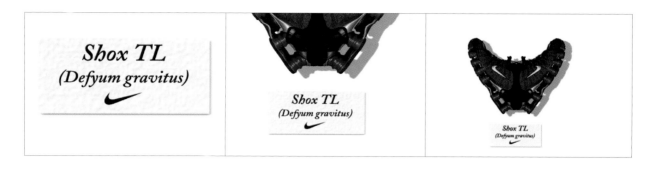

## Storyboard

Since motion design can be labor-intensive, designers must plan carefully every aspect of a piece before production begins. Once a concept is developed, the script is fleshed out with storyboard sketches and a style frame. These visual tools are essential for designing commercials, online banners, television broadcast animations, and film title sequences.

Storyboards summarize the content or key moments of an animation's events. Storyboarding also determines the flow of the storyline and suggests the major changes of action. In addition to movements, the personality, emotions, and gestures of the characters and objects are also expressed. The layout of a storyboard, similar to that of a comic strip, consists of sketches or illustrations displayed sequentially to visualize an animated or live-action piece. Notes describing camera angles, soundtrack, movement, special effects, timing, and transitions between scenes are often included.

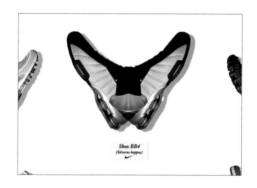

## Style Frame

The ultimate look of an animation is expressed in one or more style frames, which set the aesthetic tone and formal elements. A style frame captures many of the graphic elements used throughout the piece. The typography, colors, patterns, illustrations, and photographs chosen for the project are often included.

Storyboarding and developing style frames are creative processes that allow the designer to plan and brainstorm before the animation is realized. These tools serve as guides to production and vehicles for presentation to clients. Successful style frames and storyboards are always clearly defined and easy to interpret.

**Metamorphosis** This animated advertisement for Nike shoes, designed by Trollbäck and Company, presents golf shoes that are mounted like butterflies in a museum frame. The shoes come to life and fly away. The meaning of the scene changes as the camera moves in and out to reveal the context.

Director: Joe Wright. Designers: Jens Mebes, Todd Neale, Justin Meredith. Creative Directors: Jakob Trollbäck and Joe Wright. Editor: Cass Vanini. Producer: Elizabeth Kiehner. Client: Nike, Ron Dumas.

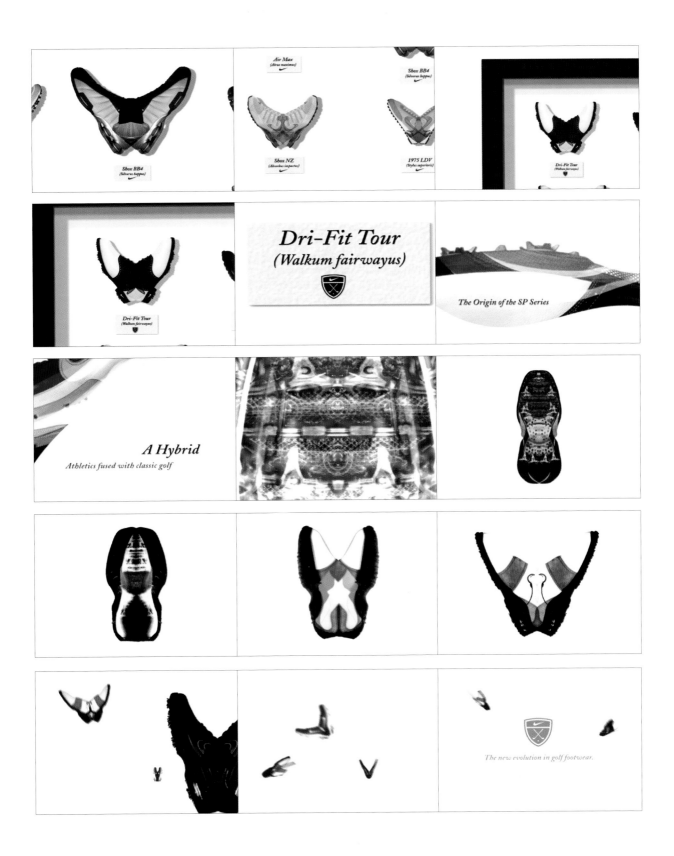

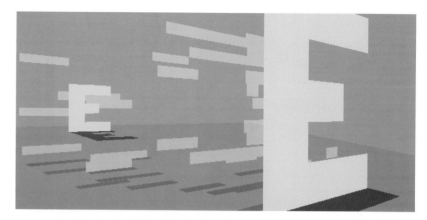

## Beyond the Timeline

Interactive logos and graphics are another aspect of motion design. Rather than devising a narrative sequence with a fixed beginning and end, the interactive designer creates behaviors. These behaviors involve change over time, just like narrative animations, but they do not occur in a fixed sequence, and they are not designed using storyboards and timelines.

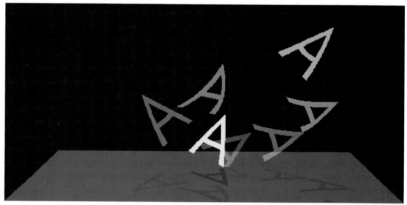

Interactive graphics are created with code, such as Flash ActionScript, Java, or Processing. Instead of working with the interface of a linear timeline, the designer writes functions, variables, if/then statements, and other instructions to define how the graphics will behave.

Interactive graphics need not be complex or hyperactive. Simple behaviors can delight users and enrich the experience of a digital interface. For example, an interactive logo on a webpage can wait quietly until it is touched with the user's mouse; instead of being an annoying distraction, the graphics come to life only when called upon to do so.

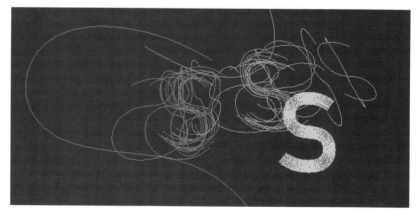

**Letterscapes** In these interactive graphics by Peter Cho, the letters dance, bounce, unravel, and otherwise transform themselves in response to mouse input. Peter Cho, 2002.

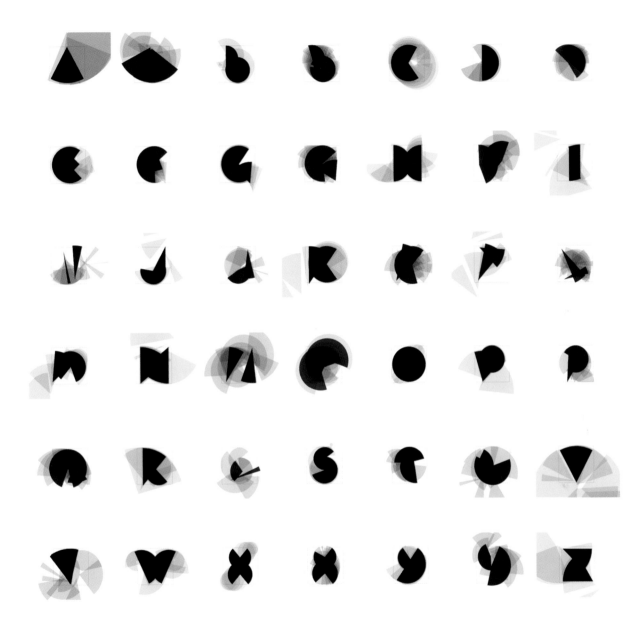

**Type Me Again** Simple pie shapes rotate
and repeat to create the letters of the
alphabet when users type in letters on their
keyboards. Peter Cho, 2000.

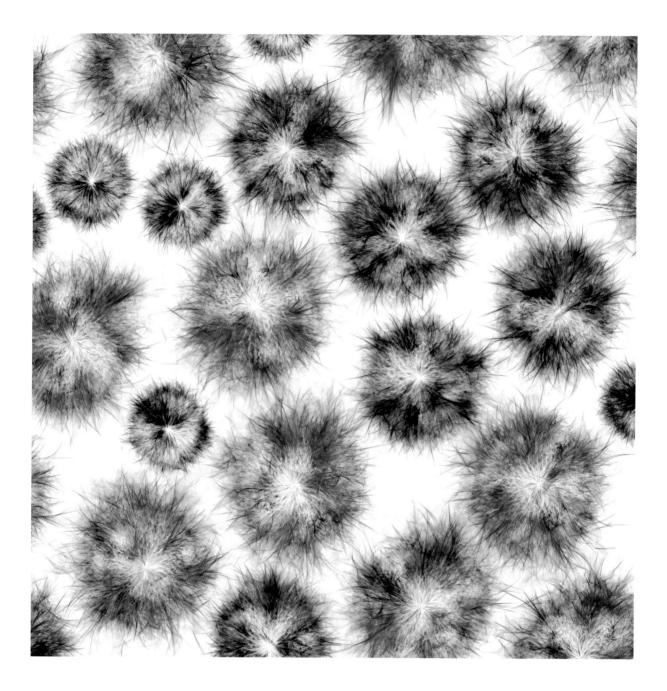

# Rules and Randomness

The idea becomes a **machine** that makes the art. Sol LeWitt

Designers create rules as well as finished pieces. A magazine designer, for example, works with a grid and a typographic hierarchy that is interpreted in different ways, page after page, issue after issue. If the rules are well planned, other designers will be able to interpret them to produce their own unique and unexpected layouts. Rules create a framework for design without determining the end results.

Style sheets employed in print and web publishing (CSS) are rules for displaying the different parts of a document. By adjusting a style sheet, the designer can change the appearance of an entire book or website. Style sheets are used to reconfigure a single body of content for output in different media, from printed pages to the screen of a mobile phone.

Rules can be used to generate form as well as organize content. In the 1920s, the Bauhaus artist and designer László Moholy-Nagy created a painting by telephoning a set of instructions to a sign painter. In the 1960s, the minimalist artist Sol LeWitt created drawings based on simple instructions; the drawings could be executed on a wall or other surface anywhere in the world by following the directions. Complex webs of lines often resulted from seemingly simple verbal instructions.

Designers produce rules in computer code as well as natural language. C. E. B. Reas, who co-authored the software language Processing, creates rich digital drawings and interactive works that evolve from instructions and variables. Reas alters the outcome by changing the variables. He explains, "Sometimes I set strict rules, follow them, and then observe the results. More frequently, I begin with a core software behavior, implement it, and then observe the results. I then allow the piece to flow intuitively from there."[1] Reas and other contemporary artists are using software as a medium unto itself rather than as a tool supporting the design process.

Designing rules and instructions is an intrinsic part of the design process. Increasingly, designers are asked to create systems that other people will implement and that will change over time. This chapter looks at ways to use rule-based processes to generate unexpected visual results.

**Unnatural Growth** Created in Processing, this work by C. E. B. Reas resembles an organic process. The forms are created in response to rules governing the behavior of an initial set of points. The work builds over time as the program runs through its iterations. C. E. B. Reas. *Process 6 (Image 3)*, 2005 (detail).

1. C. E. B. Reas, "Process/Drawing," (Statement for the exhibition at the bitforms gallery, New York, March 4–April 2, 2005).

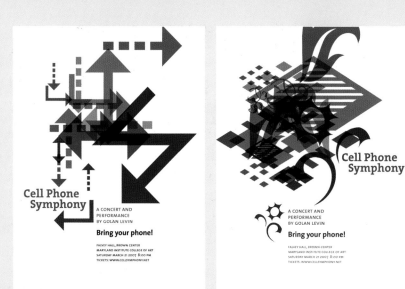

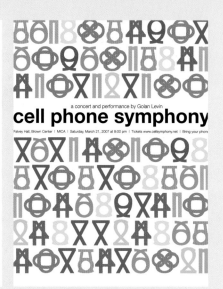

Numbers are replaced with icons from different symbol fonts. Marleen Kuijf.

Strange hieroglyphs are created by doubling and flipping each numeral. Katie Evans.

**Cell Phone Symphony** In the project shown here, students were given a list of phone numbers from which to generate visual imagery for a poster. The posters promote a "cell phone symphony," featuring music composed via interaction among the audience's cell phones.

Each poster suggests auditory experience as well as ideas of social and technological interaction. The students took numerous different approaches, from turning each phone number into a linear graph to using the digits to set the size and color of objects in a grid.

Designing the system is part of the creative process. The visual results have an organic quality that comes from random input to the system. The designer controls and manipulates the system itself rather than the final outcome. Graphic Design II. Ellen Lupton, faculty.

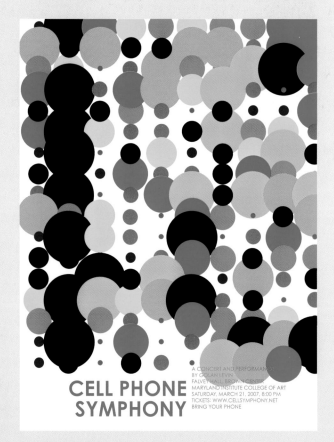

Numbers are used to set the color and size of dots on a grid. Hayley Griffin.

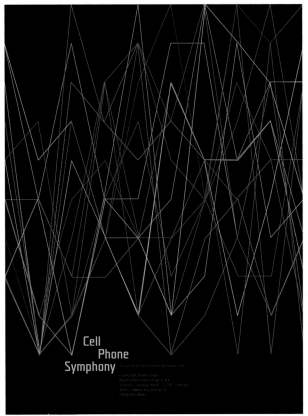

Each ten-digit number is a linear graph.
Martina Novakova.

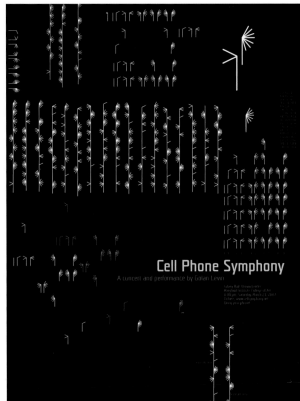

Each phone number is a twig that sprouts
marks for its digits. Martina Novakova.

Computer code is used to create a spiraling
path for each number. Jonnie Hallman.

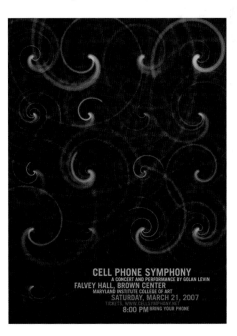

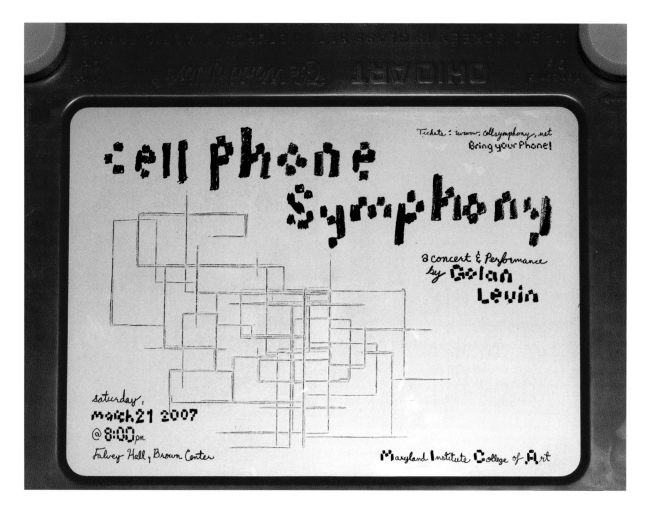

**Mechanical Drawing** The drawing was made with a child's sketching toy; the lines were created by turning the dial in response to a random list of phone numbers. The hand lettering also combines order and technology with primitive, childlike techniques. Luke Williams.

**Audio Waves** Captured from an audio editing program, the lines represent different voices speaking a list of phone numbers. Sisi Recht.

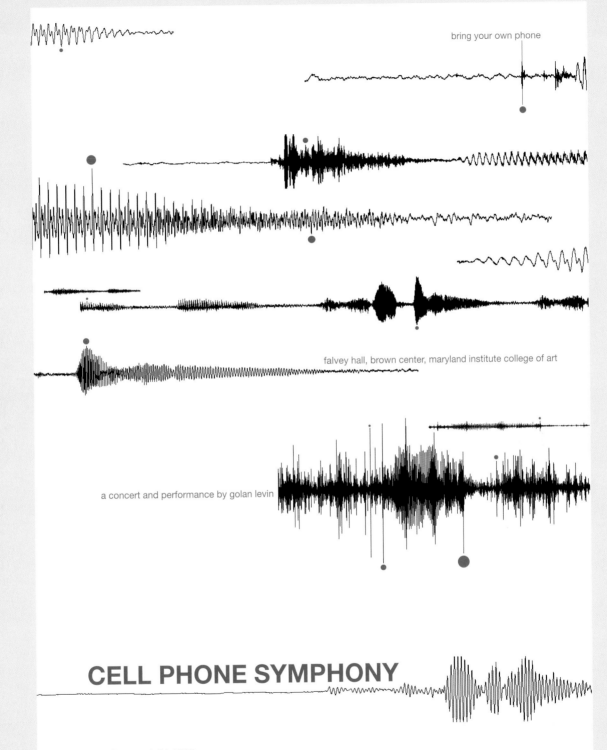

bring your own phone

falvey hall, brown center, maryland institute college of art

a concert and performance by golan levin

# CELL PHONE SYMPHONY

8:00 pm saturday, march 21, 2007

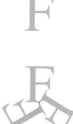

## Repeat and Rotate

Repeating and rotating forms are universal principles of pattern design. The designs shown here were created in the Processing software language. By altering the input to a set of digital instructions, the designer can quickly see numerous variations of a single design. Changing the typeface, type size, type alignment, color, transparency, and the number and degree of rotations yields different results.

```
for(int i=0;i<12;i++){
fill(0,0,0);
textAlign(CENTER);
pushMatrix();

rotate(PI*i/6);

text("F",0,0);
popMatrix();
}
}
```

Similar effects can be achieved by rotating and repeating characters in standard graphics programs such as Illustrator. Working in Processing or other code languages allows the designer to test and manipulate different variables while grasping the logic and mathematics behind pattern design.

Yeohyun Ahn

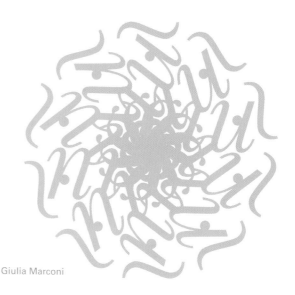

Giulia Marconi

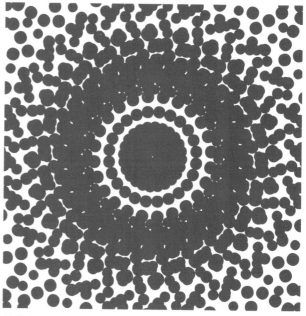

Giulia Marconi

**Rotated Letterforms** A simple code structure is used to generate designs with surprising intricacy. New designs can be quickly tested by changing the variables. Graphic Design II. Ellen Lupton and Yeohyun Ahn, faculty.

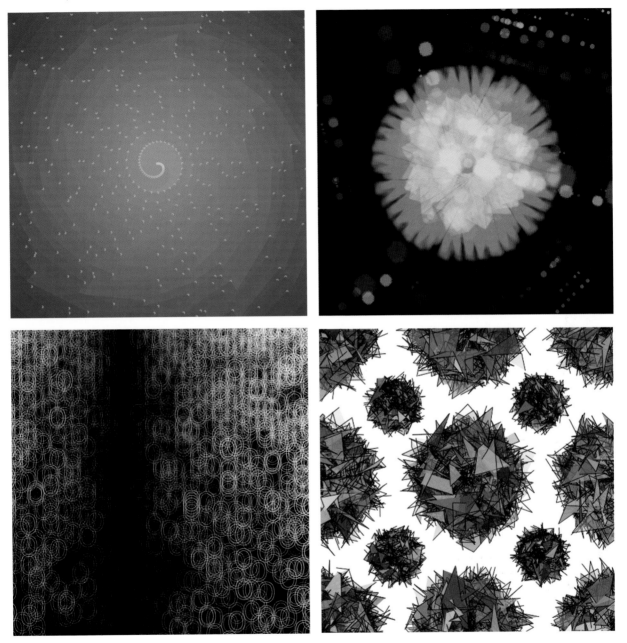

Jonnie Hallman, Shin Hyung Choi

Jessica Till, Adam Okrasinski

**Repeat and Random** One or two simple
elements are repeated using a "for" statement.
The transparency, size, or x and y coordinates
are randomized to create a sense of natural
motion. Graphic Design II. Ellen Lupton and
Yeohyun Ahn, faculty.

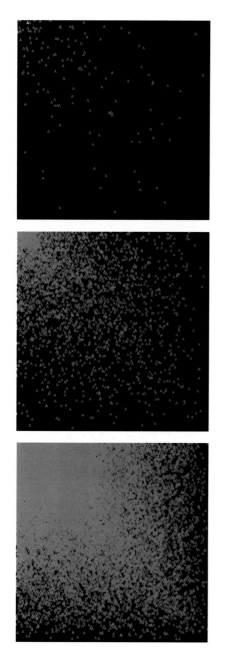

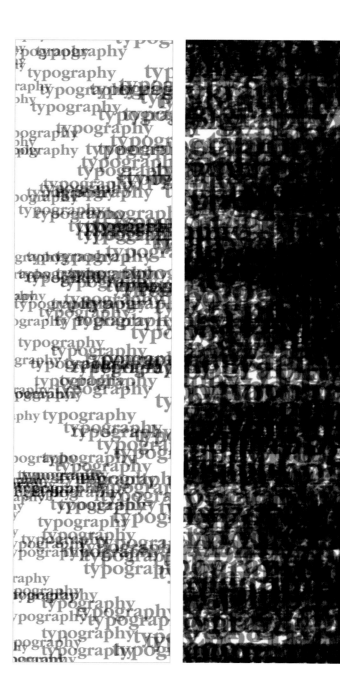

**Type Swarm** Here, the draw function in Processing has been used to randomly place the letter A on the screen, beginning from one starting point in the upper left hand corner of the screen. Yeohyun Ahn and Ryan Gladhill, MFA Studio.

**Game of Life** Using code written by Mike Davis and inspired by John Conway's Game of Life, this animation of the word "typography" uses variables with random functions, yielding a rich, soft pattern. Yeohyun Ahn and Viviana Cordova, MFA Studio.

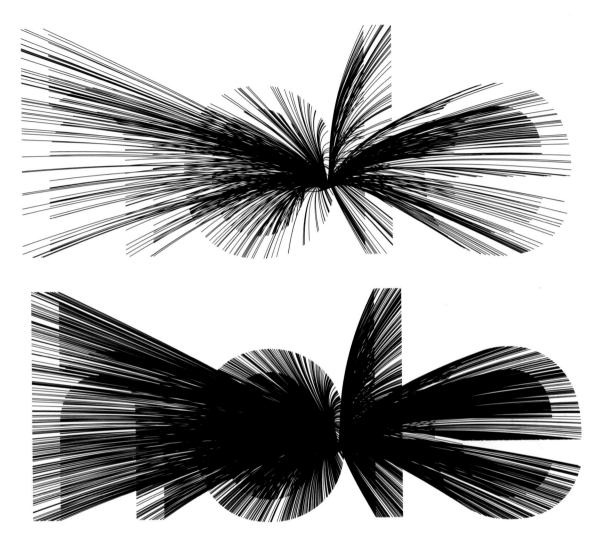

**Center of Gravity** These typographic studies
use numerous Bézier curves to describe the
edges of letterforms. Each line originates
from the center and connects to points along
the outline of the letters. The center point
and the curves can be changed to yield
different results. Yeohyun Ahn, MFA Studio.

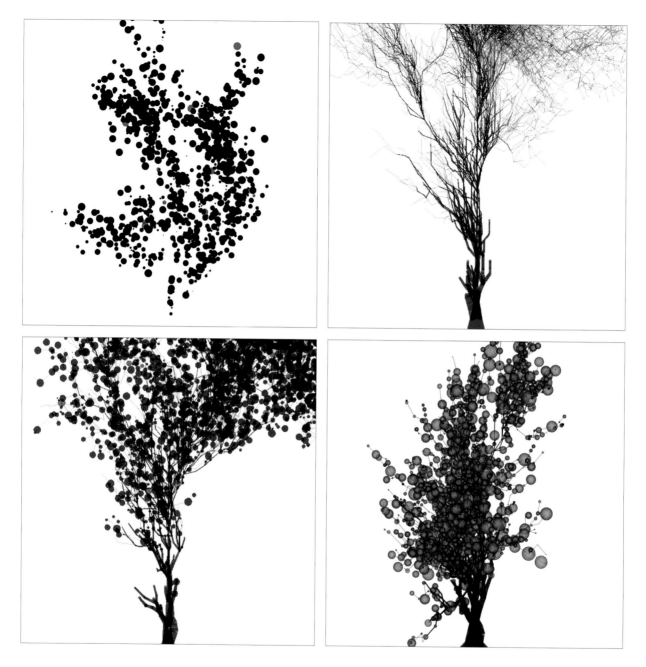

**Nature and Software** This naturalistic tree is created by software interacting with audio input from a user. Without sound the program only generates branches, but when sound is input, the tree grows leaves. The color of the leaves corresponds with the time of day. The tree grows green leaves during the day, and black leaves at night.

The piece was created using Processing with an external library, Sonia, which provides real-time frequency analysis of the microphone input. The designer created a program that generates fractals, referencing the L-system algorithm, programmed by Jer Thorp. Yeohyun Ahn, Physical Interface Design. Ryan McCabe, faculty.

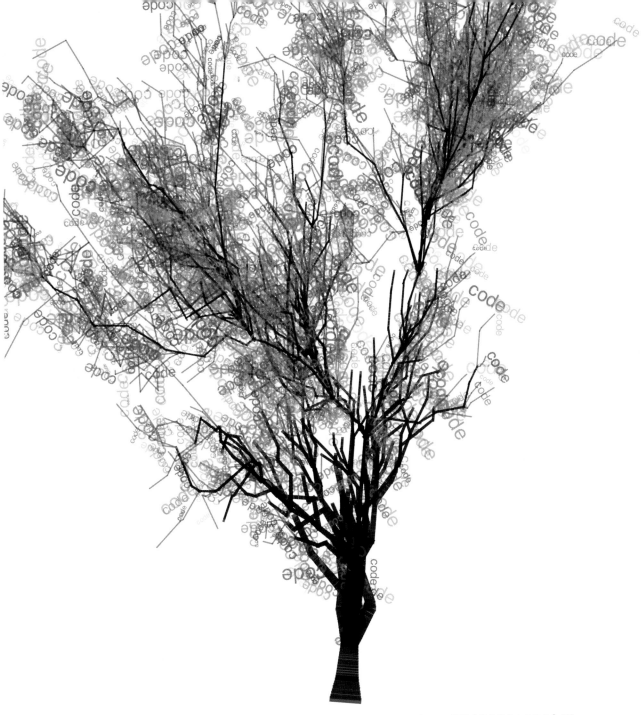

Tree = {"FF-[-F+F+F-]+[+F-F-F+]:90",
"++:5", "--:5"};

# Bibliography

## Basics

Arnheim, Rudolf. *Visual Thinking*. Berkeley: University of California Press, 1969.

Arnston, Amy. *Graphic Design Basics*. New York: Holt Rinehart and Winston, 1988.

Booth-Clibborn, Edward, and Daniele Baroni. *The Language of Graphics*. New York: Harry N. Abrams, 1979.

Carter, Rob, Ben Day, and Phillip Meggs. *Typographic Design: Form and Communication*. New York: Wiley, 2002. First published 1985.

Dondis, Donis. *A Primer of Visual Literacy*. Cambridge, MA: MIT Press, 1973.

Garland, Ken. *Graphics Handbook*. New York: Reinhold, 1966.

Graham, Lisa. *Basics of Design: Layout and Typography for Beginners*. Florence, KY: Thomson Delmar Learning, 2001.

Grear, Malcolm. *Inside/Outside: From the Basics to the Practice of Design*. New York: AIGA and New Riders, 2006.

Hofmann, Armin. *Graphic Design Manual: Principles and Practice*. New York: Reinhold, 1966.

Kandinsky, Wassily. *Point and Line to Plane*. New York: Dover, 1979.

Klee, Paul. *Pedagogical Sketchbook*. London: Faber and Faber, 1953.

Koren, Leonard, and R. Wippo Meckler. *The Graphic Design Cookbook: Mix and Match Recipes for Faster, Better Layouts*. San Francisco: Chronicle Books, 2001.

Krause, Jim. *Layout Index*. Cincinnati, OH: North Light Books, 2001.

Landa, Robin. *Graphic Design Solutions*. Florence, KY: OnWord Press, 2000.

Leborg, Christian. *Visual Grammar*. New York: Princeton Architectural Press, 2006.

Newark, Quentin. *What is Graphic Design?* East Sussex, UK: RotoVision, 2002.

Rand, Paul. *Paul Rand: A Designer's Art*. New Haven: Yale University Press, 1985.

Resnick, Elizabeth. *Design for Communication: Conceptual Graphic Design Basics*. New York: Wiley, 2003.

Rüegg, Ruedi. *Basic Typography: Design with Letters*. New York: Van Nostrand Reinhold, 1989.

Skolos, Nancy, and Thomas Wedell. *Type, Image, Message: A Graphic Design Layout Workshop*. Gloucester, MA: Rockport Publishers, 2006.

White, Alex. *The Elements of Graphic Design: Space, Unity, Page Architecture, and Type*. New York: Allworth Press, 2002.

Wilde, Richard, and Judith Wilde. *Visual Literacy: A Conceptual Approach to Graphic Problem-Solving*. New York: Watson-Guptill, 2005.

Williams, Robin. *The Non-Designer's Design Book*. Berkeley, CA: Peachpit Press, 2003.

## Code

Dawes, Brendan. *Analog In, Digital Out: Brendan Dawes on Interaction Design*. Berkeley, CA: New Riders Press, 2006.

Gerstner, Karl. *Designing Programmes*. Zurich: ABC Verlag, 1963.

Maeda, John. *Creative Code*. London: Thames and Hudson, 2004.

Reas, Casey, Ben Fry, and John Maeda. *Processing: A Programming Handbook for Visual Designers and Artist*. Cambridge, MA: MIT Press, 2007.

Reas, C. E. B. *Process/Drawing*. Berlin: DAM, 2005.

## Color

AdamsMorioka and Terry Stone. *Color Design Workbook: A Real-World Guide to Using Color in Graphic Design*. Gloucester, MA: Rockport Press, 2006.

Albers, Josef. *Interaction of Color*. New Haven: Yale University Press, 2006. First published 1963.

Krause, Jim. *Color Index*. Cincinnati: How Design Books, 2002.

## Diagram

Bhaskaran, Lakshmi. *Size Matters: Effective Graphic Design for Large Amounts of Information*. Mies, Switzerland: RotoVision, 2004.

Tufte, Edward R. *Beautiful Evidence*. Cheshire, CT: Graphics Press, 2006.

———. *Envisioning Information*. Cheshire, CT: Graphics Press, 1990.

## Grid

Bosshard, Hans Rudolf. *Der Typografische Raster/The Typographic Grid*. Sulgen, Switzerland: Verlag Niggli, 2000.

Elam, Kimberly. *Geometry of Design*. New York: Princeton Architectural Press, 2001.

———. *Grid Systems: Principles of Organizing Type*. New York: Princeton Architectural Press, 2005.

Jute, André. *Grids: The Structure of Graphic Design*. Mies, Switzerland: RotoVision, 1996.

Müller-Brockmann, Josef. *Grid Systems in Graphic Design*. Santa Monica, CA: RAM Publications, 1996. First published 1961.

Samara, Timothy. *Making and Breaking the Grid: A Graphic Design Layout Workshop*. Gloucester, MA: Rockport Publishers, 2002.

## History and Theory

Alexander, Christopher. "The City is Not a Tree." In *Architecture Culture, 1943–1968: A Documentary Anthology*, edited by Joan Ockman. New York: Rizzoli, 1993, 379–88.

Arnheim, Rudolf. *Art and Visual Perception*. Berkeley: University of California Press, 1974.

Derrida, Jacques. *The Truth in Painting*. Translated by Geoff Bennington and Ian McCleod. Chicago: University of Chicago Press, 1987.

Fish, Stanley. "Devoid of Content." *New York Times*. May 31, 2005, Op-Ed page.

Franciscono, Marcel. *Walter Gropius and the Creation of the Bauhaus*. Urbana: University of Illinois Press, 1971.

Galloway, Alexander, and Eugene Thacker. "Protocol, Control and Networks." *Grey Room* 12 (2004): 6–29.

Itten, Johannes. *Design and Form: The Basic Course at the Bauhaus and Later*. New York: Van Nostrand Reinhold, 1975.

Johnson, Steven. *Everything Bad Is Good for You: How Today's Popular Culture is Actually Making Us Smarter*. New York: Penguin, 2005.

Kepes, Gyorgy. *Language of Vision*. Chicago: Paul Theobold, 1947.

Lupton, Ellen and J. Abbott Miller. *Design Writing Research: Writing on Graphic Design*. London: Phaidon, 1999.

Manovich, Lev. "Generation Flash." http://www.manovich.net (accessed May 10, 2006).

———. *The Language of New Media*. Cambridge, MA: MIT Press, 2001.

Margolin, Victor. *The Struggle for Utopia: Rodchenko, Lissitzky, Moholy-Nagy, 1917–1946*. Chicago: University of Chicago Press, 1998.

McCoy, Katherine. "Hybridity Happens." *Emigre* 67 (2004): 38–47.

———. "The New Discourse." In *Cranbrook: The New Design Discourse*, by Katherine McCoy and Michael McCoy. New York: Rizzoli, 1990.

————. "When Designers Create Culture." *Print* LVI: III (2002): 26, 181–3.

Moholy-Nagy, László. *Vision in Motion*. Chicago: Paul Theobold, 1969. First published 1947.

Moholy-Nagy, Sibyl. *Moholy-Nagy: Experiment in Totality*. Cambridge, MA: MIT Press, 1950.

Naylor, Gillian. *The Bauhaus Reassessed*. New York: E. P. Dutton, 1985.

Rowe, Colin, and Robert Slutzky. "Transparency: Literal and Phenomenal (Part 2)." In *Architecture Culture, 1943–1968: A Documentary Anthology*, edited by Joan Ockman. New York: Rizzoli, 1993, 205–225.

Weber, Nicholas Fox. *Josef + Anni Albers: Designs for Living*. London: Merrell Publishers, 2004.

Weingart, Wolfgang. *My Way to Typography*. Baden, Switzerland: Lars Müller Publishers, 2000.

Wick, Rainer K., and Gabriele D. Grawe. *Teaching at the Bauhaus*. Ostfildern-Ruit, Germany: Hatje Cantz Publishers, 2000.

Wingler, Hans M. *The Bauhaus*. Cambridge, MA: MIT Press, 1986.

## Pattern

Archibald Christie. *Traditional Methods of Pattern Designing; An Introduction to the Study of the Decorative Art*. Oxford: Clarendon Press, 1910.

Hagan, Keith. *The Complete Pattern Library*. New York: Harry N. Abrams, 2005.

Jones, Owen. *The Grammar of Ornament*. Edited by Maxine Lewis. London: DK Adult, 2001. First published 1856.

## Time and Motion

Furniss, Maureen. *Art in Motion: Animation Aesthetics*. London: John Libbey, 1998.

Williams, Richard. *The Animator's Survival Kit: A Manual of Methods, Principles, and Formulas for Classical, Computer, Games, Stop Motion and Internet Animators*. London: Faber and Faber, 2001.

Woolman, Matt, and Jeff Bellantoni. *Moving Type: Designing for Time and Space*. Mies, Switzerland: RotoVision, 2000.

## Typography

Baines, Phil, and Andrew Haslam. *Type and Typography*. New York: Watson-Guptill Publications, 2002.

Bringhurst, Robert. *The Elements of Typographic Style*. Vancouver: Hartley and Marks, 1997.

Carter, Rob, Ben Day, and Philip Meggs. *Typographic Design: Form and Communication*. New York: Van Nostrand Reinhold, 1993.

Elam, Kimberly. *Typographic Systems*. New York: Princeton Architectural Press, 2007.

French, Nigel. *InDesign Type*. Berkeley, CA: Adobe Press, 2006.

Kane, John. *A Type Primer*. London: Laurence King, 2002.

Kunz, Willi. *Typography: Formation and Transformation*. Sulgen, Switzerland: Verlag Niggli, 2003.

————. *Typography: Macro- and Microaesthetics*. Sulgen, Switzerland: Verlag Niggli, 2004.

Lupton, Ellen. *Thinking with Type: A Critical Guide for Designers, Writers, Editors, and Students*. New York: Princeton Architectural Press, 2004.

Ruder, Emil. *Typography*. New York: Hastings House, 1971.

Spiekermann, Erik, and E. M. Ginger. *Stop Stealing Sheep and Find Out How Type Works*. Mountain View, CA: Adobe Press, 1993.

# Index

# Colophon

**Book Typography**
Univers family, designed by Adrian Frutiger, 1957

**Cover Typography**
Knockout, designed by Jonathan Hoefler, 1993–97

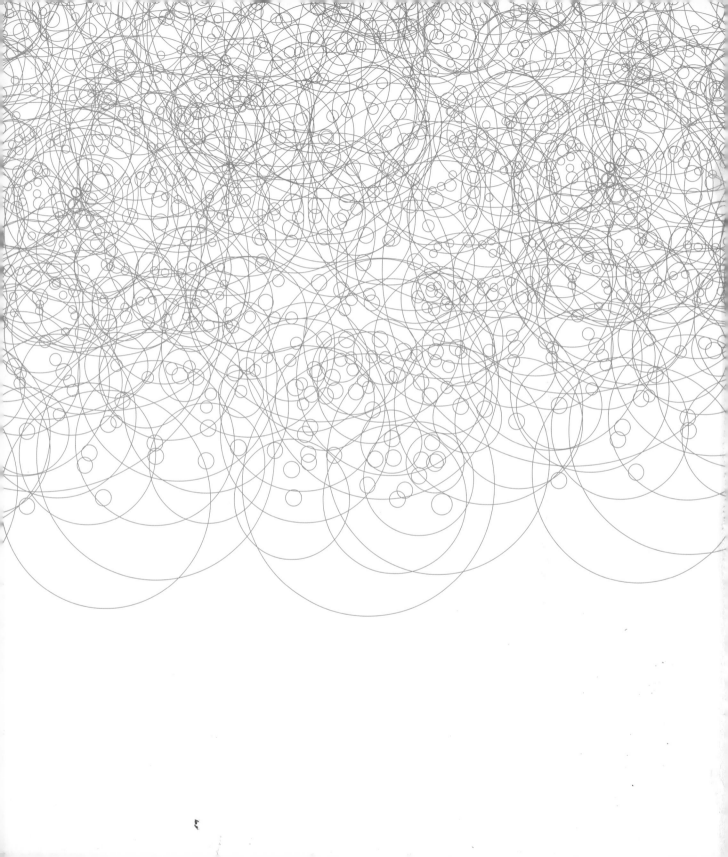